Here's How to Do Therapy

Hands-On Core Skills in Speech-Language Pathology

Second Edition

Here's How Series

Thomas Murry, PhD
Series Editor

Here's How to Treat Dementia by Jennifer L. Loehr
and Megan L. Malone

*Here's How to Provide Intervention for Children with Autism
Spectrum Disorder: A Balanced Approach* by Catherine B. Zenko
and Michelle Peters Hite

*Here's How to Do Early Intervention for Speech and Language:
Empowering Parents* by Karyn Lewis Searcy

Here's How to Do Stuttering Therapy by Gary J. Rentschler

*Here's How Children Learn Speech and Language: A Text on Different
Learning Strategies* by Margo Kinzer Courter

Here's How to Treat Childhood Apraxia of Speech by Margaret Fish

Here's How to Do Therapy

Hands-On Core Skills in Speech-Language Pathology

Second Edition

Debra M. Dwight, EdD, CCC-SLP

University of West Georgia
Carrollton, Georgia

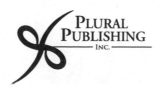

PLURAL
PUBLISHING
INC.

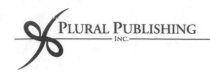

PLURAL PUBLISHING
INC.

5521 Ruffin Road
San Diego, CA 92123

e-mail: info@pluralpublishing.com
Website: http://www.pluralpublishing.com

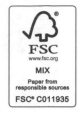

Typeset in 11/15 Stone Informal by Flanagan's Publishing Services, Inc.
Printed in the United States of America by McNaughton & Gunn, Inc.
17 16 15   2 3 4 5

Dwight, Debra M., author.
  Here's how to do therapy : hands-on core skills in speech-language pathology / Debra M. Dwight. — Second edition.
      p. ; cm. — (Here's how)
  Includes bibliographical references and index.
  ISBN 978-1-59756-565-3 (alk. paper) — ISBN 1-59756-565-2 (alk. paper)
  I. Title. II. Series: Here's how series.
  [DNLM: 1. Language Therapy—methods. 2. Speech Therapy—methods. 3. Language Disorders—therapy. WL 340.3]
  RC428
  616.85'506—dc23
                                                                    2014015316

Contents

Preface

It's difficult to measure the depth and breadth of rewards experienced by Speech-Language Pathologists (SLPs) in the daily tasks of providing therapy to clients of all ages. Sometimes rewards are in the form of inherent satisfaction in helping a young child more clearly/ accurately pronounce a once troublesome phoneme; at other times, rewards rest in the knowledge that a family is calmed by the skills brought by the SLP to a difficult communication situation following accident or injury to a loved one. Regardless of the client's communication need, the SLP's satisfaction as a habilitative or rehabilitative service provider is founded in the fact that skills needed for the job are at fingertip, thanks to various cumulative aspects of education, training, and experience. It is hoped that the information contained within this text serves as a part of the education and training that feeds into knowledgeable and prepared SLP professionals.

The first edition of *Here's How to Do Therapy: Hands-On Core Skills in Speech-Language Pathology* grew from an 11-year history of a clinical management course in which specific therapeutic skills were taught to both undergraduate and graduate students who needed to quickly and effectively learn to do therapy in preparation for initial certification in the profession. It was imperative, at that time, to identify the basic skills needed for successful intervention across broad areas of the profession including language, articulation/ phonology, voice, fluency, and resonance. The development and production of the first edition of *Here's How to Do Therapy: Hands-On Core Skills in Speech-Language Pathology* was a very satisfying creative and academic endeavor. Although maintaining the original aspects of the first edition of the text remains important, there is now an increased desire to expand the clinical application and teaching aspects of the second edition to increase and enhance user outcomes. From the beginning, readers and users of the first edition of the text reported interest, delight, and benefit from the contents of *Here's How to Do Therapy: Hands-On Core Skills in Speech-Language Pathology* for both individual and small group learning settings. Keeping in mind the positive reception of the first edition of the text, the intent of this second edition is to expand user benefits for both students and clinical supervisors by making it easier to learn/teach basic therapeutic skills based on both the content of the text and the demonstrations offered in the DVD. To this end, this second edition of *Here's How to Do Therapy: Hands-On Core Skills in Speech-Language Pathology* is designed to accomplish the following objectives for both students and clinical supervisors: (a) increase the opportunities for learning through the expansion of DVD examples and scenarios, and (b) enhance the training value of the text through the inclusion of graphic "learning points" to help promote proficiency in students' skills through systematic guides and reminders for specific skill sets. In these two ways, this second edition of *Here's How to Do Therapy: Hands-On Core Skills in Speech-Language Pathology* is seen as an endeavor borne of decades of commitment to improving skills of young professionals across broad areas of the profession in the basics of therapeutic intervention. It is hoped that readers and users agree that this second edition of the text both maintains the creative and academic aspects of the original work while also enhancing and expanding the value of the text within the clinical training arena of our profession.

Format

This text is designed to serve as a sourcebook, an easy-to read, easy-to-follow guide to enhancing foundational concepts for providing speech-language therapy services to clients of all ages, with all levels and types of speech-language disorders. This sourcebook is designed for speech-language pathology (SLP) students and professionals as a ready guide for basic, functional, practical applications of 28 underlying skills for speech-language therapy. Skills addressed in this book are cross-disciplinary in that they serve as basic skills that are fundamental for therapy across a wide spectrum of communication disorders, whether simple articulation or difficult-to-manage low incidence disorders.

Part I of the book presents definitions, relevant concepts, and information related to the basic speech-language therapy session. When possible, figures, textboxes, or exercises are provided to emphasize the concepts being taught. Additionally, 28 specific skills associated with speech-language therapy are highlighted and discussed in Chapter 6. Readers are guided through a process for learning and demonstrating each of the 28 specific skills through use of three tools that accompany the text.

1. *Therapeutic-Specific Workshop Forms (TSW Forms).* TSW forms are written in six sections to help guide learning for the skills presented, with each form designed to accompany one or more of the 28 different skills discussed in Chapter 6. Although 28 different therapeutic-specific skills are presented in Chapter 6, only 14 TSW Forms are needed to address these 28 skills because of groupings for the skills. For example, although several TSW Forms address only one therapeutic-specific skill, often two, three, and even four therapeutic-specific skills are grouped together on one TSW Form due to the nature of the skills or simply for ease in learning the skills.

2. *DVD Vignettes.* Visual demonstrations of 21 of the 28 skills presented in Chapter 6 and addressed on the TSW Forms are highlighted on DVD. For example, TSW Forms numbers 2 to 11 have DVD vignette accompaniments that address a total of 21 therapeutic-specific skills visually on DVD.

3. *Two mini-therapy sessions.* Traditional articulation and language therapy and language-based therapy are demonstrated in 20 and 11-minute DVD segments, respectively, for use in learning skills presented in both Part I and Part II of the text.

Readers are encouraged to work through the TSW Forms, and when applicable, the DVD vignette demonstrations of specific skills presented in Chapter 6 and are encouraged to view the mini-therapy sessions, all as if preparing for a theatrical production (*read, learn, practice*); after all, speech-language therapy is often a matter of "performance on demand," but often with an "impromptu script." Viewers may replay individual segments of the DVD and work through specific segments of the TSW Forms as necessary for practice and comfort in acquiring the 28 therapeutic-specific skills presented in Chapter 6 of this text. The skills acquired in Chapter 6 will be applied in the therapy progression presented in Chapter 7.

Part II of the text presents selected concepts and scripted examples of therapy sessions for five areas of the profession (language, articulation, voice, resonance, and fluency). The scripted chapters are designed to give the SLP examples of (1) how therapy proceeds from beginning to end across the three major parts of a therapy session as described in Chapter 7 of the text, and (2) what the SLP might actually say to the client to effect the kinds of responses and results desired of the client in different types of therapy. As mentioned earlier, two mini-therapy sessions on DVD add to the viewer's understanding of information presented in Part II of the text as well. As a function of learning to work, first from a given script (before eventually providing impromptu clinician-led therapeutic interactions), students and professionals learn the fundamentals of providing appropriate intervention progressions for speech-language therapy. By learning the concepts in this book in a guided, directed pattern of speech-language therapy for different disorders, students and professionals develop a better understanding of therapeutic interactions and progressions and quickly develop their own individualized intervention styles. Students and professionals typically *do not remain true to the scripts* as skills and techniques are learned and perfected, but most retain the concepts learned through guided work in providing speech-language therapy as presented in Part II of this text.

Thank you for your continued support of the objectives of this text.

—Debra M. Dwight

To Michael Sky Dwight, my granddaughter, and the generations that will follow her.
To my parents, Jerry and Valeria Maye,
My sons, Marlon and Jacob,
The Maye men: Reginal, Julius, Samuel, and Anthony,
To all of my many supporters, but especially Etta, Barbara, Glo, James, and Lydia,
and,
To my students who have given me more than I can ever repay.

To the Memory of
Renee' and Chuck, both gone too soon.

Love you much,
Debra Kim Maye Dwight
2014

PART

I

Introduction

Speech-language pathologists (SLPs) most often are exposed to a strong curriculum addressing the broad parameters of the profession (language, articulation/phonology, voice, fluency, resonance, swallowing, etc.). SLPs spend many hours devoted to addressing the specifics of therapy associated with these areas of the profession. However, several other areas of child and adult functioning found in speech-language therapy clients receive less attention during formal training for SLPs. For example, there is often little space in training programs for SLPs to address concepts related to early child development or the specifics of various recognized disability areas. SLPs who are exposed to child development and disability categories often receive that training early in undergraduate education when little relevance of these areas to the specifics of speech-language therapy is possible. Fortunately, many SLPs come to understand the relationship of child development and various disability categories to the speech-language pathology profession over the years as they engage in professional practices. For those not exposed to related areas of the profession as much as desired, Part I of this text can help.

Purposes of Part I

The purposes of Part I of this text are to (a) discuss foundational information related to speech-language therapy (Chapters 1, 2 and 3); (b) present information in related areas and global parameters of therapy in an effort to help professionals understand the impact of those areas on therapy (Chapters 4, 5, and 8); and (c) present therapeutic-specific skills and basic components of the speech-language therapy session (Chapters 6 and 7). Exercises, Figures, and Textboxes are used to help support information presented.

How to Use Part I of the Text

Chapters 1, 2, 3, 4, 5, and 8 of the text are fairly traditional in format; the reader is presented information and asked to refer to various inserts as examples or as exercises

1

designed to increase clarity. However, Chapters 6 and 7 take a less traditional presentation in that additional learning aids are required for completion of activities for these chapters. Accompanying Chapter 6 are two additional learning aids, Therapeutic-Specific Workshop Forms (TSW forms) and DVD vignettes. These two learning aids are integral to the information presented in Chapter 6. For example, 28 therapeutic-specific skills are presented in Chapter 6. As an additional aid to learning the 28 therapeutic-specific skills, students are presented with information not found in the text on TSW forms for use when learning the skills presented. Also accompanying Chapter 6 of the text are DVD demonstrations of how 21 of the 28 skills presented in the chapter actually look when applied to therapy. The 21 skills presented in DVD vignettes are incorporated as part of learning as students work through the TSW forms. For example, students will begin working through a selected TSW form and, if a DVD vignette is part of the learning for the topic presented for that form, the student will be instructed to view the DVD vignette at a point prior to completing the tasks of the TSW form. The TSW forms are presented as appendixes to the text and are labeled to match the skills presented in Chapter 6. Students should perform the following tasks in order to learn the skills presented in Chapter 6.

1. Read the information from the text in Chapter 6 for the topic selected for study.
2. Select the TSW form that accompanies the topic selected in Chapter 6.
3. Read sections A through D of the applicable TSW form.
4. View the vignette (when applicable) that accompanies the selected topic.
5. Complete sections E and F of the TSW form.

By working systematically through the information presented in Chapter 6, the TSW forms, and the accompanying DVD vignettes, students learn to demonstrate the 28 therapeutic-specific skills presented in the chapter. The TSW forms and the DVD vignettes serve as guided practice in acquiring these skills.

One learning aid accompanies Chapter 7 of the text and is felt to be foundational for learning the components of therapy presented in the chapter. Chart 7–2 presents the details of therapy progression from the beginning to the end of a session, including components, timelines, definitions, and procedures and examples of what the SLP might say in therapy. Students are encouraged to refer to this chart *often* as efforts are made to study the sequence of events that occur in therapy. Understanding the information presented in Chapter 7 and in Chart 7–2 are integral to success in providing speech-language therapy.

Finally, it is not necessary to proceed with learning all 28 therapeutic-specific skills in Chapter 6 before proceeding to the details of therapy in Chapter 7. Typically, students begin learning one or two of the therapeutic-specific skills at about the same time they are introduced to Chart 7–2, Detailed Therapy Progression. As students are introduced to the components, timelines, definitions, procedures, and examples of Chart 7–2, they are also learning selected therapeutic-specific skills in isolation. Soon, however, students begin merging therapeutic-specific skills into the progression of therapy, reading from Chart 7–2 as they learn the order of the session while at the same time practicing a new therapeutic-specific skill. For example, it is not uncommon for the clinical management instructor or clinical supervisor to assign TSW skills from Chapter 6 for practice with the greeting and rapport section of the introduction of therapy in Chapter 7. Numerous configurations for learning in that fashion are possible and Chart 7–2 lists the TSW skills likely needed for each component of the therapy session for those interested in learning skills in an integrative manner. However, also possible are more linear styles of learning and teaching whereby consecutive chapters and items within chapters are addressed in order as presented. Regardless of the choice of presentation order for learning the skills presented in Chapters 6 and 7, the content of these chapters is designed to help develop or increase skills in speech-language therapy. Let's get started!

1

Introduction: Here's How to Use This Text

Clinical supervisors and instructors, for decades, have found ways of teaching clinical skills that resulted in successful learning outcomes for speech-language pathology (SLP) students. Often, the tasks associated with teaching clinical skills to developing SLP students are time consuming and labor intensive. For every SLP student learning to do therapy, clinical supervisors and instructors expend hours of tedious lecturing, demonstrating, guiding, directing, observing, coaching, and evaluating, to name a few of the tasks required to ensure that SLP students acquire and appropriately implement the skills necessary to positively impact client outcomes in communication abilities. Each clinical supervisor and instructor responsible for helping SLPs learn the art of speech-language therapy has his or her own unique style for teaching and guiding students. However, several specific concepts and practices over the years have proven effective for helping ensure that the information presented in this text is learned easily by developing SLP students.

Teaching and Learning Pedagogy

Basic teaching *pedagogy* is the underlying philosophical beliefs and concepts that serve as foundations or guiding principles for the education of students. Often pedagogies are seen as simple and broad. The guiding educational principles such as, *"All students can learn,"* and, *"Every child deserves a chance to learn,"* are broad-based pedagogies often espoused by general educators and educational leaders responsible for teaching and learning for large groups of students in typical educational settings. However, Loughran (2013) suggested that "a pedagogy of teacher education can be viewed as the theory and practice of teaching and learning about teaching" (p. 129). Loughran's work offered more focus for educational pedagogy, and presented a type of pedagological processing that served as the foundation of this text years ago when it became necessary to very quickly teach students how to do speech-language therapy; during that time, it became clear that education pedagogy was about "the teaching–learning relationship" (Loughran, 2013, p. 135). Although, perhaps, not a typical line of conversation for speech-language pathology professionals, the concepts of teaching and learning pedagogy are crucial to the SLP clinical supervisor and instructor who carry dual responsibilities of not only operating as competent clinicians, but of also serving as the points of contact for SLP students who must quickly and effectively learn both the academics of the SLP profession, as well as the clinical applications for helping others to learn (relearn) to effectively communicate. That is an awesome responsibility, one that is not always easily accomplished (Makaiau & Miller, 2012).

The need to teach SLP students how to do therapy prompted questions such as, "What do SLP students need to know about how to do therapy, and how are those concepts best taught?", and, "What do clinical supervisors need to know and do in order to teach those concepts?" Questions of these types, and the eventual answers, led to investigations of educational pedagogy and the realization that teaching actually becomes a matter of the teaching–learning process, whereby the "teacher" is both teacher and learner. Oddly, the SLP student is placed in that same process of teacher–learner when he/she learns how to do therapy, with its inherent requirements of teaching, facilitating, or guiding the client toward communicative competence. The power of pedagogy in education is the focus it brings to the direction and purpose of education in the realms of planning, executing, and evaluating every teaching–learning aspect of the specific educational program for which the pedagogy applies. Adherence to such a pedagogy brings not only focus to educational practices, it also serves to enhance clarity, and perhaps, even purpose, for the day-to-day applications of specific practices within an educational setting or program.

Clinical supervisors and instructors responsible for the education of SLP students learning therapy are encouraged to explore pedagogies that undergird specific practices in teaching and learning that impact the content contained within this text. It is hoped that the content of this text is consistent with the professional beliefs and practices that clinical supervisors and instructors bring to the classroom when teaching clinical skills to SLP students. Furthermore, when possible, it is hoped that the management constructs outlined as suggestions for how to use this text might, additionally, serve to help clinical supervisors and instructors explore underlying pedagogies related to teaching, learning, and best practices within our profession. The following pedagogical ideals undergird both the clinical teaching strategies and suggested management of the contents of this text: *cooperative learning, interactive nature of learning,* and *critical incidents in learning.* A brief overview of each of these constructs as used in this text follows.

Cooperative Learning

Johnson and Johnson (1989, 1999) defined *cooperative learning* as the instructional use of small groups so that students work together to maximize their own and each other's learning. Although made popular in educational literature by Johnson and Johnson (1989), the concept of cooperative learning in speech-language intervention was introduced to the communication disorders profession as early as 1951 by SLP writers, researchers, and clinicians Ollie Backus and Jane Beasley. Backus and Beasley (1951) wrote:

> . . . as we have experimented with clinical practice, our theories about speech therapy have grown progressively broader in scope, more detailed in structure; such modifications in theory have resulted in certain marked differences in clinical practice.
> Such differences may be summarized as follows for purposes of this text:
>
> 1. Group instruction should form the core of learning.
> 2. Group membership should be nonsegregated in respect to kinds of speech symptoms.
> 3. The teaching situation should be structured to provide a corrective "emotional" experience.
> 4. The teaching experience should be structured in terms of those interpersonal relationships which involve conversational speech. (p. 5)

For purposes of this text, Backus and Beasley's (1951) underlying theoretical assumption related to group instruction in speech therapy learning equates to the tenets of cooperative learning as presented by Johnson and Johnson (1989, 1999). Clinical supervisors and instructors are, therefore, encouraged to consider cooperative learning when teaching therapy skills to larger groups of student learners. Two concepts serve as foundations for cooperative learning as applied to teaching the 28 therapeutic-specific skills of speech-language therapy presented in Chapters 6 and 7 of this text: *cooperative groups* and *heterogeneity within groups*.

1. *Cooperative Groups.* The clinical supervisor or instructor is encouraged to develop cooperative working or learning groups for all teaching, demonstrating, and guiding tasks associated with teaching SLP students to do therapy. To the degree possible, students are assigned to *working groups*, a cooperative learning arrangement whereby students study and learn therapeutic skills in small groups consisting of the same group members throughout the learning process. For example, students are assigned, or voluntarily form, *groups of four* early in the process of learning speech-language therapy skills; students remain in the same group for the duration of the learning process. Practice time for the groups is given in class and guided by the clinical supervisor or instructor, but other practice times outside of class are also required and expected. All group members are expected to participate in practice sessions both during and outside of class times.

2. *Heterogeneity within Groups.* For purposes of teaching therapy within the confines of this text, group membership should be heterogeneous for type of speech problems represented within the make-up of the cooperative groups as suggested by Backus and Beasley (1951). Heterogeneous groups more accurately emulate a typical interactive learning setting in that typical

societal settings for communication and speech-language learning are rarely homogeneous. For example, it is unlikely that everyone present in a social setting will have difficulty pronouncing the /s/ phoneme, or that a group of children converging for social interactions will all have difficulty with the /r/. More commonly, groups of communicators are likely to be composed of speakers with typically developing speech-language skills as well as a few speakers who may have disorders of speech-language of varying types. Of the few speakers with identified speech-language disorders, it is highly unlikely that everyone with a speech-language disorder will have the *same* speech-language disorder.

Based on prevalence indicators reported by the American Speech-Language-Hearing Association (ASHA, 2014), articulation and language disorders represent the largest categories of speech-language disorders for children during the developmental years. Within any given age range, or any given typical classroom, it is likely that children within those age ranges and within those classrooms will present with articulation and language disorders consisting of varying characteristics of the disorders rather than consisting of homogeneous characteristics. Although a practicing professional SLP certainly has a choice of homogeneous or heterogeneous grouping for intervention, for purposes of teaching therapy based on this text, heterogeneous grouping is preferred. In this way, when "clients" serve as models, the likelihood of one client actually having skills strong enough to model for another is higher. In contrast, if all clients within the group present with the same sound or concept disorder, there is little opportunity for any client to serve as a peer model, thereby lessening the interactive learning parameters of group therapy.

Interactive Nature of Learning

A second pedagogical concept that undergirds the basic tenets for the structure of this text is the ***interactive nature of learning*** wherein learning occurs through the give and take transfer of information from one person to another (Lawrence & Butler, 2010). Several researchers studied the interactive nature of the learner in areas of initial and generalized language learning (Nelson, 2011; Paul, 2011). Nelson (2011) found that students acquiring a second language learned various aspects of the target language through conversations rather than through solely writing for expressions of the concepts. Use of conversational or social exchanges in therapy is fundamental for providing a setting for clients to acquire communication interaction through social interaction activities such as typical conversational exchanges. The features of language that lend themselves to interactive learning included semantics, phonology, morphology, syntax, and pragmatics of language (content, form, and use) as presented by Bloom and Lahey (1978). The exchange noted to best promote learning of these language concepts involved one partner serving as listener, while the other partner served as speaker, and vice versa. Typical daily conversational interactions serve as examples of social interaction activities and support Backus and Beasley's (1951) concept of providing therapy within interpersonal relationships which involves conversational speech. Fox-Turnbull (2010) also discussed the positive role of conversation in a student's learning. Therefore, except for drill-based work sometimes desired to correct phoneme productions, the stimulus for basic language interactions is the sentence—or some portion, thereof. The sentence stimulus is used in an attempt to both model and elicit basic conversational structures during therapy to the degree possible.

For purposes of teaching the basics of therapy, this text is founded on the concept of the interactive nature of learning, based on conversations, whereby one member serves as group leader to facilitate teaching of skills (the student "SLP"), while other group members simultaneously serve as learners who also facilitate teaching of skills by serving as listeners, models, and evaluators (student "clients"), with each role carrying its respective responsibilities.

Interactive Roles and Responsibilities of Group Members

It is appropriate, here, to highlight information regarding beginning students' perceptions of classes that served as an important part of their education. Furr and Carroll (2003) found that,

> For students just beginning to learn to be counselors, the importance of the skill-based introductory counseling class is a dominant force in their education. Although the students' primary focus was on the development of basic counseling skills, students in this study repeatedly mentioned the importance of the experience of being both the counselor and the client in terms of dealing with the dynamics of the [therapeutic] relationship. Instructors . . . need to be alert to helping students process these interactions in addition to focusing on skill attainment. (p. 487)

For more than 20 years, the conceptualization and constructs whereby beginning SLP students have been introduced to and taught how to do speech-language therapy have been based on the elements of *cooperative learning* (Backus & Beasley, 1951; Johnson & Johnson, 1989, 1999), whereby students take responsibility for not only their own learning, but for the learning of peers within the group, as well. An effective way to achieve this shared responsibility for learning is found in the research on the *interactive* or *dynamic* nature of the therapeutic process presented by Furr and Carroll (2003).

In order to achieve the interactive aspects of group learning, groups of four members within each cooperative group are established, with each of the four members performing specific roles and responsibilities within the teaching/learning process. For example, at any given point, one group member serves as the "SLP," while the remaining three group members serve as "clients." As the "SLP" facilitates learning through direct intervention with one selected "client" (the "target client"), each of the other two "clients" are engaged in learning by serving in alternating positions as (a) peer models, and (b) peer evaluators for the target client. For example, when the student SLP is working with the target client, both remaining clients also are engaged in therapy by both serving as peer models (with the SLP's lead) for target sounds or concepts being worked on by the target client. Then, as the target client produces the target structure, both remaining clients now serve as peer evaluators (with the SLP's lead) for the target client's productions. Note, however, that engagement of remaining clients as either peer models or peer evaluators is at the discretion of the "SLP." When the SLP completes the target client's responses and corrective work, engaging the remaining clients as peer models or evaluators, at discretion, the SLP then goes to the next "target client" within the group. The former target client now becomes a peer model and peer evaluator for the current target client. In this manner, the SLP works with all clients as the target client for direct intervention, and also works with all clients indirectly as each client, in turn, becomes a peer model and/or peer evaluator.

Group members, including the student SLP, rotate roles throughout the teaching–learning process so that at any given time, one group member serves as the student SLP while the other three group members serve as the clients within the group. Once the student SLP has practiced the assigned process or skill, roles within the group are changed and another member of the group becomes the student SLP; the original student SLP now serves as a client member of the group. The roles and responsibilities of group members constantly rotate and are detailed as follows:

- Student "SLPs" lead, guide, teach, demonstrate, model, elicit, coach, evaluate, and reward

- Student "clients" respond, model, and evaluate

The group member serving as student "SLP" is responsible for leading the group through the processes of therapy by guiding the group systematically through the *Introduction*, *Body*, and *Closing* of the therapy session. In this way, the student SLP serves as facilitator of group learning for the concepts targeted in therapy. Student SLPs lead the session and guide "client" behavior by teaching, demonstrating, modeling, eliciting, coaching, evaluating, and rewarding client efforts. Student-facilitated skills were addressed by Savion (2009) and reported to be important elements in the teaching–learning process.

Each group member serving as a "client" is responsible for his or her own learning of the skills targeted for the session. However, the interactive nature of cooperative learning suggests that each client is also responsible for engaged and interactive learning in ways that support the learning of other clients in the group as well (Johnson & Johnson, 1999; Kent, 2006; Savion, 2009). Johnson and Johnson (1999) found that students learning newly introduced concepts often retained presented information better when sharing learned concepts with a peer. This peer sharing is accomplished in therapy when the target client is directed to "tell or show" another client a production of the target skills. For example, when the target client correctly produces the /k/ phoneme, the SLP might instruct the target client to, "Show Max your /k/," or "Make the /k/ for Maggie." In general education, a number of facilitative and educational presentation formats, such as Think-Pair-Share, a popular interactive or facilitative technique, and case-based teaching (basic teaching pedagogy) incorporate the concept of peer-shared learning (Dennett & Azar, 2011; Kantar, 2013; Savion, 2009; Schommer, 1990, 1993; Williams, 2011).

When peer-shared learning is applied to the interactive nature of learning in speech-language therapy, the roles of the "client" members of the group are twofold, as mentioned earlier: (a) target clients serve as learners or responders, and (b) remaining clients serve as peer models and peer evaluators. Client learners (target clients) respond to the student SLP as instructed, led, directed, or guided, based on identified needs for the client learner. However, at the same time, remaining clients also work along with the SLP to serve as peer models for other members in the group, based on the student SLP's lead. The same remaining clients also serve as evaluators of peer productions within the session, based on the student SLP's lead, as well. Roles are rotated in this way until all group members have practiced his or her designated target skill(s) and have experienced the dynamics of the therapeutic relationship by also serving as both a peer model and a peer evaluator—all within the contexts of basic conversations established by the SLP. In this way, the student SLP and all group members are constantly engaged in the teaching–learning processes of therapy to fulfill Johnson and Johnson's (1989) definition of cooperative learning: the instructional use of small groups so that students work together to maximize their own and each other's learning. More importantly, cooperative groups of four provide the experience of being both the "SLP" and the "client" within the therapeutic relationship as suggested by Furr and Carroll (2003).

Again, clinical supervisors and instructors are encouraged to establish cooperative learning groups early in the teaching–learning process when teaching large groups of students how to do therapy. Small groups are established as cooperative learning groups (Johnson & Johnson, 1999), with all learning based on interactions between and among group members who each serve different functions at given times within the learning process (Furr & Carroll, 2003) as discussed earlier in the chapter. Figure 1–1 shows a rudimentary graphic of the Interactive Nature of the Therapeutic Process with Roles and Responsibilities of Group Members.

Figure 1–1 only depicts one instance of "Remaining Clients as Peer Models and Evaluators"; however, there are typically at least two clients serving in the "remaining" peer model and evaluator roles at any given time. In fact, there could conceivably be up to three, or even four, clients serving in the remaining peer model and evaluator roles at a given time for therapy groups of four, or five students, respectively.

■ TEXTBOX 1–1. Reminder to Form Cooperative Learning Groups for the Teaching–Learning Process

> **Clinical supervisors and instructors are encouraged to establish cooperative learning groups early in the teaching–learning process when teaching large groups of students how to do therapy. Small groups are established as cooperative learning groups, with all learning based on interactions between and among group members who each serve different functions at given times within the learning process.**

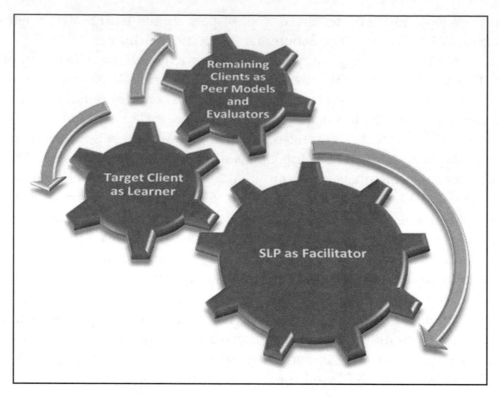

Figure 1–1. Interactive nature of the therapeutic process.

Critical Incidents in Learning

The third, and final, pedagogical concept that undergirds the basic tenets for the structure of therapy presented in this text is the concept of *critical incidents in learning*. Furr and Carroll (2003) described **critical incidents** as positive or negative experiences recognized by students as significant because of the influence on the student's development in learning how to do therapy. These researchers believed that for counseling majors, in processes with multiple parts and learning that takes place over longer periods of time, there are critical incident activities along the way that serve to significantly influence the learner's development of skills related to counseling. Similarly, close observations of developing SLP students suggested that these students also encountered experiences and activities that served as critical incident activities in the processes of learning to do basic speech-language therapy. Meyer and Land (2005) and Wilcox and Leger (2013) referred to these significant experiences in learning as "threshold" experiences in that these experiences serve to help define a student's "characteristic ways of thinking and practicing in a discipline" (Wilcox & Leger, 2013, p. 2). In the search to determine the experiences and activities that might qualify as threshold, or critical incident experiences for speech-language pathology students learning to do therapy, 18 different learning-focused activities were identified in the processes of teaching students how to do basic speech-language therapy. Although it was not clear exactly which experiences or activities served as critical incident experiences, it was clear that, while engaged in the process designed to teach the basics of therapy, something significant happened in students' learning experiences that facilitated learning to do therapy. It is important for clinical supervisors and instructors to be aware of the 18 different learning-focused activities that were found to be present in the progression of teaching basic speech-language therapy skills. These 18 different learning focused activities are presented in Figure 1–2 under three major focused activity clusters.

Although there is overlap in occurrences of the 18 different learning focused activities associated with learning basic speech-language therapy as presented in Figure 1–2, the majority of the 18 identified learning-focused activities are shown as separate elements of either (a) the Clinical Supervisor or Instructor-Focused Activity Cluster, (b) the Textbook or DVD-Focused Activity Cluster, or (c) the Interactive Learning Group-Focused Activity Cluster. It is important for clinical supervisors and instructors to grasp these three separate focal points (Supervisor-based, Textbook/DVD-based, or Interactive Group-based) for presenting and managing the aspects of teaching the 28 identified therapeutic-specific skills of therapy presented in this text (Chapters 6 and 7). For it is within the context of one or more of the 18 learning-focused activities shown in Figure 1–2 that student SLPs actually learn to do the 28 therapeutic-specific skills of basic speech-language therapy. These 28 therapeutic-specific skills are referenced later in this chapter, but for the moment, the concept of using the 18 different learning-focused activities (see Figure 1–2) to teach the 28 therapeutic-specific skills is captured in Table 1–1 (Matrix of focal points [Supervisors, Textbook, and Interactive Groups] and activities in which therapeutic-specific skills may be addressed).

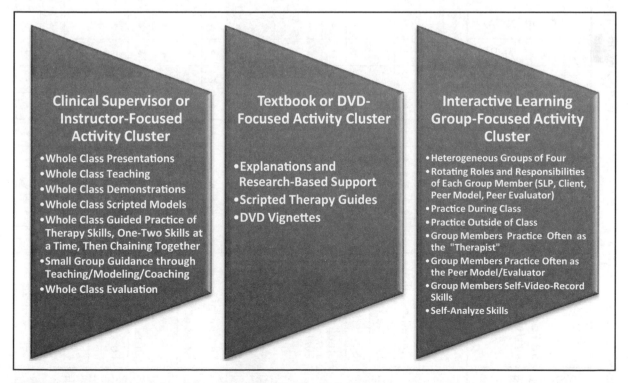

Figure 1–2. Focused activity clusters for critical incidents learning.

Table 1–1. Matrix of Focal Points (Supervisors, Textbook, and Interactive Groups) and Activities in which Therapeutic-Specific Skills May be Addressed

Focal Points	18 Focused Activities	28 Therapeutic-Specific Skills																											
		Motivation	Expectations	Enthusiasm	Animation	Volume	Seating	Proximity	Touch	Preparation	Pacing	Fluency	Alerting	Cueing	Modeling	Prompting	Modalities	Demonstrate	Questions	Wait-Time	Shaping	Verbal Praise	Tokens	Reinforcers	Feedback	Data Collect	Probing	Behavior	Trbl. Shoot
Supervisors	Presentation	•	•	•	•	•	•	•	•	•	•	•	•	•	•	•	•	•	•	•	•	•	•	•	•	•	•	•	•
	Teaching	•	•	•	•	•	•	•	•	•	•	•	•	•	•	•	•	•	•	•	•	•	•	•	•	•	•	•	•
	Demonstration	•	•	•	•	•	•	•	•	•	•	•	•	•	•	•	•	•	•	•	•	•	•	•	•	•	•	•	•
	Scripted Models			•		•						•	•	•	•	•	•	•	•	•	•	•			•		•		
	Guided Practice	•										•	•	•	•	•	•	•	•	•	•	•			•	•	•		
	Small Groups		•	•		•						•	•	•	•	•	•	•	•	•	•	•			•	•	•		
	Evaluations	•	•	•	•	•	•	•	•	•	•	•	•	•	•	•	•	•	•	•	•	•	•	•	•	•	•	•	•
Text	Supports	•	•	•	•	•	•	•	•	•	•	•	•	•	•	•	•	•	•	•	•	•	•	•	•	•	•	•	•
	Scripted Guides			•	•					•	•	•			•	•		•	•			•			•		•	•	
	DVD Vignettes			•				•	•	•	•	•	•	•	•	•	•		•	•	•	•			•	•	•	•	•
Interactive Groups	Groups of Four	•	•	•	•	•	•	•	•	•	•	•	•	•	•	•	•	•	•	•	•	•	•	•	•	•	•	•	•
	Roles in Group	•	•	•	•	•	•	•	•	•	•	•	•	•	•	•	•	•	•	•	•	•	•	•	•	•	•	•	•
	In-Class Practice	•	•	•	•	•	•	•	•	•	•	•	•	•	•	•	•	•	•	•	•	•	•	•	•	•	•	•	•
	Outside Practice	•	•	•	•	•	•	•	•	•	•	•	•	•	•	•	•	•	•	•	•	•	•	•	•	•	•	•	•
	Focus as Therapist	•	•	•	•	•	•	•	•	•	•	•	•	•	•	•	•	•	•	•	•	•	•	•	•	•	•	•	•
	Peer Tutor														•														
	Video-Record	•	•	•	•	•	•	•	•	•	•	•	•	•	•	•	•	•	•	•	•	•	•	•	•	•	•	•	•
	Self-Analyze	•	•	•	•	•	•	•	•	•	•	•	•	•	•	•	•	•	•	•	•	•	•	•	•	•	•	•	•

14

For each of the 28 therapeutic-specific skills that needs to be taught (e.g., *animation, enthusiasm, volume, proximity,* etc.), student learning appears to be greater if that skill is aligned properly and taught or presented within the confines of one or more of the above learning-focused activity clusters (Supervisor-based, Textbook/DVD-based, or Interactive Group-based), then refined in an additional learning-focused activity cluster, and finally, specifically mastered in yet another learning-focused activity cluster, as applicable. For example, the therapeutic-specific skill for *proximity* in therapy is often first introduced to students through use of the Clinical Supervisor or Instructor-Focused Activity Cluster whereby the clinical supervisor or Instructor *presents, or teaches,* the concept of proximity in a lecture to the entire class (Whole Class Presentation), followed by having the entire class physically stand or rearrange seats to *demonstrate* appropriate proximity for the therapeutic setting (Whole Class Demonstration). This type whole class presentation or teaching, then, demonstrating, is first introduced as a Clinical Supervisor or Instructor-Focused Activity. However, to continue student learning in the area of proximity, the clinical supervisor or instructor directs students to either the textbook/DVD segment on proximity, or directs students to practice proximity within Interactive Learning Group-Focused Activities. Regardless of choices for sequencing in this learning experience example, the clinical supervisor or instructor uses as many learning opportunities as possible to support student learning, and does so with full awareness that, most often, the student SLP's learning of targeted skills takes place in a variety of settings arranged for the student within and across (a) Clinical Supervisor or Instructor-Focused activities, (b) Textbook or DVD-Focused activities, or (c) Interactive Learning Group-Focused activities. It is believed that one or more of the 18 learning-focused activities will serve as critical incident activities for student SLPs as they work to develop the 28 therapeutic-specific skills across the three different focus activity clusters (Supervisors or Instructors, Textbook/DVD, or Interactive Learning Groups).

Critical Incidents in Learning to Do Speech-Language Therapy

It is not always possible to pinpoint the exact moment, nor the exact experience in learning to do therapy that can be identified as the "critical incident," the significant experience that influences an individual student's development in learning to do therapy as noted by Furr and Carroll (2003). However, during observations of student learning in the development of skills for speech-language therapy, student learning is evident. Additionally, student learning is significant and student learning, more often than not, is accurate—or at the very least—it is adequate for the initial development of skills in basic speech-language therapy.

In an attempt to localize or pinpoint those activities that students rate as critical incident activities for learning to do therapy as suggested by Furr and Carroll (2003), 60 students were given an informal survey and asked to rank each of the 18 learning-focused activities that appear in the three focused activity clusters listed in Figure 1–2 according to perceived value of the activity in helping the student learn to do therapy. Additionally, each student was asked to rank order the top three activities according to perceptions of whether the selected activity was (1) the most valuable, (2) the second most valuable, and (3) the third most valuable in learning to do therapy. Surprisingly, students indicated 15 of the 18 learning-focused activities as critical incident experiences. However, three experiences were rated as extremely valuable by student respondents. Fifty-six (56) of the 60 surveys were returned as usable for analysis. Results indicated twofold findings:

- Students rated the following activities as *valuable,* with combined results for *valuable* and *extremely valuable* also given for consideration for the power of activities in learning to do therapy:
  - *Small group teaching, guiding, coaching, or modeling by the instructor during classroom time:* 90% of students rated this activity as extremely valuable, with the percentage increasing to 98% for the combined valuable and extremely valuable ratings.
  - *Instructor's classroom demonstrations of therapy:* 85% of students rated this activity as extremely valuable, with the percentage increasing to 100% for the combined valuable and extremely valuable ratings.
  - *Verbal/scripted model by the instructor of what the "therapist" should say for the Introduction, Body, and Closing of a therapy session:* 86% of students rated this activity as extremely valuable, with the percentage increasing to 100% for the combined valuable and extremely valuable ratings.

- Students ranked the following three learning-focused activities, in order given, as the activities that qualified as the *top three* rated critical incident experiences in learning to do speech-language therapy:
  - *Instructor's classroom demonstrations of therapy*
  - *Small group teaching, guiding, coaching, or modeling by the instructor during classroom time*
  - *Verbal/scripted model by the instructor of what the "therapist" should say for the Introduction, Body, and Closing of a therapy session*

Although not generalizable to a typical population of student SLPs due to the small sample size and informal nature of the survey, clinical supervisors and instructors are, nonetheless, encouraged to note the activities designated as either (a) Clinical Supervisor or Instructor-Focused activities, (b) Textbook or DVD-Focused activities, or (c) Interactive Learning Group-Focused activities, and are encouraged to arrange classroom learning experiences in ways that provide students with opportunities to engage in each of the 18 focused activities presented in Figure 1–2. Much of the remainder of this chapter will focus on presentation of information designed to help clinical supervisors or instructors, and SLP students, benefit from engagement in these 18 learning-focused activities.

Based on years of clinical teaching experience in working with students using all three types of focused activities (Clinical Supervisor or Instructor, Textbook/DVD, or Interactive Learning Group), it is believed that, although difficult to pinpoint or project for any given student, the combined experiences of these 18 learning-focused activities together serve to achieve for each successful student the critical incidents needed for maximal learning. Let's briefly overview the tenets of each activity in which the student learner will engage in an effort to relate the 18 focused activities to the 28 therapeutic-specific skills needed to learn how to do speech-language therapy as shown in Table 1–1.

Overview of Focused Activities

Focused activities refer to clusters of activities that are centered around three different focal points that serve as foundations for the tasks that students will be learning. For purposes of this text, the three different focal points that anchor the student's learning tasks are (1) the Clinical Supervisor or Instructor, (2) the Textbook/DVD, and (3) the Interactive Learning Groups comprised of the student learners themselves. (See Figure 1–2.) Each focused activity cluster features tasks seen as important to learning to do therapy. Note that some activities occur in more than one focused cluster; this is by design, based on the nature of what—and how—the student is being asked to learn. There are some tasks that simply must be addressed from several perspectives in order to support best learning. Following is a brief overview of the three focused activity clusters with accompanying details of the type activities contained within each cluster.

Clinical Supervisor or Instructor-Focused Activity Cluster

Although not necessarily an exhaustive list, for purposes of this discussion, the Clinical Supervisor or Instructor-Focused Activity Cluster is comprised of seven different activities that clinical supervisors or instructors provide for student SLPs who are learning to do therapy. These seven activities are shown in the Clinical Supervisor or Instructor-Focused Activity Cluster in Figure 1–2 and consist of the following tasks that are conducted by clinical supervisors or instructors as basic activities designed to help the student SLP learn how to do therapy: (1) *Whole Class Presentations*; (2) *Whole Class Teaching*; (3) *Whole Class Demonstrations*; (4) *Whole Class Scripted Models*; (5) *Whole Class Guided Practice of Therapy Skills, One-Two Skills at a Time, Then Chaining Together*; (6) *Small Group Guided Practice through Teaching/Modeling/Coaching*; and (7) *Whole Class Evaluation*. Explanations and possible implementation suggestions for each of these seven activities may prove helpful to clinical supervisors and instructors.

Whole Class Presentations

Whole Class Presentations are defined as more formal lectures or presentations that clinical supervisors or instructors engage in when introducing a new skill or concept. The term "presentation," for practical purposes, may be sometimes used synonymously with the word "teach"; however, for purposes of this discussion, presentation as a concept is suggested as being separate from teaching as a concept based on the formality associated with presentations. Typically, presentations are formal orations characterized by sequenced information designed to introduce, explain, or help the listener conceptualize information within a lecture or speech type format. There is often very little intent for audience interaction with the speaker during a presentation. For example, a presentation on the concept of *"therapeutic proximity"* might call for prepared information related to the various elements of personal, communicative, and public spaces. A formal presentation on this topic that includes handouts or other media supports for the presenter is seen as appropriate. Often whole class presentations equate to an overview of general concepts to be learned in more detailed following the presentation.

Suggested Uses of Presentations. Clinical supervisors or instructors may choose to use presentations in lecture formats to introduce new therapy concepts and skills in an overview, or to move quickly from point to point in presenting work that has several sequential parts.

Whole Class Teaching

Whole class teaching is much less formal than a presentation. In whole class teaching, the clinical supervisor or instructor's objective is to ensure that students begin the task of learning the information presented in overview or presentation format. Teaching takes place in several stages with there being any number of teaching methodologies available to clinical supervisors or instructors. For example, when "teaching," a lesson might be divided as follows:

1. *Introduction, attention, or motivation,* whereby the intent is to pique the learner's interest in the lesson and help the learner focus on the selected topic. Goals and objectives of the lesson, interesting background, relevant concepts and questions, interesting uses of materials (even costumes) that help the learner focus on the topic are appropriate for this teaching phase.

2. *Direct teaching* includes uses of lectures, definitions, salient points, demonstrations, media presentations, models, and so forth, to help the learner conceptualize the foundations of the topic and connect the content to other areas of knowledge.

3. *Guided practice* may occur in two forms: (a) *whole class guided practice* is recommended when a concept is being presented for the first time. The clinical supervisor or instructor literally guides the entire class through practice of the concept or technique, step-by-step, so that everyone in the class participates as responders in unison for the first few times of practice, based on modeling/imitation, scripts, and so forth, and (b) *small group guided practice,* wherein, following apparent increased comfort with the new concept or skill as a whole class event, the class is divided into the interactive or collaborative work groups. During small group guided practice, the clinical supervisor or instructor goes from group to group, listening, guiding, and providing feedback to the groups as needed.

4. *Independent practice* is encouraged *only after the clinical supervisor or instructor determines that the group members are practicing correctly enough to be allowed to practice outside of the watchful eye of the supervisor or instructor.* This is important in that, as we will see later, if groups are allowed to practice independently, *but incorrectly*, it becomes more difficult to achieve the desired outcomes in learning.

There are, of course, numerous other approaches to teaching and learning (Brackenbury, 2012; Çakmak, 2008; Selahattin & İlknur, 2010; Tetsuo, 2011; Vajoczki, Savage, Martin, Borin, & Kustra, 2011; Wright, 2011), and each clinical supervisor or instructor may already have a preferred method or approach to teaching that may easily be continued under the structure of whole class teaching. For purposes of this discussion, whole class teaching is described as any activity that is designed to engage the entire class and help students move to progressively higher levels of awareness, understanding, and skill-building for a targeted subject or skill. In this sense, explanations, graphic representations, explorations, conversations, facilitation techniques, corrective feedback, and so forth, might all qualify as "teaching." The point here is not to lock in a clinical supervisor or instructor into a set of behaviors called "teaching," but rather to help the clinical educator understand that teaching is about sharing knowledge and helping learners (SLP student learners) navigate through the processes of learning designated skills associated with speech-language therapy. Each clinical supervisor or instructor is encouraged to seek his or her own comfort level with techniques used for teaching the designated skills for speech-language therapy identified in this text.

Suggested Uses of Teaching. Once the clinical supervisor or instructor completes any desired presentations of topics or skills, the concept of teaching begins. In fact, it is very possible to skip formal presentations for some topics, if desired, and begin student engagement with a topic in whole class teaching through uses of techniques previously mentioned: explanations, graphic representations, explorations, conversations, facilitation techniques, corrective feedback, and so forth. The basic construct to focus on is that, regardless of the topic, whole class teaching is essentially just that—teaching that is done with the whole class. For example, in working with the concept of therapeutic proximity, a presentation on the topic may include handouts, or other supports, etc., as mentioned earlier. However, in whole class teaching, the same concept may be addressed in a completely different manner. Although the clinical supervisor or instructor may, in fact, use handouts or other supports in teaching as well as in presentations, the difference in presentation and teaching becomes a matter of student engagement. Presentations are seen as passive (receptive) student engagement, whereas teaching is viewed as more interactive (or give and take) student engagement. In teaching the concept of proximity, the clinical supervisor or instructor may find conversation regarding proximity to be appropriate by leading the whole class in a discussion of the topic in the following manner:

"Let's talk about your own needs for proximity and personal space for a moment. Think about a time when you felt that your personal space was a little too small for your preferences for space—for example, at a dinner party where someone may have placed an item in a space that you privately reserved for yourself. What kind of thoughts or reactions do you remember having about the situation? Think for a moment, then, let's have volunteers share experiences."

This type of whole class teaching does not accomplish the complete goal of teaching the concept of proximity, but it does lead the entire class toward the direction of greater awareness and understanding of the concept of therapeutic proximity—and, it's far less formal than what is typically seen as a presentation. Clinical supervisors or instructors may choose to use numerous other teaching strategies (explanations, graphic representations, explorations, facilitation techniques, corrective feedback, etc.), as desired, to help accomplish the goal of helping students further conceptualize or understand new skills for learning how to do therapy.

Whole Class Demonstrations

Whole class demonstrations are appropriate when the clinical supervisor or instructor wishes to be sure that everyone in the class is exposed to the same demonstrations, examples, explanations, or applications of information that support a concept being taught. For example, to continue the work on proximity, once the clinical supervisor or instructor makes a brief presentation on the subject, then, teaches the subject through use of conversation, or exploration, and so forth, the next task in student learning might be a whole class demonstration whereby the clinical supervisor or instructor asks one student to come forward for demonstrations of effective therapeutic proximity, and how to achieve proximity in various therapeutic seating positions (e.g., side-by-side seating, across the table seating, cluster seating, etc.). In this way, everyone in the class sees the same demonstrations at the same time so that numerous repetitions of demonstrations are not necessary in smaller group work.

Suggested Uses of Whole Class Demonstrations. The majority of the 28 therapeutic-specific skills highlighted in Chapters 6 and 7 of this text can be demonstrated in whole class format, if desired. Each clinical supervisor or instructor will have his or her preferred styles and concepts of what constitutes appropriate skill levels for each therapeutic-specific skill. Whether demonstrating proximity, animation, enthusiasm, and volume, or whether demonstrating uses of therapeutic touch, each clinical supervisor or instructor brings to the whole class demonstration a wealth of possibilities. Because each clinical supervisor or instructor will have specific ways of presenting, teaching, and demonstrating skills based on personal preferences, demonstration possibilities are boundless.

Whole Class Scripted Models

A whole class scripted model is simply an activity whereby the clinical supervisor or instructor literally reads a "script," a segment from this text (Chapter 7, Chart 7–2. Detailed Therapy Progression), or from other sources, that gives students an idea of what they should sound like during therapeutic intervention. In fact, clinical educators may very well write their own script to fit specific teaching–learning needs. Regardless of the source of the script, clinical supervisors or instructors choose a skill set that students need to learn and guide the students through what that skill set sounds like in therapy by verbally modeling the skill set and having the whole class repeat the modeled segments in unison. For example, if the chosen skill set for the session is a combined animation and enthusiasm segment, the clinical supervisor or instructor reads or models a line at a time from a selected or written text (a script), and the entire class imitates or repeats the model as given—not only as given in its content, but also in its style for intonation, enthusiasm, pace, and so forth. Many students (and clinical supervisors or instructors) report feeling completely awkward in this activity. There is always a lot of laughter, sometimes a little embarrassment, and occasionally a little resistance, associated with this activity at its initial introduction. However, random comments over the years, and results of the informal survey of the 18 focused activities (mentioned earlier), suggested that scripted models were among the top three critical incident experiences that helped SLP students significantly in the development of learning to do speech-language therapy. Based on the findings of several researchers (Bisland, Malow-Iroff, & O'Connor, 2006; Kollar, Fischer, & Hesse, 2006) regarding the value of scripted information for the novice learner, the power of scripted models for the student SLP is understandable.

Scripted therapy guides may be as short as one word, as in words used for verbal praise ("Awesome!"; "Wonderful!"; "Excellent!"; etc.), or they may be as long as a sentence or short paragraph, depending on the skill being taught. Scripted therapy guides, of course, are never all inclusive, but they are typically generalizable to the therapeutic process. In fact, scripted models don't actually have to be written in that most clinical supervisors or instructors have a ready repertoire of "scripts" (what needs to be said or done) in their working vocabularies. For example, in a "scripted" therapy guide for verbal praise, the student SLP might be taught to use the phrase, "Wonderful!" in response to the client's appropriate participation in his or her turn in therapy. Verbal praise is a desirable and acceptable therapeutic skill; however, many student SLPs forget to offer verbal praise of the client's efforts during therapy, so the clinical supervisor or instructor finds it necessary to very naturally interject the "script" (unwritten) for verbal praise by modeling for the student SLP the praise, "Wonderful!" Student SLPs often simply imitate the verbal praise offered by the clinical supervisor or instructor in early learning stages of therapy, but before long, student SLPs can be observed generalizing verbal praise to include other phrases such as "Good job!" or "Way to go!" Typically, once student SLPs understand that something should be said at a certain time in therapy, for certain reasons, and in certain ways, these students first learn the given "script," then move quickly to add their own personal preferences to the situation in a generalized fashion—and this is as it should be.

The intent of a script is *not* to produce hundreds of SLPs who all sound alike, or are cloned to act the same, do the same, be the same in therapy—even though it may appear to be so in initial stages of working from a script to learn how to do therapy. Instead, the intent of the scripted therapy guides is to help with initial processing, conceptualizing, absorbing, understanding, learning, and applying skills needed for effective speech-language therapy; in this regard, the script is simply a vehicle by which student SLPs come to understand that SLP professionals use certain processes in helping to change client behavior in communication skills. Similarly, there are processes that the student SLP must master in learning to help guide the client to positive changes in communication behavior. The strength of a scripted therapy guide is that it supports the learning processes for students seeking to acquire therapy skills in simple, easy to grasp formats as novice learners.

Haring, Lovitt, Eaton, and Hansen (1978) presented four stages of learning that are relevant to this discussion: *acquisition, fluency, generalization,* and *adaptation.* A novice student operating at the *acquisition,* or beginning stage of learning, experiences learning that is slow and inaccurate. Haring et al. suggested the use of demonstrations and modeling (as in scripted therapy guides) for such learners. The use of scripts in early learning stages was promoted by several other researchers as well (Bisland, Malow-Iroff, & O'Connor, 2006; Kollar, Fischer, & Hesse, 2006; Paul, 2011; Smilkstein, 1993; Youmans, Youmans, & Hancock, 2011). As the student reaches the *fluency* stage in learning, skills start to become accurate. It is important, to the degree possible, for the learner to begin thinking about not only accuracy of skills, but speed of performances of the new skill after accomplishing fluency for new skills. Of course, for fluency of skills, first comes accuracy in the skill, then the speed of presentation or performance of skills is added. The student in *generalization* of skills is accurate with the skill, has developed skills that show increased speed with accuracy, and is learning when to appropriately apply the new skill. Through continued practice, and trial and error, the new skill becomes more accurately applied. The student in the *adaptation* stage of learning begins retaining skills over a time period, with learners showing increased accuracy in appropriately using the new skill in different settings and stimuli. As adaptation expands for the student, he/she is able to use the new skill in novel ways to problem solve across different therapeutic situations (Haring, Lovitt, Eaton, & Hansen, 1978). The belief is that, as students move from the acquisition stage of learning, with the need for models and scripted therapy guides, on into fluency, generalization, and finally to adaptation, students with solid beginnings in acquisition find it easier to move through the stages of learning to become the adapted problem-solvers that we so desire in the SLP profession. Scripted therapy guides are the beginning foundations for learning to do therapy; scripted therapy guides are *not* the desired eventual outcomes.

Suggested Uses of Whole Class Scripted Models. Whole class scripted models are very useful for helping students find their "therapeutic voice," the pitch, animation, enthusiasm levels, and intonations, students should use based on ages of clients. For example, the following greeting typically sounds completely different, depending on the age (and often, the disorder) of the client: *"Hi. It's so good to see you today."* Whole class scripted models for this greeting are often given as if the client were two different ages to show contrasts in pitch, enthusiasm, animation, and intonation: a 3-year-old, and a 40-year-old, both cognitively normal. With the clinical supervisor or instructor using a simple script to model various segments of a therapy session, such as a greeting, students are able to capture the essence of several therapeutic-specific skills very quickly.

Clinical supervisors or instructors may choose to use scripts at any given stage of learning, depending on circumstances. Due to the vast amount of skills student SLPs need to learn, maintain, generalize, and adapt, it is not always easy for the student SLP to learn skills in a linear fashion; nor is it always possible for clinical supervisors or instructors to assess skills in a linear fashion. For example, although any given skill may proceed linearly from point A to B to C, in a uniform and desired manner, the student SLP may, at the same time, also be learning another skill that is not progressing as smoothly. Thus, a student SLP may be performing as an adapted learner in the first skill, but may still be in the acquisition stages of the second, or even, third skill. In this instance, the clinical supervisor or instructor may find it necessary to interject a script or model for the second or third skill, even though the student SLP is an adapted learner for the first skill. To this end, while clinical supervisors or instructors are encouraged to monitor student progress for learning any given skill, (1) it is not always necessary to insist on linear progress in learning each skill before moving to or introducing an additional skill, and (2) it is not necessary to establish a strict 1:1 relationship between the stages of learning, or skill acquisition, and the student SLP's need for scripted therapy guides or models. Instead, clinical supervisors or instructors should be prepared to offer scripted therapy guides or models for the development of any given therapy skill regardless of where a student might be in the stages of learning other skills. This will become especially evident when working with students in small interactive groups.

Whole Class Guided Practice of Therapy Skills, One-Two Skills at a Time, Then Chaining Together

Several researchers (Bisland, Malow-Iroff, & O'Connor, 2006; Haring, Lovitt, Eaton, & Hansen, 1978) suggested that guided practice is a common teaching strategy. During guided practice, the teacher uses step-by-step instructions, demonstrations, or models to lead students through a sequence of learning events that comprise part-to-whole, or whole-part-whole learning (Backus & Beasley, 1951). For example, in this text, the Introduction section of therapy is composed of three different elements: *greeting and rapport, previous session's work,* and *collection of homework.* The Closing segment of therapy in this text consists of four different elements: *review of the objectives of the session, report of correct productions, mentioning/assigning homework,* and *rewards and dismissal.*

The clinical supervisor or instructor may find it advantageous to guide the whole class through the greeting and rapport segment of the introduction, and, once proficiency is achieved by the whole class, add on the next segment of the Introduction, then the last segment, systematically adding on, or chaining, skills in a whole class guided practice event until the entire section of therapy is more comfortable for student learners. Similarly, when guiding students through the Closing of the Session, clinical supervisors or instructors may choose to guide the whole class through the first element of the Closing, then, the second, the third, and finally, the fourth, until the whole class achieves proficiency and feels (and sounds) more comfortable with the way a typical speech-language therapy session may be closed. This sequential way of managing the verbal behaviors that accompany learning is often referred to as chaining behaviors. Chaining in learning was reported by Hulit, Howard, and Fahey (2011) to be an effective way to help students acquire and maintain larger volumes of information such as the large amounts of information SLP students are required to learn and retain when learning how to do basic speech-language therapy.

Suggested Uses of Whole Class Guided Practice of Therapy Skills, One-Two Skills at a Time, Then Chaining Together. The sequences that the SLP student needs to learn for both the Introduction and Closing of a therapy session serve as good segments for initial uses of whole class guided practice in that these segments are seen as less threatening and more fun for the novice learner. As clinical supervisors and instructors essentially use step-by-step instructions, demonstrations, or models of what various elements of therapy might look or sound like, it becomes easier for SLP students to begin to form a foundation for learning large amounts of materials quickly, one-two skills at a time. Once information is learned in small chunks, or as segmented skills, then chained together within larger whole class guided practices, students quickly become comfortable with practicing skills individually, or in smaller groups. Eventually, even the more demanding sequences of the Body of Therapy become more easily learned and absorbed when the elements of the Body of Therapy are taught in whole class guided practice of therapy skills, one-two skills at a time, then chained together.

Small Group Guided Practice through Teaching/Modeling/Coaching

Small group guided practice through teaching, modeling, or coaching is accomplished by dividing classes into groups of four student SLP learners as mentioned earlier in this chapter. Early in the training cycle (semester, quarter, year—depending on administrative arrangements of courses) the clinical supervisor or instructor allows students within the class to form cooperative groups of four that will become the "interactive learning groups" through which small group learning and interactions occur for the remainder of the training cycle. Note that the interactive learning group has its own place in student learning for a large portion of the 18 learning-focused activities as a stand-alone focused cluster. However, in this portion of the discussion, the central focus is on the clinical supervisor or instructor's work with the interactive learning group. Although, occasionally, there will be a learning group of only three members, or a learning group of five members, based on number of class members, groups of four are recommended for the basic interactive learning group for the following reasons:

1.   Forming groups of four allows student learners to better understand the interactive nature of the therapeutic process. Four members of a group allow

students to more easily study all possible roles encountered in group therapy: (a) therapist, (b) target client, (c) peer model, and (d) peer evaluator.

2. With one group member serving as the SLP, of the three members serving as clients for various learning experiences, one client is always the "target client," the one who is being taught specific objectives of the session, while the remaining two clients serve as peer models/peer evaluators to support the learning of the target client. In this way, all clients are always engaged in the therapy learning process, either as client learner, as peer model, or as peer evaluator. No client is idle as the interactive nature of the therapy session requires each client to attend and focus such that when called upon, he/she is ready to model correct structures, following the SLP's lead, or is ready to evaluate the productions of the peer client upon the SLP's request.

In situations when it is necessary to form alternate groups of three or five (rather than groups of four student SLP learners), it is preferable to form groups of five so that students more easily see the interactive nature of what therapy looks and sounds like when there are at least two peer models/evaluators, as would occur in groups of four (and possibly three peer models/evaluators, as would occur in groups of five), rather than only one peer model/evaluator as would occur in interactive groups of only three learners.

During small group guided practice through teaching/modeling/coaching, each member of the small interactive group of four is assigned a group member number: 1, 2, 3, or 4 (for groups of four, of course). Following whole group work on any given topic or skill, the clinical supervisor or instructor directs groups to gather, and assigns the task that group members will practice within the session. For ease in classroom management, typically, all groups within the class are assigned to work on the same clinical skills (for example, *Closing of the Session*), with a designated group member (by number) asked to begin the work of the session. A typical directive from the clinical supervisor or instructor to accompany this example might sound like this:

"Everyone, please get into your interactive work groups of four. Group members #3, you will serve as the "SLP" for the beginning of the class today. Please arrange the appropriate seating for your clients, and begin the small group practice session today by practicing the Closing of the Session. Everyone, once members #3 have practiced and feel comfortable with the Close of the Session, group members #4 will become the SLP for the session. Members #4, please begin your practice time for the Close of the Session, once members #3 have finished practice times. I will come around to all groups to observe members #3 for the Close of the Session, and I may be able to see some members #4 for the Close of the Session today as well. For all group members #4 not observed today, I will begin our next class session by observing your work. Group members #3, begin your practice and I'll come around for observations, teaching, modeling, coaching, and corrective feedback as quickly as possible. If there are no questions, members #3, please begin your practice for the Closing of the Session."

The clinical supervisor or instructor in the above scenario waits a few minutes for designated group members to practice the assigned skill(s) or sequence(s), then begins systematically moving among the various small groups of four within the classroom. The clinical supervisor or instructor listens, observes, teaches/reiterates, models, coaches, demonstrates, etc., as needed for not only the learning and development of the designated "SLP," but does so for the benefit of every member in that particular small group. In this way, learning becomes more interactive in that all group members help each other learn the assigned skills. They all see and hear the same model, get the same coaching, and get answers to the same question(s) at the same time, and in the same way. In helping each other understand the work of the clinical supervisor or instructor in small groups, each group member literally becomes the "teacher" of others in the group, depending on what each hears, understands, applies, and shares with others within the small interactive group format. For example, as the clinical supervisor or instructor leaves a particular small group to observe another small group, it is not uncommon to hear a member of the former group say to peer members something similar to the following: "No, no, she said we need to change . . . " At that moment of explanation or reiteration, that student learner literally becomes the "teacher" of his or her peers.

Suggested Uses of Small Group Guided Practice Through Teaching, Modeling, and Coaching. Once the clinical supervisor or instructor has presented and taught information, used whole class demonstrations, whole class scripted models, and whole class guided practice, small group guided practice through uses of teaching, modeling, and coaching (and other teaching/learning strategies) will become the foundational activity through which the student SLP learns most of the skills of how to do basic speech-language therapy. Whether learning data collection, therapeutic touch, or corrective feedback, etc., it is possible to learn all of the identified 28 therapeutic-specific skills for basic speech-language therapy within the confines of the small group guided practice opportunities.

Each clinical supervisor or instructor will determine ways that best serve to keep track of individual student SLP's progress and development during work within small group guided practice sessions. Some clinical supervisors or instructors choose more formal ways of recording/grading student progress in developing skills within the small group guided practice sessions, whereas others simply make mental notes, or jot down information that serves as indicators for the next skills that need to be addressed within the small group guided practice session. Regardless of how formal or informal the evaluation of a student SLP's development might be in the small group guided practice sessions, the major objective for the clinical supervisor or instructor during this type group work (other than student learning, of course), is to determine the degree to which students are achieving proficiency in demonstrating desired therapeutic skills for appropriate decision making regarding moving the small groups on to the next desired skill set. Although students often report feelings of nervousness when clinical supervisors or instructors come to work with them in small groups, these same students continue to report interactive small group learning to be a very powerful and sometimes fun way for student SLPs to learn the basic concepts of speech-language therapy.

Whole Class Evaluation

The final Clinical Supervisor or Instructor-Focused Activity is whole class evaluation. Each clinical supervisor or instructor will determine the values and appropriateness of whole class evaluations, depending on the nature and structure of the learning setting for the student SLP, and based on many other teaching and learning parameters. Based on teaching and learning trends in prior classes that learned to do therapy as addressed in this text, it was found that at least one lightly weighted whole class evaluation covering the components of basic therapy (components of the Introduction, Body, and Closing) may serve to help student SLPs focus, conceptualize, integrate, and apply basic learning. However, each clinical supervisor or instructor will have his or her preferred practices in both formal and informal evaluation of students' knowledge and development related to the acquisition of basic skills for speech-language therapy.

Suggested Uses of Whole Class Evaluation. Whole class evaluation of student SLPs' skills may cover as few or as many aspects of student learning as desired. Each clinical supervisor or instructor will determine evaluation needs and formats based on individual preferences and teaching circumstances.

It is important to note that, although each of the above seven Clinical Supervisor or Instructor-Focused Activities are available and recommended to clinical supervisors or instructors as activities that support student learning, not all seven activities are needed for every skill that is to be taught in the processes of learning to do therapy. Similarly, not all seven activities will be needed during each class session when student SLPs are learning to do therapy. To these ends, the successes of students learning how to do therapy are still, ultimately, dependent on the guidance and preferences of individual clinical supervisors and instructors. It is, however, hoped that the above explanations of the roles of the above seven focused activities in supporting desired outcomes is helpful. Figure 1–3 shows a graphic depiction of how a clinical supervisor or instructor might construct a typical class session using these seven activities for teaching speech-language therapy on a routine basis.

As clinical supervisors and instructors plan classroom experiences for student SLPs, the information in Figure 1–3 may be helpful for designing classroom experiences for daily practical application. However, as indicated earlier, not all possible activities will be needed for each class session. Each clinical supervisor or instructor will determine specific class content and objectives based on class needs.

Textbook or DVD-Focused Activity Cluster

When teaching student SLPs to do therapy, for purposes of this discussion, the Textbook or DVD-Focused Activity Cluster is composed of three different activities centered around this textbook and/or its accompanying DVD. These three activities are shown in Figure 1–2 as the Textbook or DVD-Focused Activity Cluster, and consist of the following tasks that

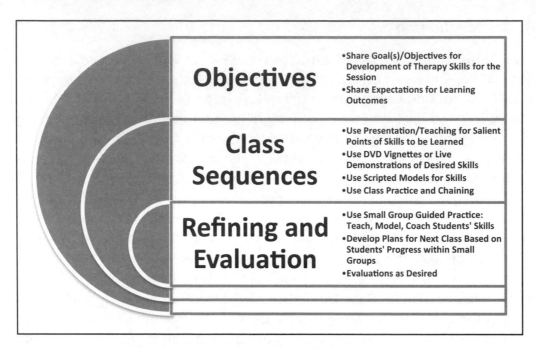

Figure 1–3. Supervisor's routine tasks for therapy skills development.

are supported by the textbook or DVD as basic activities designed to help the student SLP learn how to do therapy: (1) *Explanations and Research-Based Support*; (2) *Scripted Therapy Guides*; and (3) *DVD Vignettes.*

Explanations and Research-Based Support

This second edition of the textbook is designed to assist clinical supervisors or instructors and student SLP learners by providing explanations and an organizational schema around which central themes of the textbook are founded. For example, the textbook continues to promote student learning of 28 therapeutic-specific skills associated with speech-language therapy, and the textbook continues to provide explanations and research-based support for engaging in learning and teaching of these therapeutic-specific skills. Additionally, the expansion of information in this new Chapter 1 of the textbook is designed to add structure to how the textbook may be used to further help organize teaching and learning of the 28 therapeutic-specific skills. This is accomplished by offering 18 different learning-focused activities (Figure 1–2) in which the 28 therapeutic-specific skills presented in the text may be learned. (See Table 1–1 for a complete indication of the 18 learning-focused activities suggested for use in teaching the 28 therapeutic-specific skills.)

Suggested Uses of Explanations and Research-Based Support. Skills for learning to do speech-language therapy are found in many sources: observations, conversations, direct teaching, specific training, and even creative trial and error. Typically, no one source can be attributed to addressing the breadth and depth of skills an SLP ultimately commands over the span of a professional career. This textbook is designed to be an integral part of the SLP's early training when it is important to get a student SLP from "zero/very-little-to-something-credible" in a short period of time. The intent of the text is to present a number of different aspects of therapy designed to help student SLPs process, conceptualize, absorb, understand, learn, and apply skills needed for basic speech-language therapy. Without elaboration on technical or semantic differences in terms (process, conceptualize, absorb, understand, learn), it is hoped that this textbook, at the very least, contributes to the desired outcomes for teaching student SLPs how to do speech-language therapy. To that end, the clinical supervisor or instructor is encouraged to use the text in any ways credible for achieving targeted outcomes.

Scripted Therapy Guides

Scripted therapy guides are essentially written samples or examples of what the student SLP says in a therapeutic situation. Scripted therapy guides are included occasionally throughout Part I of the textbook, but they are a dominant portion of Part II of the textbook. These "scripts" give student SLPs parameters for what they actually say (or do) during the therapeutic exchange. Although scripted guides are included in the text, as indicated earlier in this chapter, clinical supervisors or instructors may also choose to write their own scripts for specific teaching and guided practice purposes. As indicated earlier, some "scripted" content is already a part of the clinical supervisor or instructor's repertoire and need not be actually written. Still, however, these inherent "scripts" need to be modeled for the student.

Suggested Uses of Scripted Therapy Guides. As indicated earlier, scripted therapy guides likely have the most power when used in the initial learning stages when, according to Haring, Lovitt, Eaton, and Hansen (1978), learning is slow and inaccurate (acquisition stage of learning), or when skills are accurate but slow (fluency stage of learning). Scripted therapy guides will be needed less often as student SLPs begin generalizing and adapting skills in therapy.

Textbook/DVD Vignettes

DVD vignettes are designed to provide visual support and demonstrations of 21 of the 28 therapeutic-specific skills highlighted in this textbook and shown graphically in Chart 1–2. The exact skills captured in the DVD segments of the text are outlined in Chapter 6 of this text, with guided information for student SLP engagement in activities designed to assist learning of skills noted in Chapter 6 as well. Additionally, written "workshops" to assist learners are provided in the form of appendix supports entitled, "Therapeutic-Specific Workshops" (TSW). These workshops are provided to further assist the SLP student learner with conceptualizing the processes of learning how to do therapy, and may be used in conjunction with viewing the DVD vignettes.

Suggested Uses of the DVD Vignettes. DVD vignettes and TSW forms may be used in either whole class formats, in small group work, or individually. However, DVD vignettes are not scripted to match exact content information in the book in that there is no vignette that necessarily corresponds to any given word-for-word, per-page content within the text. The DVD vignettes and the TSW formats are designed to help teach the concepts referenced within the text, particularly the therapeutic-specific skills noted in Chapters 6 and 7 of the text. It is hoped, certainly, that vignettes serve to illustrate possible occurrences of effective therapeutic scenarios from which student SLPs may learn to do therapy. Of course, none of the vignettes are promoted as "perfect" examples of therapy.

Interactive Learning Group-Focused Activity Cluster

The Interactive Learning Group-Focused Activity Cluster comprises the third and final focused activity cluster in which student SLPs might learn the 28 therapeutic-specific skills highlighted in Table 1–1. Interactive learning group is the name given to the smaller groups formed within the classroom when the clinical supervisor or instructor works with several students simultaneously in teaching student SLPs how to do therapy. *Interactive learning groups* are simply a management structure whereby students are placed in small groups to allow clinical supervisors or instructors to teach students large amounts of content and numerous therapeutic skills in a limited amount of time (see Figure 1–2). Should the clinical supervisor or instructor find that students are best taught to do therapy on an individual basis (clinical supervisor-to-student), the interactive learning group will not apply to the learning structure needed to teach therapy skills in that instance. However, several subset activities attached to the interactive learning group may still prove helpful to the individual student SLP learner. For example, clinical supervisors teach, model, and coach in small groups; these activities will be applicable to the student being taught individually (clinical supervisor-to-student) as well.

It is important to offer a guide, here, for SLP students who will be learning to do therapy, regardless of whether learning therapy on an individual basis, or learning in an interactive group. Figure 1–4 presents a simplified graphic of a focus diagram of expected learning progressions associated with learning to do therapy. Student SLPs are encouraged to refer to this diagram often as a guide to the four levels of focus when learning to do therapy. Students are encouraged to focus on (1) learning the basic components of a therapy session (Introduction, Body, Closing); (2) mastery of therapeutic-specific skills; (3) interactive nature of communication learning, and (4) client's communication skills and outcomes.

Student SLPs should begin learning therapy by focusing first on acquiring the *basic components of therapy* (Introduction, Body, and Closing, the 28 therapeutic skills, etc.). Students continue learning by *mastering* these same skills (increasing skills for both accuracy and speed of implementation). Learning is continued through focus on the *interactive nature of communication* (roles and responsibilities of all participants in the therapeutic process [SLP, target client, peer model, and peer evaluator]). Finally, the focus is on posi-

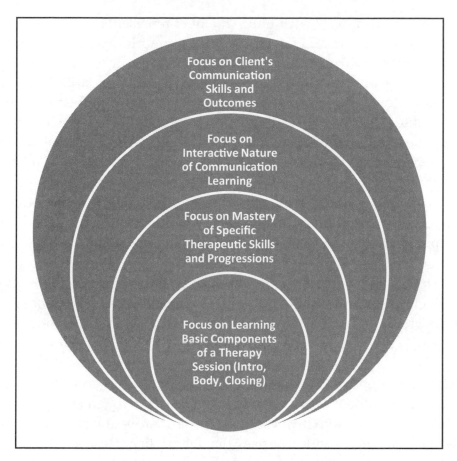

Figure 1–4. Student SLP's focus diagram of expected learning progressions.

tive impacts on the *client's communication competence and outcomes* (effectiveness of the client's communication skills). Although these levels of focus appear to be linear (and to some degree, they are), it is important for the student SLP to understand that even while learning the basic skills, the ultimate focus is always on the client's communication outcomes. (See Figure 1–4.)

When larger groups of students are simultaneously introduced to therapy, the interactive learning group has been found to be invaluable. Eight interactive learning group-focused activities are presented for the student SLP learner: (1) *Heterogeneous Groups of Four*; (2) *Rotating Roles and Responsibilities of Each Group Member (SLP, Target Client, Peer Model, Peer Evaluator)*; (3) *Practice During Class*; (4) *Practice Outside of Class*; (5) *Group Members Practice Often as the "Therapist"*; (6) *Group Members Practice Often as the "Peer Model/Evaluator"*; (7) *Group Members Self-Video-Record Skills*; and (8) *Self-Analyze Skills*.

Heterogeneous Groups of Four

Heterogeneous groups were discussed earlier in this chapter under the concept of cooperative learning. *Heterogeneous groups of four* in the context of the Interactive Group-Focused Activities Clusters refers to the makeup of the cooperative learning group in terms of heterogeneity of the "disorders" each group member represents. For example, one group member always serves as the "SLP," with the three remaining group members serving as clients. It is within the makeup of the "client" population that heterogeneity becomes important for training purposes for this focused cluster. To expand this example, typically, for heterogeneity in an articulation group, one group member will emulate a client with a specific articulation error, /r/, for example. A second client presents with an /s/ problem, while the third client works on /l/. An articulation group, whereby one client is working on /r/, another is working on /s/, and a third is working on /l/ is considered a heterogeneous group with respect to target error sounds. As mentioned earlier in this chapter and as will be seen later in the text (Chapter 7), for purposes of creating a more realistic learning and communicating environment, heterogeneity within groups is preferred over homogeneous groupings. In heterogeneous groups, it is likely that if the target client is unable to correctly produce a phoneme, another client in the group is able to correctly produce that phoneme as a peer model, following the SLP's lead. However, if all clients experience difficulty producing /s/, as would be the case in a homogeneous group for /s/ errors, then no client in the group presents as a good peer model during the early phoneme learning phases of therapy.

Suggested Uses of Heterogeneous Groups of Four. Clinical supervisors or instructors are encouraged to allow student SLP learners to establish heterogeneous groups of four for purposes of learning the interactive components of therapeutic skills. This is especially important for peer modeling within the session. Often clients (especially young children) are not impressed that the SLP is able to correctly produce a phoneme. However, it becomes much more interesting (and impressive) to the young client when his or her peer is able to correctly produce the phoneme.

Rotating Roles and Responsibilities of Each Group Member (SLP → Target Client → Peer Model → Peer Evaluator)

The roles and responsibilities of each of the four group members were presented earlier as part of a discussion on cooperative learning. However, this concept needs to be reiterated here to help student SLPs focus on the roles and responsibilities as related to any small group work that may be done outside of the classroom. Roles and responsibilities of each of the four group members within the small interactive groups rotate, depending on learner needs during practice time, both during and outside of class times. Exact structure of the small interactive groups is accomplished in the following ways:

- *Labeling of respective group members.* Once the groups of four student SLP learners are organized, each group member is assigned a group number, from 1 to 4 (1, 2, 3, or 4).

- *Rotating Roles and Responsibilities between Clients and SLP.* Each group member selects a "disorder" that he/she will emulate during the practice session—*when serving in the role of target client.* (Remember: In heterogeneous groups of four, at any given practice time, one group member serves as SLP, and the other three group members serve as clients. So, at any given time, it is only necessary for three of the four group members to emulate speech-language disorders, as the fourth member of the group will be serving as SLP.) For example, in an articulation group, group member #1 may serve as the SLP for the first practice period (usually 8–10 minutes), whereas member #2 may choose to work on /s/; member #3 may choose to work on /l/; and member #4 may choose to work on /f/. Once group member #1 has practiced being the therapist for a designated time, roles within the group change and group member #2 now becomes the therapist, while group member #1 now works on /s/ (as group member #1 had done previously); group member #3 continues working on /l/; and member #4 continues working on /f/. In the third practice rotation, roles change again, and now group member #3 becomes the SLP, while group member #1 works on /s/; group member #2 now works on /l/ (as group member #3 had done previously); and group member #4 continues working on /f/. Finally, in the fourth practice rotation, group member #4 becomes the SLP while member #1 continues working on /s/; group member #2 continues working on /l/; member #3 now works on /f/ (as group member #4 had done previously). Don't worry if keeping up with client role rotations becomes confusing. *As long as each SLP has an opportunity to work with a group of three clients, all of whom are working on different targets, the objective of learning to work in heterogeneous groups will be accomplished.*

In an example related to language-based therapy, group member #1 may serve as SLP, while group member #2 may choose to work on Mean Length Utterance (MLU) expansion, group member #3 may choose to work on vocabulary for colors; and group member #4 may choose to work on the /d/ phoneme. As outlined in the client role rotations for the above articulation example, rotations of client roles occur in the same fashion when the heterogeneous groups are practicing language therapy: as each group member practices the SLP role, the remaining three members rotate client roles so that each SLP has an opportunity to practice with three clients, with one client working on MLU expansion, one client working on vocabulary expansion for colors, and one client working on the /d/ phoneme. Of course, these selected targets (phonemes and language structures) are merely examples for the sake of clarity. In actual heterogeneous group practice, clients may choose any number of other phoneme, language structure, or even voice, fluency, or resonance combinations for practice. However, in early learning and practice stages, it is recommended that language-based therapy is limited to language and articulation objectives in order to keep initial learning more focused and easier to conceptualize.

- *Rotating Roles and Responsibilities among Clients.* By now, it should be clear that at any given time, within the heterogeneous group, one student serves as "SLP" while the other three students serve as "clients," each emulating a different "disorder." Another important thing to remember is that, more fundamentally, clients have different *responsibilities* associated with the roles within the small interactive group on another level. Each client within the small interactive group serves three different roles, with accompanying responsibilities as follows:

1. Each client is, at some point, the target client—the one with whom the SLP is working to change phonemes, language, or other behavior.

2. Each client, at some point, serves as peer model, whereby the SLP asks the peer to model sounds/language, or other structures for the target client.

3. Each client, at some point, serves as *peer evaluator,* whereby the SLP asks the peer to say/tell/show verbally or nonverbally (thumbs up, for example) how well the target client performed in producing the sounds or language structures, etc., for the target client.

Figures 1–5 and 1–6 show graphic representations of the various rotating *roles* that the student SLP holds within the group during interactive group work, and the various *responsibilities* the student SLP holds within the group during interactive group work, respectively. Several researchers found positive results in learning when students were allowed to engage in role-playing (assuming various roles) as one of the avenues to understanding (Howes & Cruz, 2009; Shapiro & Leopold, 2012).

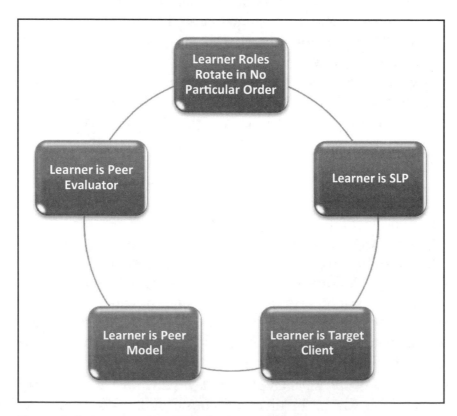

Figure 1–5. Learner roles within the interactive group.

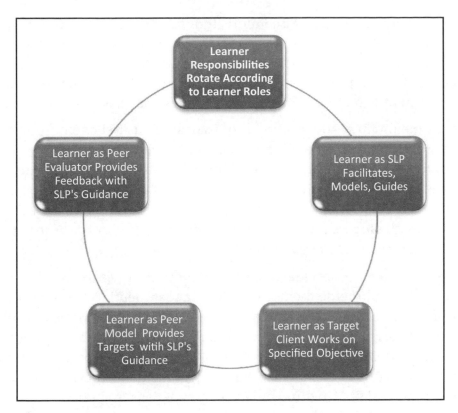

Figure 1–6. Learner responsibilities within the interactive group.

Practice During Class Times as Often as Possible

Due to the large numbers of requirements of clinical management or clinical supervision courses, it is not always possible to provide student SLPs with an opportunity to practice during each class time. However, once the interactive groups of four are established, clinical supervisors or instructors are encouraged to arrange opportunities for practice during class times as often as possible. Class time practice offers students three important advantages that impact the student SLP's learning:

1. Class time practice provides students an opportunity to refine skills in a more intimate, and less threatening learning environment. Students tend to quickly become comfortable within the small group learning setting, particularly when students are allowed to choose "group-mates." This comfort among peers typically readily translates to students becoming more comfortable learning within small groups, especially when learning challenging tasks that require lots of repetition and often result in numerous errors and false starts, particularly in early stage learning. Errors made within the small group setting, rather than those made in either whole class or individual settings, tend to be much less intimidating for student learners. Student SLPs in small groups can often be heard during small group learning activities in the following dialog: "Wait, wait, okay. I did that wrong; let me start again," with no threats of

embarrassment, or other discomforts that might occur were the performances in front of the whole class, or even worse (in students' minds), in an individual exchange with the clinical supervisor or instructor. Several researchers supported small group learning under the concept of a "safe" learning environment (Abiola & Dhindsa, 2012; Jones, Jones, & Vermette, 2013).

2. Class time practice allows small groups of students to benefit from the clinical supervisor or instructor's directed and specific teaching, guidance, or corrective feedback needed for finer points of clarity. For example, clinical supervisors or instructors may address a misunderstanding of group member #1, but all other group members benefit very quickly, as well, from clarity or corrective feedback offered by the focused attention of the clinical supervisor or instructor working within the small interactive group.

3. Class time practice provides student SLPs opportunities to quickly—and often accurately—submerge themselves into the therapeutic learning process by assuming mock therapeutic roles via role-playing as (a) clinician, (b) target client, (c) peer model, or (d) peer evaluator. Role-playing was reported by several researchers (Howes & Cruz, 2009; Shapiro & Leopold, 2012) to be a powerful learning experience, whereby, students assumed different roles simulating real life teaching or learning experiences. By assuming each of the possible therapeutic roles, with supporting responsibilities, student SLPs are essentially forced to engage in the various aspects of therapy both as clinician, and as all possible client roles (target client, client as peer model, and client as peer evaluator). Findings of the informal survey of critical learning experiences (discussed earlier in this chapter) indicated that a number of students reported serving as peer model or peer evaluator to be less critical as learning experiences than were some of the other 18 focused learning activities. Still, it is certainly hoped that role-playing as peer models and peer evaluators helps students process concepts and perspectives of the various aspects of therapy more readily.

Suggested Uses of Practice During Class Times. Once the clinical supervisor or instructor presents a concept or skill, provides whole class explanations, whole class models, etc., small group practice times are appropriate for engaging in and learning all 28 therapeutic-specific skills associated with learning to do speech-language therapy. (See Table 1–1.) Clinical supervisors or instructors make "rounds" from group to group within the classroom setting, teaching, guiding, coaching, and providing corrective feedback, but ultimately, the small groups teach themselves by working cooperatively with each other. One very nice serendipitous result of small group work, often, is a bonding or interdependence among group members. Within small interactive groups, group members not only assume responsibility for their own learning, but group members often support the learning of others in the group under the concept of interdependence.

The interdependence that often emerges during focused small group work is akin to the Backus and Beasley (1951) suggestion that "the teaching situation should be structured to provide a corrective 'emotional' experience" (p. 5). For example, in the small interactive group, each group member works to learn and habituate his or her skills, but often, each member of the group also works to help others in the group successfully demonstrate therapeutic skills as well. However, because of the strength of possible interdependence, or the possible emotional experience attached to small interactive group learning, whether during class practices, or outside of class practices, a word of caution regarding group dynamics is warranted: It is sometimes possible for one group member to carry enough influence over other group members to essentially destroy correct learning opportunities for others. Clinical supervisors, instructors, and group members themselves need to guard against, and correct, situations whereby one group member essentially leads the other group members astray regardless of amount of corrective feedback received from the clinical supervisor or instructor during in-class practice sessions. In situations such as this, typically, a general discussion of group dynamics is sufficient. However, occasionally, groups may need to be reconfigured by the clinical supervisor or instructor to achieve proper learning balance for all group members.

Practice Outside of Classes as Often as Possible

Groups should practice together outside of classes as often as possible—but **not** *until therapeutic skills have sufficiently developed within the group members during in-class practices and demonstrations.* This caution is added because it becomes easy—and often detrimental—for group members to practice *incorrectly* outside of the clinical supervisor's or instructor's guidance. Clinical supervisors or instructors are, therefore, cautioned to be aware of the negative practice effect of small interactive group work and guard against groups rushing to prematurely practice as a group outside of class in order to accomplish an assignment.

Suggested Uses of Practice Outside of Classes. Small groups should practice outside of classes only when overall proficiency in group skills supports *correct* practice. To this end, group members should become comfortable with the idea of asking clinical supervisors or instructors to evaluate *group readiness* for practicing outside of the classroom.

Group Members Practice Often as the "Therapist"

The concepts of both *heterogeneous groups of four* and the *roles and responsibilities of interactive groups* were presented earlier in the discussion of the Interactive Learning Group-Focused activities. However, there is a need for practicing as the "therapist" as often as possible. Ideally, this practice is done in conjunction with other group members serving as clients. However, it is possible for any individual group member to actually practice his or her "therapy script" alone, without benefit of "clients," once the individual group member understands the therapist's roles and responsibilities. Using the scripted language from Chart 7–2 of the textbook (Detailed Therapy Progression), the individual group member is able to practice the "therapist's" part of an intervention session based on imagined client responses, similar to the way an actor/actress might practice his or her part in a stage or film production.

Suggested Uses of Group Members Practicing Often as the "Therapist." It is suggested that group members practice the role and responsibilities of the therapist as often as possible, both with and without the group. Practicing with the group was discussed in the section on *Rotating Roles and Responsibilities of Each Group Member* (above). However, individuals may practice separate from the group by standing in front of a mirror (or other feedback mechanisms) and verbally reading aloud through the Detailed Therapy Progression (Chart 7–2). Student SLPs are reminded that practicing alone often yields the same effect as working in small interactive groups in that similar feelings of awkwardness (and sometimes, frustration) are often present when first attempting practicing alone. Still, however, student SLPs are encouraged to try this method of practice as an added possibility to increase opportunities to practice as the therapist as often as possible.

Group Members Practice Often as the Peer Model/Evaluator

Peer models are clients who are called upon by the SLP to give models of how sounds or other structures are produced. Peer models, themselves clients in the therapy session, work to support the target client's learning—upon the therapist's command. *Peer evaluators* are clients who are called upon by the SLP to give the target client feedback regarding the accuracy of his or her productions. Peer evaluators, themselves clients in the therapy session as well, work to support the target client's learning—upon the therapist's command. All clients in the therapy session rotate between serving as the target client (the client who is the direct/immediate recipient of the therapist's intervention), peer model, or peer evaluator. In all instances, the objectives of the peer model and peer evaluator are to support the learning of the client serving as the target client. In serving to help other clients learn, however, peer models and peer evaluators are still engaged in communicative learning.

Suggested Uses of Practicing as the Peer Model/Evaluator. In that the therapist guides the responses of the peer model and peer evaluator during the therapy session, the greatest value of practicing the roles of peer model/evaluator is in helping student SLPs further understand the processes of the interactive nature of therapy: one client works on his or her targets or goals, while the remaining clients serve as either peer models or peer evaluators, on a rotating basis, to help support learning for the client working on targets/goals. This peer-shared learning, however, supports the learning of the peer models and peer evaluators as well (Savion, 2009).

Group Members Self-Video-Record Skills

Lasting impressions of therapy skills are often obtained through visual self-recordings of group work. Video recording each individual group member in the role of therapist is encouraged for its value in serving as a good feedback mechanism to help each group member learn to do therapy.

Suggested Uses of Group Members Self-Video-Record Skills. Analysis of Table 1–1 (Matrix of Focal Points and Activities) suggests that all of the 28 therapeutic-specific skills may be addressed through use of video-self-recording, depending, of course, on the specific nature of the therapy goals/objectives. Student SLPs are encouraged to self-record in the role as therapist in an effort to improve therapeutic skills.

Group Members Self-Analyze Skills

Interactive group members may self-analyze skills development in two ways: (1) use of cognitive processes for task analyzing skill development of each of the 28 therapeutic-specific skills (or parts, thereof), and (2) self-analysis of the self-recorded video session. Once group members self-record skills, it is important to self-analyze, individually, the results in efforts to assess desired outcomes in skills attainment. Although it was noted above that all of the 28 therapeutic-specific skills may be addressed through use of video-self-recording, depending, of course, on the specific nature of the therapy goals/objectives, it is more feasible for the student SLP to select a subset of the 28 therapeutic-specific skills for analysis for any given video-recording effort. In this regard, the student SLP may choose to analyze skill development for selected skills, rather than attempting to self-analyze all of the 28 therapeutic-specific skills at a given time.

Suggested Uses of Group Self-Analysis. Individuals within groups may benefit from self-analysis of therapy skills development for any selected therapeutic-specific skill. Once a skill is selected, student SLPs may use several sources for evaluative comparisons of skills development: clinical supervisor or instructor's feedback, Textbook/DVD descriptions or demonstrations, and findings or results of self-recorded video sessions. Mistakes are a common part of the therapy learning process; mistakes are expected. Whether using cognitive processes for task analyzing skills development of selected therapeutic-specific skills, or self-analyzing self-recorded video sessions, the value of self-analysis is, ultimately, in the information gathered from the processes of scrutiny of performances, both subjective and objective, for skills development for student SLPs learning how to do therapy.

Overview of the 28 Therapeutic-Specific Skills

Although the 28 therapeutic-specific skills were presented earlier in this chapter (see Table 1–1), an additional treatment of these skills needs to be highlighted. The list below contains the 28 therapeutic-specific skills from Table 1–1, grouped together in ways that are easy to teach and easy to comprehend. The skills in bold print represent the skills addressed on the DVD accompaniment to the textbook. Notice that on some lines, several skills are not only listed together on the line, but several are also in bold print, indicating that these skills are grouped together and demonstrated in respective DVD vignettes. More discussion of the 28 therapeutic-specific skills follows in Chapters 6 and 7; however, the following list for indicating the skills is offered simply to help with clarity of thinking as student SLPs begin preparations for learning the skills. The 28 therapeutic-specific skills include:

1. Motivation
2. ☽ **Communicating Expectations**
3. ☽ **Enthusiasm, Animation,** and **Volume** in the Therapeutic Process
4. ☽ **Seating Arrangements, Proximity,** and **Touch** in the Therapeutic Process
5. ☽ **Preparation, Pacing,** and **Fluency** for Therapeutic Momentum
6. ☽ Antecedents: **Alerting Stimuli, Cueing, Modeling,** and **Prompting**
7. ☽ Direct Teaching: **Learning Modalities,** Describing/Demonstrating, **Questioning,** and **Wait-Time**
8. ☽ Stimulus Presentation: **Shaping (Successive Approximations)**
9. ☽ Positive Reinforcers: **Verbal Praise, Tokens,** and **Primary Reinforcers**
10. ☽ **Corrective Feedback** in the Therapeutic Process
11. ☽ **Data Collection** in the Therapeutic Process
12. Probing in the Therapeutic Process
13. Behavioral Management in the Therapeutic Process
14. Troubleshooting in the Therapeutic Process

Each of the above skills are further presented in discussion and applications in Chapter 6. As student SLPs work to accomplish the 28 therapeutic-specific-skills, the list above serves as a quick review of skills, the possible grouping of skills, and shows skills that are presented in DVD format (indicated by the media symbol ☽).

Welcome to This Text

The suggestions offered in this chapter should help with the application of the information presented in this text. A final note related to the use of cooperative learning and interactive groups is important here. Cooperative learning and interactive group arrangements for student learning have been successfully used for over 20 years with several hundred students, with approximately 16 inadequate student presentations in culminating demonstrations using these techniques. Interestingly, in each of the poorer performing student presentations, each student in respective groups presented therapy in the *same incorrect manner*, using the same incorrect techniques and therapy sequences, with the same incorrect degree of details, thereby, with each poorer performing student demonstrating the power of cooperative learning within interactive groups, but doing so in *negative* rather than *positive* student outcomes. Additionally, in each instance of poorer performing student SLP learners, it was easily determined that lack of student successes stemmed from identifiable faults: (1) students did not received enough corrective feedback during small interactive group class time practice from the clinical supervisor or instructor, (2) students began practicing outside of the classroom *before* obtaining enough skills to *practice correctly* outside of the classroom, or (3) there was one group member who wielded enough persuasive power as to essentially lead the other group members astray regardless of amount of corrective feedback received from the clinical supervisor or instructor during in-class practice sessions.

Regardless of prior experiences in teaching/learning therapy skills, the concepts presented in this text should support continued successes and gratification in SLPs interested in learning more about basic therapy skills. So, to all students and practicing clinicians, welcome to this book and to its encouragement for your continued best performances in a career as an SLP professional. "Showtime!"

References

Abiola, O. O., & Dhindsa, H. S. (2012). Improving classroom practices using our knowledge of how the brain works. *International Journal of Environmental & Science Education, 7*(1), 71–81.

American Speech-Language-Hearing Association. (2014). *Speech-language disorders and the speech-language pathologist.* Retrieved March 19, 2014, from http://www.asha.org/careers/professions/sld.htm

Backus, O., & Beasley, J. (1951). *Speech therapy with children.* Cambridge, MA: Riverside Press.

Bisland, B. M., Malow-Iroff, M. S., & O'Connor, E. A. (2006). *Instructional practices among alternatively certified elementary teachers.* Paper presented at the American Educational Research Association Annual Convention, San Francisco, CA.

Bloom, L., & Lahey, M. (1978). *Language development and language disorders.* New York, NY: John Wiley & Sons.

Brackenbury, T. (2012). A qualitative examination of connections between learner-centered teaching and past significant learning experiences. *Journal of the Scholarship of Teaching and Learning, 12*(4), 12–28.

Çakmak, M. (2008). Concerns about teaching process: Student teachers' perspective. *Education Quarterly, 31*(3), 57–77.

Dennett, C. G., & Azar, J. A. (2011). Peer educators in a theoretical context: Emerging adults. *New Directions for Student Services, 133,* 7–16.

Fox-Turnbull, W. (2010). The role of conversation in technology education. *Design and Technology Education, 15*(1), 24–30.

Furr, S. R., & Carroll, J. J. (2003). Critical incidents in student counselor development. *Journal of Counseling & Development, 81,* 483–489.

Haring, N. G., Lovitt, T. C., Eaton, M. D., & Hansen, C. L. (1978). *The fourth R: Research in the classroom.* Columbus, OH: Charles E. Merrill.

Howes, E. V., & Cruz, B. C. (2009). Role-playing in science education: An effective strategy for developing multiple perspectives. *Journal of Elementary Science Education, 21*(3), 33–46.

Hulit, L. M., Howard, M. R., & Fahey, K. R. (2011). *Born to talk* (5th ed.). Boston, MA: Pearson.

Johnson, D. W., & Johnson, R. T. (1989). *Cooperation and competition: Theory and research.* Edina, MN: Interaction Book.

Johnson, D. W., & Johnson, R. T. (1999). Making cooperative learning work. *Theory into Practice, 38*(2), 67–73.

Jones, K. A., Jones, J. L., & Vermette, P. J. (2013). Exploring the complexity of classroom management: 8 components of managing a highly productive, safe, and respectful urban environment. *American Secondary Education, 41*(3), 21–33.

Kantar, L. D. (2013). Demystifying instructional innovation: The case of teaching with case studies. *Journal of the Scholarship of Teaching and Learning, 13*(2), 101–115.

Kent, B. (2006). What does it take to facilitate? *Kairaranga, 7*(Special Issue), 59–63.

Kollar, I., Fischer, F., & Hesse, F. W. (2006). Collaboration scripts—A conceptual analysis. *Educational Psychology Review, 18*, 159–185.

Lawrence, M. N., & Butler, M. B. (2010). Becoming aware of the challenges of helping students learn: An examination of the nature of learning during a service-learning experience. *Teacher Education Quarterly*, Winter 2010, 155–175.

Loughran, J. (2013). Pedagogy: Making sense of the complex relationship between teaching and learning. *Curriculum Inquiry, 43*(1), 118–141.

Makaiau, A. S., & Miller, C. (2012). The philosopher's pedagogy. *Educational Perspectives, 44*(1–2), 8–19.

Meyer, J. H. F., & Land, R. (2005). Threshold concepts and troublesome knowledge (2): Epistemological considerations and a conceptual framework for teaching and learning. *Higher Education, 49*, 373–388.

Nelson, C. (2011). The complexity of language learning. *International Journal of Instruction, 4*(2), 93–112.

Paul, R. (2011). *Language disorders from infancy through adolescence* (4th ed.). St Louis, MO: Mosby Elsevier.

Savion, L. (2009). Clinging to discredited beliefs: The larger cognitive theory. *Journal of the Scholarship of Teaching and Learning, 9*(1), 81–92.

Schommer, M. (1990). Effects of beliefs about the nature of knowledge on comprehension. *Journal of Psychology, 82*, 498–504.

Selahattin, A., & İlknur, Ö. (2010). Prospective teachers' skills in planning and applying learning-teaching process. *US-China Education Review, 7*(3), Serial No. 64, 34–41.

Shapiro, S., & Leopold, L. (2012). A critical role for role-playing pedagogy. *TESL Canada Journal, 29*(2), 120–130.

Smilkstein, R. (1993). Acquiring knowledge and using it. *Gamut*, Published by Seattle Community College District (Washington), pp. 2–7.

Tetsuo, H. (2011). The concept and effectiveness of teaching practices using OPPA. *Educational Studies in Japan: International Yearbook, 6*, 47–67.

Vajoczki, S., Savage, P., Martin, L., Borin, P., & Kustra, E. D. H. (2011). Good teachers, scholarly teachers and teachers engaged in scholarship of teaching and learning: A case study from McMaster University, Hamilton, Canada. *The Canadian Journal for the Scholarship of Teaching and Learning, 2*(1), Article 2, 1–27.

Wilcox, S., & Leger, A. B. (2013). Crossing thresholds: Identifying conceptual transitions in postsecondary teaching. *The Canadian Journal for the Scholarship of Teaching and Learning, 4*(2), Article 7, 1–12.

Williams, L. B. (2011). The future of peer education: Broadening the landscape and assessing the benefits. *New Directions for Student Services, 2011*(133), 97–99.

Wright, G. B. (2011). Student-centered learning in higher education. *International Journal of Teaching and Learning in Higher Education, 23*(3), 92–97.

Youmans, G., Youmans, S. R., & Hancock, A. B. (2011). Script training treatment for adults with apraxia of speech. *American Journal of Speech-Language Pathology, 20*, 23–37.

2

Basic Considerations for the Therapeutic Process

Introduction

This discussion is designed to help the speech-language pathology student and professional focus on concepts that are fundamental and foundational to service provision in the profession. Some discussions are specific to the speech-language pathology profession, but others are general and so broadly founded as to be applicable to almost any chosen profession. Students and professionals are encouraged to revisit often the concepts discussed in this chapter during professional practice.

Artistry in Speech-Language Pathology

There is something that continues to be magical in ways a good speech-language pathologist (SLP) does his or her therapy. SLPs are scientists, firmly rooted in the academics across many areas of study, yet watching a good SLP at work makes it clear that something beyond science is operational. That "something" can only be explained as simple artistic flair—for lack of a more creative expression. Good SLPs have somehow found effective ways to mesh, layer upon layer, the knowledge and requirements of the sciences with the caring expressions of the humanities, and the skills of a well-trained craftsman to emerge as skilled artisans, masters in the art of helping clients with communicative skills. Most typically do not view speech-language therapy as being akin to artistry. Yet, SLPs daily *perform* the acts of positively impacting clients, in some way, to improve communication. SLPs, of course, are versed in research-based knowledge in the profession, and SLPs embrace best practices in the everyday performances of duties as speech-language pathology professionals. However, at the juncture of research and practical application of basic tenets of the profession is the concept of "the art of speech-language therapy."

Rarely have SLPs discussed the art of speech-language therapy. Typically, the focus is on knowledge, skills, techniques, competencies, models, and theories of the profession. SLPs try to ensure that professional practices are firmly grounded in accepted research and best practices. Research is necessary for ensuring accuracy in understanding the anatomical, physiological, and neurological structures and functions being manipulated for positive communicative change in clients. But once these structures and functions are understood, it is up to the professional to incorporate the best from learning theories, and from physical, behavioral, and social sciences to effect appropriate change in the client's skills. Research tells us the *what* of speech-language therapy: *what* structures, *what* functions, *what* client goals to address in therapy. However, practical application helps us with the *how* of the profession: *how* best to implement techniques appropriate for a specific client's needs, and *how* best to attain the desired outcomes for our clients. The merging of the *what* and the *how* of our profession is, in fact, no less than *artistry*. This **artistry**, the artistic quality, or effect, on workmanship (*Merriam-Webster's*, 1993) is illustrated in Figure 2–1.

Practicing SLPs are encouraged to focus on research-based knowledge of the profession, for we need that foundation. Equally important, however, is the need for SLPs to focus on appropriate applications of techniques and methodologies for excellence in therapy. For SLPs to achieve increased levels of excellence in therapy, we must find ways to interface research with practical application; artistry is that interface. The development and execution of artistry in therapy often equates to the difference between the speech-language pathology professional assessed as "good in therapy" and one judged as "excellent in therapy." It is hoped that this text will help to promote excellence in therapy.

"Showtime!"

Showtime is an underlying guiding concept whereby clinicians come to understand the significance of excellence in providing therapy to clients. In the theatrical world, rallies of "*Showtime!*" or "*The show must go on!*" are heard often. Although the SLP's work is not designed to entertain in the way that a traditional Broadway show might, it is important

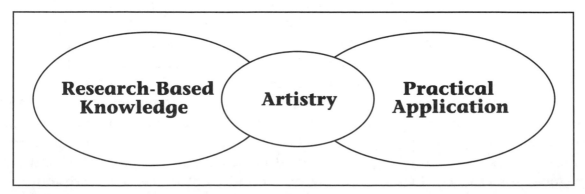

Figure 2–1. Artistry is the bridge between research-based knowledge and practical application in speech-language therapy.

for SLPs to understand that we provide a valuable service to clients whose communicative competence depends on our professional skills. We are charged with the mammoth task of providing therapy services to clients to the best of our professional abilities at all times. Of course, there are perhaps times when SLPs feel ill prepared to provide speech-language therapy: we get sick, and sickness should be attended; we have personal traumas and tragedies, and those must be addressed. The underpinning of our work, however, should be the concept that clients receive the best possible speech-language therapy at all times. The SLP's commitment to providing the best possible therapy equates to the rally of the performing artist who, without hesitation, musters the performing troupe with the cry, "*Showtime!*" Similarly, when it is time to provide speech-language therapy services, SLPs are expected to "perform" with precision and excellence as we serve our clients. We train tirelessly to acquire skills to serve clients. We observe them, read about them, research them, and write about them. We assess them, and we analyze and interpret data on them. With the kinds and amounts of investments SLPs make in understanding client behavior and client needs, how can we be expected to offer less than our best when it comes to therapy for the client? The answer is, "We cannot give the client less than our best!" Now, how different are speech-language pathology and performing art? Certainly, different in many aspects; yet, not at all different when it comes to "Showtime!"

Speech-Language Therapy and Task Analysis

Aspiring SLPs observing speech-language therapy for the first time often are overwhelmed with the dynamics of a typical therapy session. Within the constructs of a given group therapy session, the clinician talks to clients, clients talk to the clinician, and clients talk to each other. Clinicians lead, guide, model, direct, facilitate, collect data, encourage, and reinforce efforts, to name some of the skills used during a typical therapy session. All of these skills are demonstrated under the auspices of **therapeutic interaction**, a highly responsive and fluid exchange between clinician and clients during therapy; often the beginning professional is not sure just *what* is being observed. No wonder beginning SLPs feel intimidated at the thought of eventually taking the responsibility for providing therapy services on their own! Although initially uncomfortable with the thought of providing therapy services, new professionals, through guided practice in therapy skills, become not only comfortable with taking the lead as a practicing SLP, but eventually excel in the methods and techniques of speech-language therapy.

SLPs are taught to negotiate the path from beginning level practices to professional competence in therapy through a series of experiences designed to promote successful mastery of therapeutic skills. This mastery is accomplished through use of **task analysis**, a behavioral concept whereby tasks, or skills, are broken down into component parts in order to learn the parts separately; then the parts are put back together to demonstrate the target or required tasks (Hallahan & Kauffman, 2000). By task analyzing each segment of therapy, developing the skills required for successful implementation of that segment, then putting those skills together to demonstrate the entire target sequence, SLPs learn the art of demonstrating or performing the basic skills of speech-language therapy. Hulit, Howard, and Fahey (2011) referred to this type segmentation for learning new skills as chaining, whereby large volumes of information are broken into smaller segments for initial learning, then segments are put together to form the full sequence of the newly learned skill.

Skills for Speech-Language Therapy

Many talents, skills, techniques, and a broad knowledge base for the profession comprise the constellation of proficiencies that SLPs demonstrate. Several researchers (Hegde & Davis, 2005; Low & Lee, 2011; Paul & Cascella, 2007) presented helpful information regarding the skills needed by SLPs in the clinical setting. Hegde and Davis (2005), for example, discussed the importance of broad-based knowledge that SLPs need regarding the profession. For purposes of this discussion, there are two broad-based skill areas that SLP professionals must demonstrate when providing speech-language therapy: *interpersonal communication skills* and *therapeutic-specific skills*. **Interpersonal communication skills** are the personal behaviors or interactions used for engaging others. Interpersonal communication skills emerge in various forms during various stages of child development (Adams & Wittmer, 2001). These skills include characteristic traits such as empathy, friendliness, politeness, honesty in feedback, and appropriate nonverbal interactions (eye contact, body language, proximity, etc.). Some students are considered to be "a natural" for therapy because they possess interpersonal communication skills (Conderman, Johnston-Rodriguez, & Hartman, 2009) appropriate for speech-language therapy, whereas other students must be taught interpersonal communication skills in addition to being taught the therapeutic-specific skills for therapy. In cases in which an SLP student must be taught appropriate interpersonal communication skills that are perceived as appropriate for therapy, clinical supervisors or instructors must, then, work through training levels to help students acquire those skills on a case-by-case basis. However, essentially every student SLP is taught therapeutic-specific skills in that such teaching is the essence of clinical training in the communication disorders discipline.

 Therapeutic-specific skills are fundamental core professional skills necessary for effective speech-language therapy. Typically, because of their importance to clinical effectiveness, therapeutic-specific skills are taught and learned in relation to their applications in speech-language therapy, although many of the skills apply across other disciplines. Regardless of how well-versed students are in interpersonal communication skills, all students studying the discipline of communication disorders must be taught therapeutic-specific skills. As a point of encouragement, beginning SLPs should understand that *all skills demonstrated in speech-language therapy are learned skills*. Whether students must be taught both interpersonal communication skills *and* therapeutic-specific skills, or need only to be taught the therapeutic-specific skills related to therapy, SLPs learn all skills and eventually demonstrate them, one by one, without difficulty through use of task-analysis activities. The therapeutic-specific skills that should be present within the context

TEXTBOX 2–1. Twenty-eight therapeutic-specific skills important to speech-language therapy. Ten DVD vignettes (media symbol ☉) highlight 21 of these skills listed in bold italics.

- Motivation in the Therapeutic Process
- ☉ *Communicating Expectations*
- ☉ *Enthusiasm*, *Animation*, and *Volume* in the Therapeutic Process
- ☉ *Seating Arrangements*, *Proximity*, and *Touch* in the Therapeutic Process
- ☉ *Preparation*, *Pacing*, and *Fluency* for Therapeutic Momentum
- ☉ Antecedents: *Alerting Stimuli*, *Cueing*, *Modeling*, and *Prompting*
- ☉ Direct Teaching: *Learning Modalities*, Describing/Demonstrating, *Questioning*, and *Wait-Time*
- ☉ Stimulus Presentation: *Shaping (Successive Approximations)*
- ☉ Positive Reinforcers: *Verbal Praise*, Tokens, and **Primary Reinforcers**
- ☉ *Corrective Feedback* in the Therapeutic Process
- ☉ *Data Collection* in the Therapeutic Process
- Probing in the Therapeutic Process
- Behavioral Management in the Therapeutic Process
- Troubleshooting in the Therapeutic Process

of speech-language therapy, regardless of goals, are presented in Textbox 2–1 and are discussed in more detail in Chapter 6.

Once an SLP commands appropriate use of the skills listed in Textbox 2–1, in conjunction with the broad-based knowledge of the profession per disability area (articulation/phonology, language, voice, fluency, resonance, swallowing, etc.), excellence in therapy becomes not only possible, but probable.

These 28 therapeutic-specific skills were presented in Chapter 1 and are more fully explained in Chapter 6. However, they are being presented here as a reminder of their importance to learned effectiveness in providing appropriate speech-language therapy to clients.

Therapeutic Mindset

Mindset is a mental disposition or attitude that predetermines one's responses to and interpretations of situations (*Webster's II*, 1996). *Therapeutic mindset* for the SLP is the mental disposition or attitude that predetermines the SLP's responses to and interpretations of situations that occur within therapy sessions. It is the therapeutic mindset that guides the SLP to continuously assess stimuli, responses, and all other interactions of the therapeutic process and to act, or respond, accordingly. For example, when a client is asked to respond to the SLP's speech model and the client's response is *correct*, the SLP must be aware of and follow up with one or more of several possible options. Similarly, when the client's response to a given stimulus is *incorrect*, the SLP must be aware of and follow up with one or more of several possible, but different, options. *The awareness of the options and the preparedness to select and implement the appropriate option for the situation is a function of therapeutic mindset.*

To further illustrate the impact of therapeutic mindset, think of a family preparing for a long-anticipated camping trip. Plans must be made and implemented; dozens of details must be addressed. Safety as well as fun should be considered. Although plans are made and exacted, alternatives in cases of emergencies must be identified. The therapeutic mindset is no less requiring. Plans for therapy must be made; details of structures or concepts elicited in therapy, how they are elicited, and what is expected as acceptable client responses must be addressed. Client and clinician safety, and, certainly, some element or desire for improved communication as an outcome must be considered. Finally, alternative strategies, or techniques, in the event therapy does not proceed as planned, must be identified. This parallel between a camping trip and speech-language therapy is, of course, an oversimplification of the therapeutic process. However, it serves to help illustrate the idea that, for the SLP, providing speech-language therapy is, most often, much more than meets the eye. When therapy is executed well, there are so many more elements or aspects involved than can be seen by the untrained observer. The SLP gives these elements of therapy proper focus, in large part, due to therapeutic mindset—the awareness, anticipation, planning, executing, evaluating, adjusting, and readjusting of sequences of occurrences in therapy to achieve positive therapeutic outcomes are all functions of therapeutic mindset.

Developing Therapeutic Mindset

There are three important elements of therapeutic mindset: *anticipation*, *evaluation*, and *interaction*. To develop the therapeutic mindset needed to provide effective speech-language therapy, the SLP must become proficient in thinking through and anticipating the possibilities of therapy. Additionally, each phase, step, or communicative occurrence in therapy must be evaluated and supported with the proper response or interaction. Following is a brief discussion of each element of therapeutic mindset:

* **Anticipation as Part of Therapeutic Mindset.** SLPs must learn to consider, predict, or anticipate, at all times, the possibilities of events ranging from best to less-than-ideal case scenarios. This range of possibilities traverses a broad span to include everything from the client's lack of understanding of, or interest in, his or her role in the required exchanges of therapy, to the client's actual production of the desired response and all points between. Of course, it is not probable that the SLP might predict, anticipate, and prepare for every conceivable therapeutic sequence or occurrence; however, it is hoped that the SLP is familiar with

and anticipates the *probable* sequences based on client status and established therapeutic outcomes. Does a good, or even excellent, SLP ever anticipate incorrectly the probable responses to known stimuli in therapy? The answer is, "Yes, of course." However, therapeutic mindset continues to rule and the SLP quickly, even in the face of unexpected client responses, evaluates the situation, and adjusts accordingly.

- **Evaluation as Part of Therapeutic Mindset.** Once a therapeutic event takes place, the SLP must quickly and accurately evaluate the quality, correctness, and acceptability of that therapeutic event. The evaluative process is based on comparisons of the client's productions to the prescribed, established, or desired outcomes. To the degree that there is consistency with the client's productions, and the prescribed, established, or desired outcomes, the SLP evaluates or judges the response as within acceptable response ranges and communicates this information to the client. However, as client responses venture farther from the established outcome, and the SLP correctly assesses that the outcome was not achieved, the SLP must communicate to the client that the outcome was not produced. For all responses, the SLP must indicate, to the degree possible, aspects of client responses that were correct, and why, as well as aspects in error, and why. The quick identification of the exact nature of difficulties for client responses is not always an easy task, but is a task that the SLP must, nonetheless, embrace to provide effective speech-language therapy.

    An investigative or questioning entity forces the SLP to repeatedly ask, "What is correct about this response?" or "What is causing the difficulty in obtaining the correct response?" Although not stringent in the sense of empirical research, the investigative or evaluative element of therapeutic mindset requires the SLP to remain focused on questioning both the stimuli and the responses in therapy. For example, when asked to produce the /r/ phoneme following a correct model in the beginning stages of therapy, the client may (a) produce the sound correctly, or as modeled, or (b) produce the sound in any number of unacceptable configurations. Certainly, the client's correct production of the /r/ following the SLP's correct model is desired. However, the SLP must be aware that (a) /r/ may be a difficult phoneme to accurately teach, and (b) even when the teaching strategy is accurate, any number of client variables (history of production, physical limitations, learning difficulty, lack of motivation, etc.) may negatively impact the client's ability to correctly produce /r/ in the beginning stages of therapy. Although the SLP works for correction of /r/ early in therapy, it is understood that a number of phenomena may, in fact, impede the correct production of the sound or phoneme. When difficulty in correct production of /r/ arises, as often happens, the SLP must then begin the task of evaluation: questioning, investigating, and analyzing client responses to determine which of several possible variables may be negatively impacting the client's ability to correctly produce the phoneme. In this scenario, the SLP's questioning, investigating, and analyzing of reasons for the variance in the production of /r/ illustrates the evaluative quality of therapeutic mindset. In a different scenario, perhaps, even in this same /r/ example, following several sessions of therapy, the SLP may well expect or anticipate the correct production of /r/ following a correct model. The evaluative mindset exists even when productions are correct. When responses are correct, however, the questioning, investigating, and analyzing of responses are designed to examine why the sounds were produced *correctly*. The SLP communicates findings regarding correct responses to the client so that client learning and repeated correct productions are promoted and encouraged. In behavioral terms (Low & Lee, 2011), then, it is just as important for the SLP to evaluate the elements of *correct* productions as it is to investigate the elements of *incorrect* productions.

- **Interaction as Part of Therapeutic Mindset.** Regardless of client responses, the SLP must be prepared to act, interact, or respond in a manner appropriate for sustaining the therapy session. This *ready-to-respond* mode is attributable to the SLP's interactive skills in therapy. Once the SLP understands the role of interaction in the therapeutic process, the exchanges of client and clinician acting on each other, every detail of therapy becomes important to both the client and the clinician: the SLP's words and actions in therapy impact therapy, and the client's communicative behaviors impact therapy. Operating under a therapeutic mindset, the SLP's seemingly random interactions such as questioning the quality of the client's weekend activities are not at all "random," but rather are designed to evaluate the client's targeted communicative skills. In fact, this same line of questioning might be used to note the client's expressive language, phonological skills, conversational pitch, intensity, fluency, or other skills, depending on the identified learning outcomes. For this reason, SLPs are encouraged to "see with broader eyes" the possibilities for interactions that transpire within the confines of a given therapy session. Of course, seeing broadly is more difficult for students in the early stages of training when both knowledge base for the profession and therapeutic mindset are limited. In time, however, students are expected to interface the knowledge of the profession with therapeutic mindset to more readily identify objectives within a given therapy session. SLPs develop the therapeutic mindset through practice and exercises in the use of *anticipation, evaluation,* and *interactions* within the therapeutic setting. (An opportunity to compare less exemplary mindset with more exemplary mindset is provided in Textbox 2–2A and Textbox 2–2B, respectively.)

Often, beginning SLPs observing therapy in the first days and weeks of exposure to the speech-language pathology profession are unable to identify the subtleties of anticipation, evaluation, or interaction within a typical therapy session. However, with opportunity to work through scenarios such as the ones in Textboxes 2–2A and 2–2B, in conjunction with guided observations and guided practices, inexperienced SLPs soon are able to identify the elements of the therapeutic mindset (anticipation, evaluation, interaction) when exemplified in therapy.

■ TEXTBOX 2–2A. Scenario A: Less exemplary therapeutic mindset.

Scenario A:
Less Exemplary Therapeutic Mindset

Try to identify the elements or exchanges related to anticipation, evaluation, or interaction that make this scenario **less exemplary** of appropriate therapeutic mindset. (A few notes will be added to help you identify weaknesses within this scenario.) List your findings regarding the SLP's work in the Reader Comments section and write a summary statement of your overall impressions of the work in the Summary Comments section.

SLP	Client	Reader Comments
Goal: Production of plurals. Maggie, tell me, "I see two books." (SLP has not thought of how client might produce the plural for *books*.)		
	I see two book.	
Let's see. Um, you didn't quite get it. Ah, let's try again, and make sure you say all the parts this time, okay? Tell me, "I see two books." (SLP may recognize as an evaluative element of therapy that the /s/ phoneme is missing in the plural production of *books*, but does not communicate this to the client.)		
	I see two book.	
Okay, Maggie, tell me, "/s/."		
	/s/.	
Very good; now let's be sure to put the /s/ sound on the end of "books," okay? Like this, "books," okay?		
	Okay.	
Let me hear you say, "books."		
	Books.	

continues

■ Textbox 2–2A.   *continued*

SLP	Client	Reader Comments
Very good, Maggie. Now let's say the whole thing, "I see two books."	I see two books.	
Very good. I see two books.		

Summary Comments for Scenario A

■ Textbox 2–2B.   Scenario B: More exemplary therapeutic mindset.

Scenario B:
More Exemplary Therapeutic Mindset

Try to identify the elements or exchanges related to anticipation, evaluation, or interaction that make this scenario **more exemplary** of appropriate therapeutic mindset. (A few notes will be added to help you identify strengths within this scenario.) List your findings regarding the SLP's work in the Reader Comments section and write a summary statement of your overall impressions of the work in the Summary Comments section.

SLP	Client	Reader Comments
Goal: Production of plurals. Maggie, tell me, "I see two books."		

SLP	Client	Reader Comments
(SLP has thought of how client might produce the plural for *books*.)		
	I see two book.	
Good trying, Maggie; you got most of it. You said, "I see two book" but you left off the /s/ at the end of "books." (SLP recognizes as an evaluative element of therapy that the /s/ phoneme is missing in the plural production of *books*, and communicates this to the client.) Listen for the /s/ at the end of "books" again: "books." Now you try; let me hear /s/.		
	/s/.	
Good /s/. Your tongue was in exactly the right place to make a clear, crisp /s/. Now, let's take the /s/ and put it at the end of the word "books." Tell me "books."		
	Books.	
Great, Maggie. Good /s/, good "books." When we put the /s/ at the end, it means more than one book. Excellent! You said, "books." Now, let's put that word back into your sentence, very slowly. Tell me, "I - see - two - books." (The SLP holds up a finger for each word as it is spoken, both during the SLP's model and during Maggie's response, to help Maggie process the number of words needed.)		
	I - see - two - books.	

continues

■ TEXTBOX 2–2B.   *continued*

SLP	Client	Reader Comments
Very good, Maggie. You said, "I - see - two - books." You got the /s/ for the plural exactly right on the end of books. "I - see - two - books." Excellent work!		
Summary Comments for Scenario B		

Role of the Speech-Language Pathologist in the Therapeutic Process

It is possible to use dozens of descriptors to indicate the role of the SLP in therapy; among the possibilities are the following words: *helpful*, *supportive*, *facilitative*, *communicative*, *guiding*, *encouraging*, and *prompting*. Although the SLP is charged with the task of helping the client improve communication skills, ultimately the SLP does not simply *correct the communication disorder*, but instead serves in a role that *helps the client improve communication skills* (American Speech-Language-Hearing Association, 2001). The word *facilitator* is used to refer to this *helping* role, with SLPs expected to excel in facilitation skills.

Facilitation skills promote or accentuate student learning. Several researchers studied the use of facilitation skills among regular educators (Kent, 2006; McGee, Menolascino, Hobbs, & Menousek, 1987; Savion, 2009). Menolascino, Hobbs, and Menousek (1987) found that teachers classified as excellent "facilitative" teachers conducted long conversations with their students, were natural, spontaneous, sensitive, individualized, and less constraining. These teachers used more encouragement and humor, and they clarified strategies. Mirenda and Donellan (1986) noted that the communicative styles of facilitative teachers were marked with fewer topics and rare usage of direct questions. SLPs are encouraged to emulate these facilitation practices in the therapeutic process by striving to (a) develop a conversational communication style of therapy (Backus & Beasley, 1951); (b) avoid the temptation to "teach by testing," and (c) structure questions that are more open-ended, as opposed to "yes–no" questions.

Interpersonal Demeanor in Therapy

It was mentioned earlier in this chapter that some students are "a natural" for therapy because they already possess interpersonal communication skills that are important for speech-language therapy. Students considered to be a natural for therapy routinely incorporate several characteristics of good communication into their everyday interactions with clients. Samovar and Mills (1986) noted 10 different characteristics of communication, and although it is not necessary to expound on each of these within this discussion, it is noteworthy to relate several of these characteristics to the SLP. Samovar and Mills (1986) indicated that **communication** is a response-seeking, two-way symbolic, yet real-life process; they added that communication is a receiver phenomenon, and is a complex, transitory, continuous, and contextually based event. Those who negotiate interactions well enough to honor all or most of these characteristics of communication are likely viewed as effective communicators; those who do not may be viewed as less effective, poor, inept, awkward, or possibly even crass communicators. Samovar and Mills (1986) discussed five different types of communication interactions: intrapersonal, interpersonal, small group, public speaking, and mediated communication. Each type of communication has its importance; however, of particular note for our discussion are interpersonal communication skills, particularly as exemplified by the SLP.

SLPs need to bring good interpersonal communication skills into the therapy setting; the basic elements of good communication must be emulated before the SLP begins the process of direct speech-language therapy. For example, it is important that the SLP considers the personality and basic needs of the client as a function of interpersonal communication skills before beginning actual speech-language therapy with the client. Interpersonal communication skills are important, also, in working toward therapeutic objectives. As interpersonal communication skills are exercised within the therapeutic interaction, the SLP is encouraged to consider the elements of good communication and to practice these elements as part of therapeutic interaction. Within the practice of good elements of communication lies the interpersonal demeanor required to propel speech-language therapy. SLPs are, therefore encouraged to work to continuously improve effectiveness of communication skills through improvements of following basic skills as suggested by Hommes (2012):

(a)   listening skills (attending, questioning, paraphrasing, reflection of feelings, summarizing)

(b)   regulating skills (opening and closing a conversation, defining goals, clarifying unclear expectations)

(c)   assertive skills (requesting, rejecting requests, giving an order, rejecting an order, criticizing, responding to criticism) (online source)

Jackson and Woolsey (2009), additionally, found that increasing the engagement of students through uses of "problem-based learning, participation in workshop-type learning activities, peer mentoring and teaching, and increased uses of technology" (p. 8) often served to support development of clinical skills. It is believed that among these clinical skills are effective communication skills that support eventual development of therapeutic effectiveness.

Nonverbal Behaviors and Emotional Affect in the Therapeutic Process

Nonverbal behaviors exhibited by the SLP in therapy are important for client success. Eye contact, facial cues, proximity, body language, and other nonverbal communicators all impact the outcomes of therapy, and as such, should be controlled by the SLP as part of interpersonal communication skills. Along with nonverbal communication behaviors comes the concept of *emotional affect*. Nicolosi, Harryman, and Kresheck (2004) described **affect** as the "feeling, emotion, mood, and temperament associated with a thought" (p. 5). The importance of emotional affect was studied decades ago when Krathwohl, Bloom, and Bertram (1964) determined that attending, responding, valuing, organizing, and characterizing information were all integral to learning. Adding to this concept, Johnson, Musial, Hall, Gollnick, and Dupis (2005) noted that "an unavoidable part of instruction is consideration of students' attitudes and beliefs, because the affective elements are related to classroom behaviors" (p. 437). Although not responsible for classroom behavior of students, as Johnson et al. (2005) noted, SLPs, nonetheless, are responsible for the affective behaviors of clients in therapy. To this end, SLPs are encouraged to (a) learn to manipulate indicators of appropriate therapeutic affect (joy, excitement, enthusiasm, animated pitch, volume, etc.), and (b) learn to "read" the affective behaviors of clients in order to determine attitudes, beliefs, feelings, emotions, moods, and temperaments associated with the client's work during speech-language therapy. Exercise 2–1 is provided as a reminder of common affective behaviors.

Just as the SLP is able to "read" the graphics and label the emotions in Exercise 2–1, so are clinicians encouraged to "read" the affective behaviors of clients in therapy. This is, however, a two-way street. Many clients are able to "read" the faces and body language of the SLP during therapy as well. For this reason, SLPs are further encouraged to *practice often exemplifying each of the following emotions, using only facial expressions, or other nonverbal communications: excitement and encouragement.* These two emotions are among the feelings that SLPs will need to exemplify in therapy, both verbally and nonverbally.

Simple exercise to focus on common affective behaviors. Label each of the graphics below using the following possible terms: *excited, sad, angry, happy.*

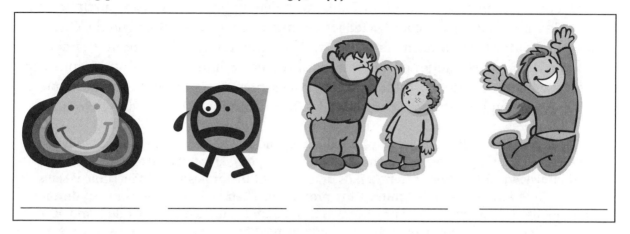

Professionalism

For purposes of this discussion, **professionalism** is a characteristic style, practice, or habit for personal and professional presentation, representation, and general demeanor. *Webster's II* (1996) further defined professionalism as professional standing, techniques, attributes, or ethics. Professionalism is a learned trait, but often it is easier to buy into or live up to professionalism and professional ethics and character, or traits, if personal integrity is consistent with the requirements of professionalism. Discussions in this text are not designed to evaluate or teach personal integrity. However, students are encouraged to assess whether traits of personal character (beliefs, ideals, etc.) are consistent with the concepts of professionalism and to work toward alignment of these entities.

Professional Appearance

Professional appearance is affected by dress, hairstyle, and personal grooming choices. Each of these areas of personal management impacts the SLP's overall presentation and is considered worthy of discussion.

Dress

Personal choices in the area of dress are more varied and relaxed than they were even a decade ago. As professionals, we must constantly balance our *preferred personal dress* with *required professional dress*, even though indicators suggest that *required professional dress* standards may be somewhat more relaxed than in prior years. Sometimes that balance is not easy, especially among young professionals who quickly indicate that they do not have the funds for a professional wardrobe. Although the cost of clothing is often expensive, it should be noted that frequently a student's ability to purchase a professional wardrobe is hampered not by limited financial means, but by preferred choice. For example, for the price of a pair of jeans, sneakers, and a T-shirt, a student might just as easily purchase a pair of dress slacks, or skirt, an unconstructed jacket, and a top, or dress shirt and tie. Often one professional outfit (or "uniform," as some students grudgingly refer to professional dress) is enough for the early stages of a professional career. Although each training program, employer, or SLP professional ultimately determines interpretations of standards for professional dress, individual SLPs are encouraged to think through the following accounts.

> Julie and Janet were both nationally accredited and licensed speech-language pathologists who owned a joint private practice in a thriving metropolis. They seemed to be well-trained and knowledgeable of the current trends and issues in the profession. Their clinical skills were well within acceptable limits of the profession. Their clients came from within the metropolitan area where their practice was located and consisted of 60% adult and 40% child or adolescent clients who were either private paying or were seen for insurance reimbursement. The office seemed to be located in a good area and was well maintained. Julie and Janet seemed positioned for a thriving business. Yet, within 2 years, community support for their business waned, and despite massive advertisement campaigns, they closed their business within 27 months of opening.

> Megan and Mollie also began a speech-language pathology partnership in a thriving metropolis at about the same time as did Julie and Janet. In fact, Megan and Mollie's situation paralleled Julie and Janet's scenario almost exactly. However, there was one notable difference: Julie and Janet received their clients and provided therapy wearing relaxed and casual clothing. Their clothing was, in essence, not dissimilar to what typical college students wear, whereas Megan and Mollie made a point to always dress more professionally in either slacks or skirts and lightweight jackets or in commercially available uniforms (sometimes called "scrubs"); they received and served their clients that way, even small children with whom they were often on the floor. Of course, there is no definitive way to say that dress impacts the public's perceptions of professionalism. It was, however, interesting to note that with all things being equal between the two practices, and the only notable difference being dress, that Megan and Mollie were still in business eight years later.

Perhaps dress does not make that much difference in a professional practice, but one SLP working in skilled nursing facilities and other medical settings reported, without reservation, that she is received and treated more professionally by staff and clients in those settings when she is more professionally dressed (L. K. Kendrick, personal communication, September 21, 2004). SLPs are, therefore, encouraged to consider professional dress at all times of professional practice.

Hairstyle

Hairstyles are subject to the same variability in personal preference as is dress among SLPs. For therapeutic intervention, hair length and color does not seem to matter as long as color is viewed as more traditional in nature. What does seem to impact therapy, however, is hair that falls over the face enough to cover one or both of the SLP's eyes. SLPs are encouraged to refrain from wearing hairstyles that cover, or partially cover, the eyes because of the loss of communication that results when the eyes are not visible to the client for communication interaction. Years ago, rumor had it that a college professor teaching clinical courses required students to cut their hair, if a long hairstyle was worn. Of course, nothing was further from the truth. In fact, the professor merely asked students to find ways to wear the hair so that it did not fall into the face, particularly over the eyes, during therapy. One negative aspect of hair in the SLP's face is the distraction of having to constantly brush it back from the face, a motion that is sometimes viewed as nervousness or uncertainty. Today, that same professor is careful to make sure students understand that cutting the hair is not necessary, but that keeping hair out of the face, particularly away from the eyes, is important.

Personal Grooming Choices

The personal grooming choices that we bring into the therapeutic setting are areas for discussion. For example, the fragrances that we wear during therapy may matter to some clients who have sensory sensitivity issues. Choices of neckties may make a difference in clients' attention and focus skills; the same may be true if the SLP chooses loud, flashy, flowery, plaid, or otherwise busy patterns in clothing. Additionally, SLPs are encouraged to avoid revealing or provocative clothing during therapy because of the distractive nature of such attire. Along these lines, SLPs are encouraged to rethink personal choices for wearing large dangly earrings; noisy bracelets; tongue, nose, lip, or eyebrow jewelry during therapy sessions because of the distractive nature of such jewelry during therapy. Additionally, good oral hygiene practices are important for the SLP because of the proximity often needed for modeling phonemes or other speech-language targets.

Excellence as a Hallmark of Therapy

A resurgence of excellence in productivity in the United States began in the late 1970s and early 1980s, led largely by the automobile industry (Iacocca, 1984). Education soon followed with school reform, school restructuring, and school improvement movements (Rauhauser & McLennan, 1994). Today, the "No Child Left Behind" (NCLB) law of 2001 with its emphasis on reading, leads the thrust for excellence in education in the United States. *Excellence*, as applied to speech-language therapy, is the achievement of therapy to a level of exceptional quality. As a hallmark, excellence becomes the standard by which clinical performances are measured. SLPs are urged to adopt a position of excellence for all aspects of therapy.

Time-On-Task as a Hallmark for Excellence

Cotton and Savard (1981) defined *time-on-task* as the time when students are attending to a learning task and are attempting to learn. School improvement research indicated powerful findings regarding time-on-task in relationship to student achievement (Cotton & Savard, 1981; Walberg, 1988; Wyne & Stuck, 1979). According to researchers, time-on-task interactive activities with a teacher produced greater student achievement than other types of time-on-task activities (Walberg, 1988). Researchers reported that time-on-task is needed for learning, but no definitive time for specific learning to occur was reported; this nondefinitive time span suggested possible broad ranges for required time to learn a concept or activity. Because SLPs have limited time to teach new concepts, or change client behavior, professionals are encouraged to take a *minutes-matter attitude*, a way of thinking about time-on-task during speech-language therapeutic intervention, in honor of the school improvement research. Minutes matter! It matters how many minutes we devote to small talk, when that is not our objective, and it matters how much time we spend getting out, setting up, and putting away materials for therapy. Time spent interacting in on-task behaviors in therapy with clients is limited; minutes matter! (Time commitments within the therapy session are discussed further in Chapter 7.)

Summary

SLPs work along an imaginary line between knowledge-based research and practical application of techniques and skills within the profession; artistry serves as the bridge between research and practical application for the SLP professional. Working under concepts such as *"Showtime!"* and the therapeutic mindset, the SLP professional is encouraged to work toward a "hallmark of excellence" by demonstrating both interpersonal and therapeutic-specific skills integral to the therapeutic process.

Learning Tool

1. Write a brief statement regarding your concept of "artistry" in speech-language pathology.

   _____

   _____

   _____

   _____

2. List and briefly discuss three elements of the therapeutic mindset for speech-language pathologists.

_____

_____

_____

_____

3. Peer Interaction: Interview three class members to gather their thoughts about professional dress as related to perceived professionalism. Develop a summary statement of findings based on discussions with peers and enter the statement here.

_____

_____

_____

_____

References

Adams, S. K., & Wittmer, D. S. (2001). "I had it first": Teaching young children to solve problems peacefully. *Childhood Education, 78*(1), 10–17.

American Speech-Language-Hearing Association. (2001). *Scope of practice in speech-language pathology.* Rockville, MD: Author.

Backus, O., & Beasley, J. (1951). *Speech therapy with children.* Cambridge, MA: Riverside Press.

Conderman, G., Johnston-Rodriguez, S., & Hartman, P. (2009). Communicating and collaborating in co-taught classrooms. *Teaching Exceptional Children Plus, 5*(5), 1–17.

Cotton, K., & Savard, W. G. (1981). *Time factors in learning.* Portland, OR: Northwest Regional Educational Laboratory (ED 214706).

Delmar Learning. Iacocca, L. A. (1984). *Iacocca: An autobiography.* New York, NY: Bantam Books.

Hallahan, D. P., & Kauffman, J. M. (2000). *Exceptional learner: Introduction to special education* (8th ed.). Boston, MA: Allyn & Bacon.

Hegde, M. N., & Davis, D. (2005). *Clinical methods and practicum in speech-language pathology* (2nd ed.). New York, NY: Thomson.

Hommes, M. A. (2012). Effects of a self-instruction communication skills training on skills, self-efficacy, motivation, and transfer. *European Journal of Open, Distance and e-Learning, 1,* (Online, no page numbers).

Hulit, L. M., Howard, M. R., & Fahey, K. R. (2011). *Born to talk,* (5th ed.). Boston, MA: Pearson.

Iacocca, L. (1984). *Iacocca: An autobiography, with William Novak.* New York, NY: Bantam Books.

Jackson, C. A., & Woolsey, J. D. (2009). A different set of classrooms: Preparing a new generation of clinicians. *Forum on Public Policy,*

Online: http://forumonpublicpolicy.com/spring09papers/archivesspr09/Jackson.pdf

Johnson, J. A., Musial, D., Hall, G. E., Gollnick, D. M., & Dupis, V. L. (2005). *Introduction to the foundations of American education* (13th ed.). Boston, MA: Pearson Education.

Kent, B. (2006). What does it take to facilitate? *Kairaranga, 7*(Special Issue), 59–63.

Krathwohl, D. R., Bloom, B. S., & Bertram, B. M. (1964). *Taxonomy of educational objectives: The classification of educational goals handbook II: Affective domain.* New York, NY: David McKay.

Low, H. M., & Lee, L. W. (2011). Teaching of speech, language and communication skills for young children with severe autism spectrum disorders: What do educators need to know? *New Horizons in Education, 59*(3), 16–27.

McGee, J. J., Menolascino, F. J., Hobbs, D. C., & Menousek, P. E. (1987). *Gentle teaching.* New York, NY: Human Science Press.

Merriam-Webster's Collegiate Dictionary (10th ed.). (1993). Springfield, MA: Merriam-Webster.

Mirenda, P., & Donellan, A. (1986). Effects of adult interaction style versus conversational behavior in students with severe communication problems. *Language, Speech, and Hearing Services in the Schools, 17*, 126–141.

Nicolosi, L., Harryman, E., & Kresheck, J. (2004). *Terminology of communication disorders: Speech-language-hearing* (5th ed.). Baltimore, MD: Lippincott Williams & Wilkins.

Paul, R., & Cascella, P. W. (2007). *Introduction to clinical methods in communication disorders.* (2nd ed.). Baltimore, MD: Brookes.

Rauhauser, B., & McLennan, A. (1994). *America's schools: Meeting the challenge through effective schools research and total quality management.* Lewisville, TX: Authors.

Samovar, L. A., & Mills, J. (1986). *Oral communication: Message and response* (6th ed.). Dubuque, IA: William C. Brown.

Savion, L. (2009). Clinging to discredited beliefs: The larger cognitive theory. *Journal of the Scholarship of Teaching and Learning, 9*(1), 81–92.

Walberg, H. J. (1988). Synthesis of research on time and learning. *Educational Leadership, 45*, 76–86.

Webster's II New Riverside Dictionary (Revised ed.). (1996). Boston, MA: Houghton Mifflin.

Wyne, M. D., & Stuck, G. B. (1979). Time on-task and reading performance in underachieving children. *Journal of Reading Behavior, 11*, 119–128.

3

Foundations for the Therapeutic Process: Overview

Introduction

"The overall objective of speech-language pathology services is to optimize individuals' ability to communicate and/or swallow in natural environments and, thus, improve their quality of life. This objective is best achieved through the provision of integrated services in meaningful life contexts" (American Speech-Language Hearing Association [ASHA], 2001, p. I–26). To this end, SLPs are held to the highest professional standards and monitored by an internationally respected professional, scientific, and credentialing association, the American Speech-Language Hearing Association (ASHA). ASHA's mission is empowering and supporting audiologists, speech-language pathologists, and speech, language, and hearing scientists through advancing science, setting standards, fostering excellence in professional practice, and advocating for members and those they serve (ASHA, 2014b). As of early 2014, ASHA represented more than 173,000 members and affiliates working as SLPs; audiologists; and speech, language, and hearing scientists in the United States and internationally (ASHA, 2014a).

The speech-language pathology profession is solidly founded on principles of professional ethics, and so, too, is the therapeutic process founded on those same ethics. Those entering the profession are encouraged to embrace concepts of professional ethics and to emulate and espouse those ethics during training and in all aspects of professional endeavors, thereafter. Professional ethics should resound throughout speech-language services within the context of the therapeutic process.

The Therapeutic Process Defined

The term *therapeutic process* in its purest sense involves procedures designed to heal or cure. Although speech-language therapy services are often closely aligned with the medical profession, particularly when speech services are offered in hospitals and medical clinics, "speech-language pathologists work to improve quality of life by reducing impairments of body functions and structures, activity limitation, participation restrictions, and environmental barriers of the individuals they serve" (ASHA, 2001, pp. I–28). SLPs are not likely viewed as healing or curing in the strict sense of the definition of therapeutic process. Rather, SLPs prevent, diagnose, habilitate, rehabilitate, and enhance the skills, activities, structures, and functions of clients (ASHA, 2001). For purposes of this discussion, the **therapeutic process** is defined as broad-based professional procedures, activities, and interactions with clients designed for the intervention of communication disorders. This definition takes into account a wide array of professional responsibilities including assessing, planning, implementing, and evaluating procedures for speech-language therapy services. Additionally, a wide array of peripheral activities and concepts associated with providing speech-language services (discussed in Chapter 8) also accompanies the therapeutic process and must be managed as well by the SLP.

Basic Confidence and Trust in the Therapeutic Process

Webster's defines trust as "firm reliance in the honesty, dependability, strength, or character of something or someone" (1996, p. 723). Federal, state, and local laws guide and govern the legalities associated with providing a service to the public through laws or ordinances often overseen by governmental licensing boards. However, it is through individual professional presentation and effort that the SLP comes to be trusted by his or her clientele for providing the best possible services. That trust, of course, must be earned and is only garnered through the SLP's consistent efforts in providing the highest quality and best services possible to those he or she serves. For the SLP to secure the trust of clients, the clinician must first build his or her own confidence in the profession and in the services being provided to the client. Development of the SLP's confidence in the therapeutic process is actually the first step in engendering the client's trust in the therapeutic process.

Increasing the SLP's Confidence in the Therapeutic Process

The beginning SLP often feels overwhelmed when trying to understand the basic tenets of the profession. This feeling often results in the beginner's lack of confidence in his or her abilities to eventually adequately perform the skills and tasks of an SLP professional. Even during courses of study when students are performing well, they often continue to agonize that they will never be able to learn all that they must in order to perform as a professional responsible for services to clients. This apprehension in transitioning from SLP student into SLP professional is understandable, and, perhaps, even typical. The knowledge and skills required of aspiring SLPs are vast (ASHA, 2014), and the credentialing process is grueling. Thus, a healthy respect for the levels of both training and practice standards is appropriate for the beginning student SLP. However, even experienced SLPs admit to feeling less than completely comfortable with clients with whom they have less experience, and veteran SLPs are still sometimes uncomfortable with new and emerging technologies associated with services offered in our profession. These feelings, too, constitute understandable reactions and interpretations by the practicing SLP professional.

Even though it is understandable that students, and even practicing professionals, may occasionally feel less than comfortable with providing certain types of therapies to various clients, it is important that the student, and the professional alike, understand that his or her confidence in the therapeutic process is an essential and foundational element in that therapeutic process. As professionals, we need to develop confidence that (a) the information given, the techniques used, and overall directions in which we are leading our clients are, in fact, the best available; (b) the outcomes toward which we are working are valid for the client; and (c) we as professionals possess the skills and knowledge to obtain those outcomes. Understandably, time and experience are required to impact levels of confidence in clinical skills across broad-based services. However, even beginning students are encouraged and coached toward building trust in what they know and understand in order to positively impact the therapeutic process. Students are encouraged to (a) gather information, (b) interpret findings by bridging findings with known information, and (c) develop conclusions with appropriate rationales early in training and to continue those practices even as seasoned and experienced professionals.

Through repeated exercises in systematic questioning, hypothesizing, analyzing, testing, and reaching conclusions, students begin to understand concepts related to the profession, but more importantly, they begin to build confidence in their own skills in determining appropriate directions and arriving at appropriate conclusions for client management. Exercise 3–1 provides a practice opportunity to help the student develop confidence in emerging skills for making the kinds of decisions required for the SLP to develop confidence in the therapeutic process. Typically, once the SLP works through four or five imagined client profiles (presented in Exercise 3–1), the understanding of and confidence in the therapeutic process begins to take shape for the student as exemplified by increases in fluency when discussing cases, increases in comprehensively considering all aspects of the client's profile, and increases in speed for completing the exercise. *Although only one exercise template is given at Exercise 3–1, the student is encouraged to develop at least five scenarios as prescribed in Exercise 3–1 over the next several days.*

In addition to the exercise in Exercise 3–1 designed to help develop the SLP's confidence in the therapeutic process, the following activities help foster confidence.

- *Read client files from beginning of therapy to dismissal* to develop a "sense" of how therapy proceeds in actual cases.

- *Talk to former clients,* if available, to hear their views on how therapy helped them (occasionally peers and classmates were enrolled in speech-language therapy as children and have no reservations in sharing remembered experiences).

Developing the SLP's confidence in the therapeutic process.

Gather Information

Develop a profile for an imagined client by filling in the Imagined Client Profile below. You may use general information remembered from clients seen in observation experiences, or you may recall general information regarding the performances of clients from prior class experiences or discussions. If desired, pair with a peer to help develop the Imagined Client Profile. Enter the age, gender, disorders, speech-language assessment results, and so forth, for your imagined client in the spaces below.

Develop an Imagined Client Profile

Age of Client: _____

Gender of Client: _____

Documented Disorder(s): _____

Suspected Disorder(s): _____

Speech-Language Assessment Results: _____

    Receptive Language Age: _____   _____

    Expressive Language Age: _____   _____

    Articulation/Phonology Skills: _____

    Fluency Skills: _____

    Voice Skills: _____

    Resonance Skills: _____

Probable Cognitive Skills: _____

- *Develop a relationship with professionals for observations in the same setting* periodically so that familiar clients, and their progress, are seen over a period of time.

The discussion of confidence in the therapeutic process, thus far, has focused on the concept of *helping the SLP develop confidence in the process of therapy, itself.* However, it is imperative that the SLP develops confidence in his or her abilities to appropriately serve clients as well. Hegde and Davis (2005) noted that:

> Confidence in your ability to help your client is an important characteristic to develop. You will probably be nervous when you first talk with your clients but it is important that you make a good impression. You will often be the first clinic person to contact a client. The client must believe that you are capable of providing quality clinical services. Also,

Exercise 3–1 *continued*

Interpret Findings

Think about the information entered for the Imagined Client Profile above. Determine whether the profile you have developed for the imagined client represents a person with (a) normal speech-language skills, (b) a mild disorder, (c) a moderate disorder, or (d) a severe disorder. Check the box that matches your interpretation for the level of the client's speech-language difficulty and enter the explanations for your interpretation in the spaces below.

❑ Normal speech-language skills: (Explain) _____

_____

_____

❑ Mild speech-language disorder: (Explain) _____

_____

_____

❑ Moderate speech-language disorder: (Explain) _____

_____

_____

❑ Severe speech-language disorder: (Explain) _____

_____

_____

Develop Conclusions and Recommendations

Develop a conclusion or summary statement about the client's needs for intervention based on whether the client has a mild, moderate, or severe speech-language disorder. Tell why you think the intervention is needed for the client, or why you think the intervention is *not* needed for the client.

Is therapy indicated for the client?

Yes: _____ If yes, tell why: _____

_____

_____

No: _____ If no, tell why not: _____

_____

_____

your clients must believe they are important to you and trust that you will do all you can to help them. A large part of this trust is developed as you initially establish rapport with your clients. (p. 78)

There are several things the SLP can do to build confidence in his or her ability to serve the client and, at the same time, build the client's trust in the clinician's skills.

- *Think about, and practice a communicative style to introduce yourself.* This action may seem awkward, or unnecessary, but this practice often proves more helpful for presenting a professional demeanor than expected. The most classic cases of professional awkwardness when this detail is left undecided or unaddressed occur most often in relation to ages when (a) younger SLPs find themselves unsure of how they would like to be addressed by older clients, or (b) SLPs of similar ages as the clients feel uncertain of how they would like to be addressed by age-level peers. Occasionally, the SLP's name, itself, is difficult for clients to pronounce, making it somewhat awkward for the client when first meeting the SLP. For example, often the SLP first introduces him or herself by customary name, realizes that the requirement for pronouncing the name further magnifies the client's discomfort with his or her communication difficulty, then hurriedly changes the introduction to a less difficult form of the name to increase client comfort. Of course, the SLP is not encouraged to change his or her name for the sake of client comfort, but certainly, the professional is encouraged to think through the options for personal introductions prior to meeting the client for the first time. Examples of introductions include:

  "Hi, I'm _____."

  "Hello, my name is _____."

  "Good morning. It's very nice to see you. I'll be your therapist today; my name is _____."

  "Good morning, Mr. Maye, I'm *very-long-or-difficult-to-pronounce name*, the clinician for your speech and language services. You may call me _____."

  The possibilities are endless, of course, but it is advisable to select *an introduction style that best suits you, and practice it often before meeting your first client.*

- *Practice your handshake.* Select a partner who will give you feedback regarding the appropriateness of your handshake for business communications. Avoid handshakes that are too loose or too tight in touch, handshakes in which only the fingers and not the full palm are engaged, or handshakes in which the palm is extended down or extended upward.

- *Practice appropriate business eye contact.* Appropriate business eye contact focuses on the face, in what is called the "triangle of eye contact," a gaze beginning at the outer corner of the communicating partner's eyebrow, horizontally across to the outer corner of the opposite eyebrow, diagonally down to the chin, then diagonally up to the outer corner of the eyebrow for the original starting point. If one gazes anywhere within that imaginary triangle, the communicating partner perceives that eye contact is made. Note, however, that the acceptable time for business and even social eye gaze in the United States is only about 3 to 5 seconds, after which time, the gaze is broken by looking slightly away, perhaps over the partner's shoulder, or slightly downward, then back to the face for another 3 to 5 seconds. Eye gazes that are too short or too long often make the communicating partner uncomfortable and may negatively impact the client's trust in the therapeutic process.

- *Be sure you are comfortable in appropriate professional clothing* for therapy. (See Chapter 2 for a brief discussion on professional dress.)

- *Become familiar with the intake data and other information available for each client.*

- *Become familiar with other forms you will need to fill out during the session with your client.*

- *Plan well for all aspects of your contact with the client* (therapy space, proper operations of materials and equipment needed for the session, questions and other communications necessary for the session, client comfort for room temperature, bathroom breaks, and so forth. Equip the therapy room with tissues and trash cans that might be needed for medically fragile or other clients, etc.)

- *Actually practice the session*, and mentally walk through each aspect of the contact with the client, beginning with your introduction of yourself, through the final good-bye as you walk the client to the appropriate waiting or exit area at the end of the session. (Always know when and where the next session is scheduled, and remind the client of that appointment as you end the session.)

- *Determine if contact with caregivers will be possible*, and if so, practice interactions and communications with them as well.

- *Know the payment arrangements for services* and be prepared to direct the client or caregiver to the appropriate person(s) for taking care of financial arrangements for services, if any. Although you may *feel awkward, do not act awkward* in discussing money matters with the client or caregiver to the degree that you have the knowledge and authority to do so.

- *Practice the therapeutic process* as if someone will be taking notes on every aspect of your performance because, essentially, someone is: your client, his or her caregiver, and likely, your supervisor as well.

Increasing the Client's Trust in the Therapeutic Process

Clients occasionally express interest in the broad-based legislative or professional ethical principles that undergird professions offering various services. For example, most patients are aware of the American Medical Association (AMA) and the physician's professional relationship to it. However, few clients are aware of ASHA and the SLP's professional relationship to it. The practicing SLP should remain cognizant of not only ASHA's Code of Ethics and the approved standards of the profession, but should also share with clients the basic principles and standards promoted by ASHA as a way of helping clients establish trust in the individual SLP professional and in the communication disorders profession as a whole. The Code of Ethics of the American Speech-Language Hearing Association (2010r) consists of a Preamble, and four Principles of Ethics. The principles address a wide range of professional responsibilities and include respective rules for SLP professionals regarding treatment of clients, research subjects, professional competence, and relationships with colleagues and collaborative professionals. (A copy of ASHA's Code of Ethics may be retrieved at http://www.asha.org/policy on most search engines.)

In addition to sharing the ASHA Code of Ethics with clients as a way of helping to instill or build client trust in the therapeutic process, SLPs may also choose to highlight various federal and state laws that impact services to clients. Numerous special education and civil laws affect services to clients with communication disorders. However, several laws are far-reaching and should be noted by the SLP professional as integral, even foundational, for the services provided to speech-language pathology clients. Following are some of the laws that impact speech-language services to children.

1. *The Education for All Handicapped Children Act (EHA) (PL 94-142), 1975.* This was the first federal law mandating free and appropriate public education for all children with disabilities (Hallahan & Kauffman, 2000). Under provisions of this law, children were assessed, placed, and served categorically and noncategorically, with *Speech Impaired* serving as one of the categories under which children received free, appropriate services under the prescription of an Individualized Education Plan (IEP). The IEP is a federally mandated document that details specific information regarding several aspects of services for the child, including the status of the child's disorder, the recommended services, amount of time prescribed for the services, and other information for addressing the disorder.

2. *EHA Amendment: Preschool and Infant/Toddler Programs (PL 99-457), 1986.* This amendment was considered to be a "downward extension" of PL 94-142 to include free and appropriate public education for children ages 0 to 5 years. Children ages 3 to 5 years most often were seen in schools for speech-language services under the IEP as a result of this EHA Amendment. However, PL 99-457 instituted services for children with disabilities, including speech-language services, ages 0 to 3 years in Early Intervention (EI) programs under the prescription of the Individualized Family Service Plan (IFSP).

3. *EHA Amendment: Individuals with Disabilities Education Act (IDEA) (PL 101-476), 1990.* This amendment changed considerably the components of the original EHA law of 1975 by (a) changing the name to IDEA, (b) providing transportation services, (c) extending eligibility to children with autism and traumatic brain injury (TBI), (d) adding assistive technology devices and services for children with disabilities as prescribed by the IEP, and (e) extending provisions of the least restrictive environment (LRE), the aspect of EHA, 1975, that allowed children, to the degree possible, to be educated in regular classrooms with nondisabled peers. SLPs continued services for children in

schools under the IEP. Children with autism and TBI became eligible for speech-language services according to the IEP under this amendment.

4. *Goals 2000: Educate America Act (PL 103-85), 1993.* This Act was a broad-based federal law that established eight goals for education in the United States. These goals addressed (a) the child's readiness to learn; (b) increases in high school graduation rates to 90%; (c) achievement testing in grades 4, 8, and 12; (d) continuous development for teachers; (e) national prominence in math and science; (f) adult literacy and global competence; (g) drug-free schools; and (h) school–parent partnerships. Children with special needs were included along with children in general education classes as beneficiaries of the law. SLPs continued to serve children in both regular and special needs classrooms under this law.

5. *Improving America's Schools Act (PL 103-382), 1994.* This law was an amendment to the *Elementary and Secondary Education Act of 1965, (ESEA)*. It appropriated funds for improving education across broad parameters that included staff development for teachers and eliminating ability grouping for children. SLPs continued services to students in both regular and special needs classrooms under this law.

6. *IDEA Amendment: Individuals with Disabilities Education Act (PL 105-17), 1997.* This amendment extended LRE, extended consideration of assistive technology devices on the IEPs of all children with disabilities, and added orientation and mobility services for children who are blind or visually impaired or other children needing such services. SLPs continued services for children in schools according to the IEP under this amendment.

7. *No Child Left Behind (NCLB) Act (PL 107-110), 2001.* This legislation provided states an opportunity to account for the Adequate Yearly Progress (AYP) of all students enrolled in public schools, including students with disabilities. Schools failing to post AYP for a certain percentage of its students, including students with disabilities, for two consecutive academic years are identified as "needing improvement," with structured plans for how to improve the school required. The law requires schools to look at the performances of all children, not just the ones performing at average or above average levels. SLPs continue to serve children in schools impacted by the NCLB law and must meet standards of the law as "highly qualified" professionals.

8. *IDEA Amendment: Individuals with Disabilities Education Act (PL 108-446), 2004* is due to be reauthorized in 2014, likely subsequent to this publication. The 2004 amendment of IDEA made substantial changes to the historical law. Among the changes were (a) adding the concept of "highly qualified" for special education professionals, consistent with the NCLB Act of 2001, (b) piloting the "reduction of paperwork" process, (c) extending services to mobile populations, (d) impacting assessments to line up with the Elementary and Secondary Education Act of 1965 (ESEA), and (e) changing compliance to focus on student achievement rather than procedures. SLPs continued services in schools under

this new amendment. SLPs are encouraged to survey for the 2014 amendment to IDEA as it becomes available and to gather from its changes all aspects of the law that impact the SLP profession for daily practices of business.

Other laws also impact speech-language pathology and should be considered important to the services provided by SLPs and as additional legislative foundation for helping clients develop trust in the therapeutic process. These laws, *Section 504 of the Rehabilitation Act of 1973 (Section 504)*, and the *Americans with Disability Act (PL 101-336), 1990 (ADA)* supported the equitable treatment and rights to services for clients regardless of whether an IEP or an IFSP was in place for the client, regardless of whether the client was in school, and regardless of age of the client. Although the SLP may not be fully competent in interpreting every aspect of the laws that impact speech-language pathology services to clients, it is important that the SLP professional not only recognizes the existence and intent of these laws, but it is important that he or she informs the client, or caregivers of the client, of client rights under applicable laws. By making clients aware of the laws that govern speech-language services, it is hoped clients will both better understand the laws and be more willing to entrust their speech-language needs to the clinician. ASHA (1999) published *Guideline for the Roles and Responsibilities of the School-Based Speech-Language Pathologist* that included further information regarding most of the laws highlighted here. SLPs, particularly those in school settings, are encouraged to refer to this publication often as additional support for helping build client trust in the therapeutic process. Textbox 3–1 illustrates a scenario of the ways in which the SLP may help increase the client's trust levels for the therapeutic process using information suggested in this section of the chapter.

Once the SLP begins to help the client build trust in the therapeutic process (see Textbox 3–1), that trust will need to be continued and nurtured throughout the duration of therapy with the client. Most often, sustained trust in the therapeutic process is accomplished by well-trained, well-organized professionals who take interest in the progress and welfare of their clients and who find ways of communicating this information to the client.

■ Textbox 3–1.   Developing the client's trust in the therapeutic process.

Developing Client's Trust in the Therapeutic Process

Clinician	Client
Good morning, Mr. Sams. My name is Pamela and I will be working with you today for speech services.	
	Good morning.

Clinician	Client
Before we actually begin the speech work, I'd like to take a few minutes to share with you some information regarding our services and the communication disorders profession, in general.	
	Okay.
Our clinic is privately owned by three other speech-language pathologists, James, Charles, Lydia, and myself. We are all licensed by the state to provide speech-language services to the public. Additionally, we each hold recognized professional certification in our field, the Certificate of Clinical Competence, affectionately known as the Cs, from our professional association, the American Speech-Language Hearing Association, ASHA for short, located in Rockville, Maryland. ASHA is respected worldwide as a credible professional organization with over 173,000 members currently working in the profession. If at any time you'd like to know more about the communication disorders profession, or more about ASHA, feel free to ask, or you may simply type in *asha* under a search engine on your computer, and I believe you will find quite a lot of information that's available to the public. Is everything clear so far?	
	I think so.
Great. I'd like to also tell you, Mr. Sams, that many of the clients who come to us exhibit disabilities in one or more areas of functioning. Our office recognizes the requirements of Section 504 of the Rehabilitation Act of 1973 and the Americans with Disability Act of 1990.	

continues

■ **TEXTBOX 3–1.**   *continued*

Clinician	Client
Please inform us if something appears to be inconsistent with the requirements of these laws as we provide services to you in our facility. I'm placing handouts regarding these federal laws in your *Welcome Packet* for your review. Also included in your *Welcome Packet* is basic introductory information about our agency, or mission, and philosophy. A statement regarding confidentiality related to the services we provide for you is also included. Any questions so far?	
	No, it all seems clear.
Excellent. Now, let me explain the services we will provide for you today, and we'll get started. You have already filled out for us several forms that we keep on file for you. Those forms include basic intake information, a case history, and the Health Insurance Portability and Accountability Act (HIPAA) forms, and others (Golper & Brown, 2004). Today we will conduct a complete screening of your speech, language, and hearing skills, including in-depth diagnostic assessments of any areas shown to need additional evaluation following the screening. Any questions before we begin?	
	No.
Let's get started then. I will explain each step of our work today so that the procedures are clear to you.	
	Okay.

The Therapeutic Relationship

Stone (1992) discussed a systems approach to resolving relationship problems in communication disorders treatment. She found that well-functioning relationships are characterized by "open communication and a respect for different beliefs and feelings. Roles and rules are clear, flexible, and appropriate to the participants' abilities and needs. When necessary, such relationships will change to meet individuals' needs" (p. 301). Stone (p. 301) listed the following six concepts regarding relationships:

1. *Participants in a relationship are interdependent.* (For example, the client and the clinician are affected by each other.)

2. *Interaction patterns are shaped and sustained by all participants in a relationship.* (For example, each person in the therapy session impacts the entire group.)

3. *Relationships have rules based on patterns of behavior and expected roles.* (For example, each person has an idea of how he or she expects other members of the group to behave within the group.)

4. *Rule violation and change are stressful in an established relationship.* (For example, consistency in interactions keeps anxiety low because everyone knows what to expect. Stone noted that persons with strong intrapersonal and interpersonal skills will be able to change within a relationship more readily than persons with more limited skills in these areas.)

5. *People in a relationship communicate about the nature of the relationship as well as about actions and events.* (Stone believed that *behaviors* are indicators of how people in the group feel about the relationship, but it is believed that *verbalizations* may be used to communicate about the nature of the relationship as well.)

6. *Relationships interact with larger systems and are affected by them.* (For example, Stone noted that the larger systems that affect a clinical relationship include families, schools, administrations, and clinics.)

Several other researchers (Conderman, Johnston-Rodriguez, & Hartman, 2009) discussed the importance of communication skills in relation to co-workers and suggested the following communication skills for improving collaborative environments in the workplace: "I-messages, Sandwich Techniques [beginning with two positive statements, giving the note of concern, and ending with an invitation to find a solution], Paraphrases, Summarizations, Open-ended Questions, Closed Questions, Seed Planting, Response to Affect, and Word Pictures" (p. 13). SLPs are encouraged to acknowledge that the therapeutic relationship is dependent on the quality of interpersonal and intrapersonal communications exhibited by group members. When communications among and between group members become problematic, it is up to the SLP to assess and redirect the dynamics of the communication in order to provide effective therapeutic interactions for the benefit of all clients.

Occasionally, behavior intervention or management is required to establish or reestablish effective therapeutic interactions. In these cases, the SLP is encouraged to seek techniques aimed at increasing compliance and reducing resistance (Brooks, 1991). Regardless of the techniques deemed necessary to promote and maintain the therapeutic relationship, the SLP should remember that the primary reason for addressing the dynamics of the therapeutic relationship is to maximize progress in therapy. In situations when an appropriate therapeutic relationship cannot be established, maintained, or regained, the SLP is encouraged to consider appropriate referral sources for the client in an effort to provide continuous quality support for the client, even if the client then becomes another SLP's responsibility.

Referrals to Other Professionals

Often, the SLP finds it necessary to refer a client to other professions (medical, educational, psychological, etc.). Occasionally, speech-language therapy does not progress as expected, and the SLP must explore causes for the lack of appropriate progress. In other cases, the client's progress is as expected, but it is simply time to add or explore the possibilities of addressing related issues that were previously identified, but placed on the back burner in favor of addressing more pressing or immediate communication needs initially. In either case, the SLP should discuss the possibility of the referral with the client, then establish contact with the receiving professional in order to bridge the various aspects of the referral. For example, if the client is referred to an occupational therapist after 3 to 4 months of intervention with the SLP, this referral should be discussed with the client, and appropriate appointments and follow-up efforts made to ensure that the referral services are both correct for the client and are instituted or initiated for the client. This is especially important if speech-language services continue to be necessary during or after the referral period. Shipley and McAfee (2005) offered a Sample Referral for Medical Evaluation for evaluation of laryngeal or vocal pathology. However, the components of that referral easily transfer for SLP referrals to other professions. For example, Shipley and McAfee developed the referral form consisting of the following elements:

1. Title of the form
2. Demographic information for the client
3. Salutation to the receiving professional
4. Indication of when and why the SLP evaluated the client
5. Status of the client's skills during assessment
6. Findings of the SLP assessment
7. Indication of prior intervention efforts
8. Request for professional evaluation of the client by the receiving professional
9. Enclosure of the form the SLP would like the receiving professional to complete
10. Instructions for returning the enclosed form to the referring SLP

11. Closing note of appreciation to the receiving professional

12. Signature, address, and telephone lines for the referring SLP

Using these basic components of a referral to other professions, the SLP should be able to adequately devise appropriate referral requests to medical, educational, or other professions. As mentioned earlier, the SLP should be prepared to follow up on all referrals made to other professions to help ensure proper management of client needs.

Summary

Simply put, the therapeutic process for the speech-language pathology profession is founded on professionalism. That professionalism is guided by the professional standards of ASHA and is undergirded by numerous state and federal laws regarding professional services to the public. Knowledge of both ASHA guidelines and federal laws helps promote client trust in the therapeutic process. However, the SLP also must address issues related to his or her confidence in (a) the therapeutic process itself (the belief that the process works), and (b) confidence that he or she has the professional skills to exact the aspects of the therapeutic process for benefit of clients. SLP confidence and client trust both develop over time and are nurtured within the context of the therapeutic relationship. SLPs are encouraged to invest daily in developing and improving the therapeutic relationship.

Learning Tool

1. Retrieve a copy of ASHA's Code of Ethics. Read it, and list 10 relevant items addressed in the Code.

_____

_____

_____

_____

2. Briefly discuss salient points of three laws that apply to SLPs providing services to the public, for children or adults.

_____

_____

_____

_____

3. List five things an SLP might do to foster his or her confidence in the therapeutic process.

_____

_____

_____

_____

References

American Speech-Language-Hearing Association. (1999). *Guidelines for the roles and responsibilities of the school-based speech-language pathologist.* Rockville, MD: Author.

American Speech-Language-Hearing Association. (2001). *Scope of practice in speech-language pathology.* Rockville, MD: Author.

American Speech-Language-Hearing Association. (2010). *Code of ethics [Ethics].* Retrieved from http://www.asha.org/policy

American Speech-Language-Hearing Association. (2014a). *About the American Speech-Language-Hearing Association (ASHA).* Retrieved from http://www.asha.org/about/

American Speech-Language-Hearing Association. (2014b). *Certification standards for speech-language pathology frequently asked questions: General information.* Retrieved from http://www.asha.org/certification/2014-Certification-Standards-for-SLP/

Brooks, A. R. (1991). Clinical exchange: Behavior problems and the power relationship. *Language, Speech, and Hearing Services in the Schools, 22,* 89–91.

Conderman, G., Johnston-Rodriguez, S., & Hartman, P. (2009). Communicating and collaborating in co-taught classrooms. *Teaching Exceptional Children Plus, 5*(5), 1–17.

Golper, L. A. C., & Brown, J. E. (Eds.) (2004). *Business matters: A guide for speech-language pathologists.* Rockville, MD: American Speech-Language Hearing Association.

Hallahan, D. P., & Kauffman, J. M. (2000). *Exceptional learner: Introduction to special education* (8th ed.). Boston, MA: Allyn & Bacon.

Hegde, M. N., & Davis, D. (2005). *Clinical methods and practicum in speech-language pathology* (2nd ed.). New York, NY: Thomson Delmar Learning.

Shipley, K. G., & McAfee, J. G. (2005). *Assessment in speech-language pathology: A resource manual* (3rd ed.). New York, NY: Thomson Delmar Learning.

Stone, J. R. (1992). Resolving relationship problems in communication disorders treatment: A systems approach. *Language, Speech, and Hearing Services in the Schools, 23,* 300–307.

Webster's II New Riverside Dictionary (Rev. ed.). (1996). Boston, MA: Houghton Mifflin.

4

Learning Theories Related to Speech-Language Intervention

Introduction

Learning theories have broad applications to numerous disciplines, including speech-language pathology. Yet, the study of learning theories is rarely included as an integral part of clinical training for SLPs. Whether working with the developing child or an adult client recovering from a stroke, it is important for the SLP to be aware of possible supports and barriers to therapy, based on learning theory research and practice, that impact client progress. For example, consider the patient who has a fluency disorder with presenting difficulties with repetitions and prolongations. The SLP's skills for working with the client with a fluency disorder are strengthened if basic concepts about not only fluency, but also about learning in relationship to the client's general abilities, are understood and considered during speech-language therapy. Although it is not important that SLPs spend hours learning and regurgitating comparisons and contrasts between learning theories, it is helpful for clinicians to be aware of major concepts regarding learning and learning theories related to client successes.

Learning Defined

Numerous researchers devoted large segments of their careers to learning and learning theories (Bruner, 1960; Dewey, 1910; Piaget, 1954; Skinner, 1953; Vygotsky, 1978), with each defining learning in slightly different ways. In recent years, Oakes and Lipton (2003) defined *learning* as "the processes and mental structures by which people accumulate experiences and make them into new meanings" (p. 44). Although more than two dozen orientations, explanations, and theories of learning exist (Merriam & Caffarella, 1991), four orientations to learning will be highlighted because of their broad-based applicability to the speech-language pathology profession:

1. the behavioral orientation to learning
2. the cognitive orientation to learning
3. the humanistic/experiential orientation to learning, and
4. the social orientation to learning.

Although overlaps and indistinct lines of division may be noted among these orientations at various points of discussion, each orientation takes a different view of the learning process, and SLPs are encouraged to consider these different views of learning in relation to client needs.

The Behavioral Orientation to Learning

The behavioral orientation to learning addresses the study of overt behaviors that can be observed and measured (Good & Brophy, 1990). Ivan Pavlov, a Russian psychologist widely known for his experiment in conditioning a dog to salivate by ringing a bell, developed the concept of *classical conditioning*, whereby a neutral stimulus becomes associated with a conditioned response (Pavlov, 1926). Most notably, Pavlov used food, an unconditioned stimulus, paired with the ringing of a bell, a neutral stimulus, to elicit a conditioned response, salivation in the dog. Pavlov also introduced the concepts of *conditioning, stimulus generalization, extinction,* and *discrimination* in relation to classical conditioning, giving rise to principles that would later be known as behaviorism.

Behaviorism as a psychological construct was presented by John B. Watson who wrote a paper entitled, "Psychology as a Behaviorist Views It" (Watson, 1913). Watson was the first American to embrace Pavlov's work, and he believed that practice strengthens learning.

Another American behaviorist, B. F. Skinner, suggested that the mind is viewed as a "black box," in the sense that an individual's response to a stimulus can be observed quantitatively as a result of stimulus-response relationships without consideration for thought processes that occur in the mind (Skinner, 1953). Skinner was well known for this "black box" concept in behaviorism. Most notable of Skinner's behavioral concepts for SLPs was his work in **operant conditioning**, a method of changing behavior in which a reinforcer/reward is offered the subject immediately following the production of a desired response (Nicolosi, Harryman, & Kresheck, 2004). Skinner believed that the individual "operates" or "behaves" in a certain way, receives a reward for that operation/behavior, and eventually establishes a bond between behavior and reward. For example, in speech-language therapy, a client responds to a stimulus presented by the clinician and correctly says the /s/ sound; the clinician offers a reward (verbal or nonverbal); the client is expected to perform the behavior (correctly producing /s/) to receive the reward; however, in time, the client is expected to perform the behavior (correct production of /s/)

without a reward. Skinner also introduced the concepts of *positive reinforcement*, *negative reinforcement*, *punishment*, *behavioral shaping*, and *reinforcement schedules* as important to behavioral concepts.

Behaviorists believe that "the school environment must be highly organized and the curriculum based on behavioral objectives, and they hold that knowledge is best described as behaviors that are observable" (Johnson, Musial, Hall, Gollnick, & Dupuis, 2005, p. 345). The behavioral orientation to learning produced several concepts and techniques routinely used by SLPs during speech-language intervention, including imitation, shaping (successive approximations), and cueing and prompting. Several researchers believe that, in general, the teaching of speech, language, and other communication skills can be accomplished through uses of the behavioral-oriented perspective for teaching (Low & Lee, 2011). Further application for speech-language intervention using the behavioral orientation to learning suggests that SLPs (a) state objectives, and break them into sequential steps, (b) provide cues and prompts that guide clients to desired behavior, and (c) use rewards (such as stickers) or natural communication consequences (such as being understood by the listener) to reinforce the desired behavior.

The Cognitive Orientation to Learning

Cognitive theorists view learning as "involving the acquisition or reorganization of the cognitive structures through which humans process and store information" (Good & Brophy, 1990, p. 187). A major promoter of the cognitive theory of learning was Swiss psychologist, Jean Piaget, who developed most of his theory of cognitive learning based on observations of his three children. Piaget developed the stages of cognitive development ranging from birth throughout adulthood and indicated that, as the child goes through various stages of "cognitive readiness," learning may occur. Although much of Piaget's work was done in the 1920s, it was not until 1960, when George Miller and Jerome Bruner established the Harvard University Center for Cognitive Studies, that Piaget found prominence in the United States (Good & Brophy, 1990).

Although many aspects of the cognitive orientation to learning impact the SLP's work, among the cognitive concepts typically viewed as valuable on an everyday basis for the SLP are the four stages or periods of cognitive development from Piaget's work. Piaget (1954) described the development of children's thinking as progressing through four **developmental stages**, periods of time during the growth process in which thoughts, behaviors, and feelings of an individual remain relatively the same. Piaget noted that the developmental stages begin at birth and traverse throughout adulthood. Following are brief descriptions of Piaget's stages of cognitive development:

Sensorimotor Period: This stage ranges from birth to age 2 years. Piaget characterized this stage of development as consisting of motor reflexes in beginning phases, from birth to about 1 year. However, children's physical interactions with objects in their world eventually dictate this phase of development from ages 1 year to 2 years. During this period, the child learns through touch and movement throughout the environment.

Preoperational Period: This stage includes ages 2 years to 7 years and is characterized by acquisition of representational skills in areas of language, mental imagery, and drawing, with the greatest increases occurring in language during this stage (Siegler, 1991). During this period, due to representational thought, a broomstick easily becomes a "horse" for the child.

Concrete Operations Period: Piaget determined that the concrete operations period of development lasts from 7 years to 12 years of age, during which time the child learns mental transformations for quantity and time. For example, prior to this stage of development, a child viewing a tall, narrow glass with 8 ounces of liquid and a shorter, wider glass with 8 ounces of liquid believes that the taller glass contains more liquid. However, once the child transitions into the concrete operations period of cognitive development, he or she is able to understand that, regardless of configuration of the container, 8 ounce quantities are the same across containers. Toward the end of this period, the child begins taking points of views of others, humor escalates, and the child positions to transfer into adult-like thought.

Formal Operations Period: This period begins at around age 12 years and continues throughout life. The characterizing achievement in this stage is the child's ability to "reason on the basis of theoretical possibilities as well as concrete realities" (Seigler, 1991, p. 21). Hypothetical thought becomes possible.

Piaget viewed three mental processes, processes that are important to SLPs, as crucial for the child's progression from one developmental period to another: *assimilation, accommodation,* and *equilibration.* **Assimilation** refers to a person's ability to transform incoming information so that it fits with his or her existing way of thinking. For example, a 4-year-old boy who had no concept of middle-age impacts on the body, but understood other realities, was noted to ask his uncle, "What are you doing with that basketball in your stomach?" then, also noticing the uncle's balding head, added, "And why do you cut your hair that way?" The child of 4 years was beginning to understand what the representation of a basketball inside a stomach might look like, and he understood the effects of haircuts. However, the child at that age had no mental representation for middle-age girth, and no mental concepts for patterned baldness. The child's mental task of *assimilation* was to make what he was seeing in his uncle fit a 4-year-old's knowledge base and way of thinking.

Piaget (1954) referred to **accommodation** as the way in which a person adapts his or her way of thinking regarding new experiences. For example, a man who grew up in a community that viewed a woman as aggressive if she worked outside of the home may find himself adjusting his thinking, *accommodating,* when his wife or daughter chooses to find a job. An interesting point regarding assimilation and accommodation was reported by Seigler (1991) when he noted that assimilation and accommodation mutually influence each other.

Finally, **equilibration** encompasses both assimilation and accommodation and refers to the overall interaction between existing ways of thinking and new experiences (Seigler, 1991). Piaget (1954) suggested that equilibration occurs in three phases such that when children are satisfied with current modes of thought, *equilibrium* exists. Then, when they become aware of shortcomings in their thinking, they become dissatisfied and enter a state of *disequilibrium*. Finally, children adopt a more advanced way of thinking that eliminates the shortcomings of the prior way of thinking, and enter into, now, a heightened state of *equilibrium*.

Siegler (1991) attributed the success and longevity of Piaget's work to several factors. Siegler noted:

1. Piaget's theory communicates an almost tangible sense of what a child's thinking is like.

2. Piaget's theory addresses topics that have been of interest to parents, teachers, scientists, and philosophers for hundreds of years.

3. Piaget's theory is of exceptional breath, covering an unusually broad age span—the entire range from infancy through adolescence.

4. Piaget had a gift for making interesting observations (1991, p. 18).

Other key concepts of the cognitive orientation to learning involve (a) the *Three-Stage Information Processing Model*, from which we take the concepts of *sensory input* and *short-term* and *long-term memory*; (b) *learning **schema***, whereby new information is compared to existing cognitive structures; and (c) *learning effects* such as practice, transference, mnemonics, and processing effects (Good & Brophy, 1990).

The cognitive orientation, along with Piaget's periods of cognitive development, is a broad-based and effectual orientation for educators' treatments of instruction and learning. The cognitive orientation to learning is important to SLPs for several reasons: (a) it establishes expectations for typical cognitive behavior, (b) it provides a point of reference against which the client's developmental data may be compared, and (c) it provides support and direction for programming expectations for individual clients.

Humanistic/Experiential Orientation to Learning

Psychologist Abraham Maslow was considered to be the father of humanistic psychology. He believed that experience is the primary phenomena in human learning (Patterson, 1973). Maslow believed that the development of human potential, dignity, and worth are ultimate concerns, and he maintained that human motivation is based on a hierarchy of needs including—from lowest to highest order needs—physical, safety, love/belonging, esteem, knowledge/understanding, aesthetic, and self-actualization; Maslow believed that learning actually takes place at the level of self-actualization (Combs, 1982). When applied to schools, Maslow's Humanistic Theory of Learning relates to a wide spectrum of activities and rationales for school structure, operations, and instruction. For example, physiological needs are addressed by school lunch programs, attention to temperatures in the building, and regularly scheduled bathroom breaks; safety is addressed by use of sound discipline practices; love/belonging is addressed by teachers and administrators who are supportive and show appreciation for students; self-esteem is addressed by promoting self-control; knowledge/understanding is addressed by a curriculum that is intellectually challenging; aesthetic is addressed by maintaining clean, pleasant-smelling classrooms; and self-actualization is addressed by helping students connect learning to meaningful experiences in "real life" exercises. Maslow believed that learning (self-actualization) was more difficult if the lower order needs were not first met, at least to some degree. For example, Maslow believed that it is more difficult for a child to learn when he or she is hungry, that it is more difficult for a higher order need (self-actualization) to occur when a lower order need (physical) is unmet.

Carl Rogers, American psychologist, believed in experiential learning as well. His views on self-actualization (Rogers, 1951) impacted education in several ways. Rogers believed that (a) learning takes place when the topic is relevant to the interests of the student, (b) learning proceeds faster when the threat to self is low, and (c) self-initiated learning is the most lasting and pervasive (Rogers & Freiberg, 1993). Rogers' theory of learning emerged as an integral part of the humanistic education movement (Patterson, 1973). In fact, the concept of an emotionally "safe" learning environment was addressed by Jones, Jones, and Vermette (2013) who found that relationships between teachers and students were an essential part of "creating a highly effective community of learners" (p. 24).

The concepts promoted by Maslow (1954) and Rogers (1951) are helpful across several aspects of the SLP's efforts. Incorporating components of the humanistic/experiential orientation into intervention plans may help the SLP in (a) creating physical climates to meet clients' needs during intervention, (b) maintaining a supportive emotional climate for clients, and (c) developing challenging and meaningful activities for client progress throughout therapy.

The Social Orientation to Learning

Russian psychologist Lev Vygotsky was noted for the development of the social learning theory (Crawford, 1996; Hausfather, 1996). Vygotsky believed that social interactions, more than biological and cultural impacts, profoundly influence cognitive development. Vygotsky believed that development was dependent on lifelong social interactions and that social interactions are the foundation for cognitive development. "Vygotsky believed very strongly that language is a social and cultural phenomenon that is centrally involved in the development of thinking and that cognitive development is profoundly influenced by cultural and social environments" (Lefrançois, 1994, p. 76). Vygotsky (1962) further believed that individuals learn on two levels: (a) initially through social interactions with more competent persons, and (b) gradually developing more self-directed learning as a result of teacher or peer guidance.

Application of Vygotsky's theory within the classroom (Crawford, 1996) dictates that students are seated at tables or clustered desks for small group, peer instruction, and collaboration, with instruction designed to promote and encourage student interaction and collaboration. The application of the social orientation to learning in speech-language therapy generated techniques such as description, self-talk, parallel-talk, expansions, and extensions for early child intervention (Hegde, 2008). Further application of the social orientation for learning for the SLP equates to (a) structuring at least part of the client's therapy within small groups and (b) designing intervention to include peer interaction in the form of peer modeling and peer evaluation of responses. These concepts align well with cooperative learning (Johnson & Johnson, 1989, 1999), and with Backus and Beasley's (1951) suggestions to arrange speech-language therapy in conversational groups that create an emotional experience for clients (presented earlier in Chapter 1).

Conclusion Regarding Learning Theories for Speech-Language Pathology

Certainly, the brief overviews just discussed do not begin to detail the breadth of the learning theories highlighted; a lifetime of work is not easily encapsulated within the framework of a few brief statements. However, through consideration of the basic and primary concepts presented within the constructs of each theory, it is hoped that the SLP is able to implement an intervention program that adequately reflects the awareness of how traditional and emerging interventions may be impacted by one or more possible learning theories. It is believed that in so doing, the SLP comes to better understand rationales for teaching, establishes better parameters for outcome expectations, and assesses, more effectively, client behavior. Exercises 4–1 and 4–2 are designed to help the SLP professional more fully process the impact of learning theory on the therapeutic process.

Exercise 4–1.

Quiz: Match learning theory orientation and researchers to speech-language therapy practices.

> Read statements/questions 1–10, and select the letter(s) of the most appropriate theorist(s) from the Answer Pool; place the letter(s) in the space to the left of the statement/question.
>
> **Answer Pool: A.** Maslow **B.** Pavlov **C.** Piaget **D.** Rogers **E.** Skinner **F.** Vygotsky **G.** Watson
>
> *(Possible answers are on the last page of this chapter. Several answers may be correct based on rationales.)*
>
> 1. _____ Group therapy is valuable for communication learning.
>
> 2. _____ Great sound; you put your lips together exactly right! Two stickers for you.
>
> 3. _____ Jared, repeat that sound five times.
>
> 4. _____ Watch my lips as I say these words for you.
>
> 5. _____ Raise your hand when you hear the sound.
>
> 6. _____ Let's work on your 4-year-old sounds today.
>
> 7. _____ Jules, name three things that have wheels.
>
> 8. _____ Let's get you seated near the light and away from the air conditioning vent.
>
> 9. _____ Who likes the circus? Everyone? Wonderful, we'll start there.
>
> 10. _____ Kay, tell Anthony how these are different.

Exercise 4–2.

Quiz: Match name of learning theory to speech-language therapy practices.

Read statements/questions 1–10, and select the letter(s) of the most appropriate theory(ies) from the Answer Pool; place the letter(s) in the space to the left of the statement/question.

Answer Pool: A. Behavioral   **B.** Cognitive   **C.** Humanistic/Experiential   **D.** Social

(Possible answers are on the last page of this chapter. Several answers may apply, depending on rationales.)

1. _____ Wow! Joe, you got 97% correct production today. Here's a star for your therapy chart; only three more stars and you'll have enough for video check-out! Way to go!

2. _____ Syreeta, tell José how well he did with that sound.

3. _____ SLP: "Remember. What should you do when you see the green light?"
Client: "I should continue holding the /s/ for five seconds."

4. _____ Sakiko, tell Travis what you're working on in therapy.

5. _____ Lydia, repeat the /l/ sound five times; let Maggie see where your tongue is.

6. _____ You guys are almost 12 years old! That's great. Everyone is working on idioms today.

7. _____ Julius, let me hear the "motor boat" sound.

8. _____ Find three things that are the same.

9. _____ Everyone, get a good night's sleep, so you'll be ready to work hard in fluency camp tomorrow.

10. _____ Samuel, you're having a difficult time sitting quietly today; let me move you closer to me so that I can help you.

Learning Styles: Client and Clinician Applications

The information in the following sections is intended for both client and clinician consideration. Although SLPs take responsibility for addressing learning style possibilities of clients, SLPs are also encouraged to think of their own learning style in an effort to enhance awareness and increased probabilities of clinical effectiveness related to learning styles research.

Smith (1982) defined learning styles as the "the individual's characteristic ways of processing information, feeling, and behaving in learning situations" (p. 2). A *learning style* is the way in which an individual receives, processes, and internalizes new and challenging information (Dunn, 2000). The theory behind learning styles is that different individuals perceive and process information differently, based on inherited traits, family upbringing, and environmental exposures and demands. Learning styles are typically classified according to a number of parameters. However, two points of view have particular importance to the SLP: (a) *processing style* (global/synergetic or analytical) and (b) *preferred modality* (visual, auditory, or tactile/kinesthetic).

Global/Synergetic and Analytical Processing Styles

Dunn (2000) noted that individuals who are considered to be *global* or *synergetic learners* are people who prefer learning from a whole-part-whole format, seeing the whole unit first, then breaking the unit into parts as needed, then reconstructing back to the whole. Global or synergetic learners often prefer to work in an environment with soft lighting, and informal seating. Global learners often simply want to know the "bottom line," without regard for the processes of all the steps it takes to get there. People with a global processing style of learning tend to need breaks, snacks, mobility, and sound for best learning. Of course, the global learner has the ability to learn in environments with characteristics other than those just listed, but the *preferred* style is more closely aligned with those indicators.

Dunn (2000) described **analytical learners** as people who prefer to learn in a step-by-step fashion, sequentially. Analytical learners often prefer to work in an environment with bright light and formal seating. These learners prefer working in a quite environment, with little distraction, and little snacking. Analytical learners prefer step-by-step linear progressions that are easily catalogued into discrete units. For example, the analytical learner interested in learning a new dance typically asks a peer to demonstrate the dance by telling or showing what happens first, then second, then third, and so forth, wanting to understand the steps, one after the other, as individual units, whereas a global learner typically asks the peer to demonstrate the steps from beginning to end as a whole movement sequence. However, as with the global learner, analytical learners are capable of learning under other conditions, with the characteristics indicated above serving as the *preferred* learning parameters for the analytical learner. (See Textbox 4–1 for further illustration.)

Visual, Auditory, and Tactile/Kinesthetic Preferred Modalities

Each learner receives and processes information through several channels or learning modalities. Kolb (1983) indicated that learning styles are determined by the combinations of ways in which a person perceives and processes incoming information. The ways in which information may be received primarily involve the visual, auditory, and tactile/kinesthetic learning modalities (Dunn & Dunn, 1978), although an additional area of stimulation, vestibular stimulation, was discussed in relation to sensory integration and intervention with clients with sensory integration needs (Ayers, 1972). Nicholosi, Harryman, and Kresheck (2004) defined *modality* as any sensory avenue through which information may be received.

■ TEXTBOX 4–1.   Illustrations of global/synergetic learners.

Jacob's mother, Mrs. Richards, brought home a TV and DVD player for his 13th birthday. When she arrived home with the new units, Jacob's best friend, Harold, was at the Richards' home looking over old comic books with Jacob. Mrs. Richards asked the boys to go out to the garage, bring in Jacob's birthday present, and set up the units in Jacob's bedroom. The boys were delighted and saw it as a chance to do something fun together. Mrs. Richards began evening chores, leaving the boys to the task at hand.

About 25 minutes later, Mrs. Richards heard Harold saying to Jacob, "No, we have to read everything first." A few minutes later, she noticed that Jacob was going back and forth between the family room and his bedroom every few minutes. After another 10 minutes, Harold left the house without saying good-bye to Mrs. Richards. Jacob then came to his mother and told her that he was afraid his friendship with Harold was over. Mrs. Richards asked why Jacob thought that, and he recounted the following scenario.

> Jacob and Harold worked well together in taking the TV and the DVD player out of the packing boxes, but once that was done, they started to disagree on how to connect the units. Jacob reported that Harold wanted to read every single word on the instruction sheets for both the TV and the DVD player before beginning, and Jacob became frustrated with doing it that way. Jacob remembered that the Richards had another TV and DVD player exactly like the one they were trying to assemble, so he made a few trips to the family room, looked at how those units were hooked up, came back to the bedroom, and began the assembly based on the units in the family room. Harold was continuing to read the step-by-step instructions, protesting that Jacob should not do anything until he finished reading. Jacob ignored this advice and continued the assembly, checking the units in the family room to be sure he was doing it correctly, and before Harold finished the reading, the units were correctly assembled and operating properly. Harold became furious and stormed out of the house. "Harold was furious with me mom, and the worst part is that I don't even know what happened to upset him; I'm really afraid I've lost my friend," Jacob lamented.

Mrs. Richards, an educator, comforted her son by encouraging him to give Harold a little time to calm down. "You haven't lost your friend," she explained. "What happened is that the two of you simply disagreed on how to assemble the TV and DVD player because you have different learning styles. Harold is an analytical learner; it's important for him to read everything, and precede sequentially, one step at a time, to arrive at the finished product. Whereas you are a global/synergetic learner; you like getting to the bottom line and having an idea of where you are going as quickly as possible. One way is not necessarily better than the other; they're just different. You haven't lost a friend; you simply discovered that the two of you approach things differently, that's all. Harold will be back," Mrs. Richards noted. Within the next several days, Harold was again visiting. That was 20 years ago. Jacob and Harold are still friends, and occasionally they still work on projects together, each in his own way.

Research in the area of learning styles began as early as the 1970s (Atkinson, 1989; Dunn, 1981; Dunn & Dunn, 1978; Keefe, 1979; Knowles, 1978; Mickler & Zippert, 1987). Since inception, educators began incorporating concepts related to how differences in learning modalities impact the ways the learner takes in and processes information. Following is a brief description of the primary learning modalities and an example of learners preferring each particular channel.

Auditory Modality: The auditory modality relates to the hearing channel for receiving information. The auditory learner prefers hearing verbal directions, enjoys group discussion, rarely takes notes in class, and often studies with instrumental music in the background. (See Figure 4–1 for additional information for working with the auditory modality.)

Visual Modality: The visual modality relates to the visual channel for receiving information. The visual learner prefers written information such as handouts; visual representations of concepts such as graphics, mind-mapping, or other schematic representations; takes copious notes to review and study; and uses color as a learning aid. (See Figure 4–2 for additional information for working with the visual modality.)

1. Auditory learners in the classroom pose a challenge to teachers because often these learners appear to be uninterested in the lesson: they take sparse notes, if any at all, and they often look away when the teacher is talking, especially if the teacher also is looking at the auditory learner. Clients with preferred auditory modality often find visual presentations distracting; when presenting information to this client, be sure that competition from visual information, even your facial features, are not distracting. For example, in teaching and describing phases of therapy, the auditory client may be more comfortable looking away rather than at the source of the auditory stimulus.

2. Auditory learners enjoy working with audio-recorded stimuli.

3. Auditory learners often repeat what was said to them for clarity and processing.

4. Auditory learners often enjoy soft instrumental music playing in the background when extended time-on-tasks or extended concentration are required.

Figure 4–1. Tips for working with clients using the auditory modality.

1. Visual learners usually watch intently what the teacher does.

2. Visual learners learn well from demonstration, modeling, and imitation methods of instruction.

3. When working with a visual learner, be sure to demonstrate accurately and completely the skills you want learned; any portions demonstrated poorly or incompletely will be imitated by the visual learner in the manner presented.

4. Visual learners enjoy the use of colors and high stimulus items in teaching and learning.

Figure 4–2. Tips for working with clients using the visual modality.

Tactile/Kinesthetic Modality: The tactile/kinesthetic modalities actually address two modes of learning related to how the body processes information: **tactile**, relating to a sense of touch, and **kinesthetic**, relating to a sense of movement originating from sensory end organs in muscles, tendons, joints, and sometimes the ear canals (Nicolosi et al., 2004). The tactile/kinesthetic learner prefers hands-on manipulatives, the opportunity to get up and perform, walk, or in some way experience the application of a concept in motor ways. For example, if teaching colors, tactile/kinesthetic learners might enjoy working with large sheets of fabrics in different colors, waving the fabrics as they move about the room, talking about the experiences of how the sheets feel when waved, and so forth. (See Figure 4–3 for additional information for working with the tactile/kinesthetic modality.)

Percentages vary for the number of persons classified as preferring a specific learning modality. However, Dunn and Dunn (1978) were among the first researchers to report findings in this area. They found that approximately 30% of students are classified as audi-

---

1. Tactile/kinesthetic learners prefer handling materials related to the subject matter. For example, if introducing the concept of *fruit*, allow the client to hold and manipulate a piece of fruit (real or model) while the information is being presented.

2. Tactile/kinesthetic learners enjoy drawing, tracing, and assembling and constructing items/objects. Art activities work well for tactile/kinesthetic learners. However, the SLP should exert caution in this regard during therapy sessions because of the amount of time such activities detract from time-on-task for specified objectives of therapy. For example, cutting, coloring, and pasting activities take a lot of time to complete and should be used only when directly related to an objective addressing such activities.

3. Tactile/kinesthetic learners typically respond well to touch as cues and prompts in therapy. However, SLPs should limit touch for cues and prompts during therapy to acceptable zones for communicative touch for those clients who are not offended by touch; the face, chin, throat, shoulder, upper arm, and upper back are considered to be areas acceptable to touch for cueing and prompting during the therapeutic process. Occasionally, when **cluster seating** is used for young children (semicircle seating for groups in which the SLP's knees are close to the clients' knees, either sitting in chairs, or sitting on the floor without a table between clinician and clients), touching the child on the knee for cueing and prompting is considered to be acceptable therapeutic touch. Again, however, SLPs are encouraged to be observant of clients who, for whatever reasons, do not appear to prefer touch from the clinician during therapy and to find alternative ways of cueing and prompting the client, for example, calling the client's name or presenting a visual cue.

4. SLPs should constantly monitor clients, even those judged to be tactile/kinesthetic learners, for the possibility of "sensory overload," too much feedback to the tactile/kinesthetic system as a result of a therapeutic activity. For example, in prekindergarten and kindergarten classrooms, students are often encouraged to trace letters in sand, on sandpaper, or on other high sensory materials. This may not present a problem for many children, but for some, the feedback to the fingertips is too strong, and the child becomes overloaded with sensory input. The result of overstimulation of this type for a young child is often nausea, and possibly even regurgitation.

Figure 4–3. Tips for working with clients using tactile/kinesthetic modalities.

tory modality learners, 40% as visual modality learners, and 30% as tactile/kinesthetic modality learners. Dunn and Dunn (1978) indicated that most students have a dominant preferred learning modality and a secondary learning modality as well. For example, a student may prefer a visual modality as the primary mode of receiving information and may prefer a tactile/kinesthetic modality as the secondary mode of receiving information. If students are unable to receive information through the preferred modality, information is lost, unless the secondary modality is able to compensate for the lack of stimulation of the primary modality. Regardless of the student's preferred learning modality, research indicates that students learn faster and easier when taught in their primary learning modality (Dunn & Dunn, 1978; McCarthy, 1987).

The greatest difficulty for ensuring that students are taught in their primary preferred modality for learning is the fact that teachers often teach in their own preferred learning modality without regard to student learning modality variability (Barbe & Milone, 1981). Wallace (1995) found that teachers in the Philippines most often taught in an auditory modality because the teachers themselves preferred the auditory modality, when, in fact, their students least preferred the auditory modality for learning. In a more recent study, Thompson, Orr, and Thompson (2002) reported that, most often, teachers teach according to the way they learn. Dunn and Dunn (1978) indicated that the modality most often neglected in the classrooms in general was the tactile/kinesthetic modality, particularly for older students, after third grade. Although there was no research to suggest the number of SLPs subscribing to a particular learning modality, research indicated that a large number of preservice teachers preferred the visual modality for learning new information (Sloan, Daane, & Giesen, 2004). Interestingly, according to Dunn (2000), learning style preferences often are developmental and may change over time, as the individual ages.

The adult learner often perceives that addressing information presented in one fashion or another makes the information easier to absorb and remember (Mickler & Zippert, 1987). The adult often seeks out learning opportunities that cater to preferred learning modalities and avoids learning situations that do not honor his or her preferred learning modality. However, children, especially young children, often fail to process that a particular learning modality is preferred, and even if they recognize a preferred style, children are often powerless to control how information is presented to them in the learning arena. Lemire (2001) indicated that learners appeared to be roughly balanced along the one-third lines of distinction for classification as one-third visual, one-third auditory, and one-third tactile/kinesthetic and suggested that teachers design instruction with this balance between modalities. For this reason, teachers are often introduced to strategies designed to help them structure lessons with elements of auditory presentation (verbal instructions, lectures), visual presentation (charts, graphs, handouts, use of color), and tactile/kinesthetic presentation (models, artistic or scientific creations) for each concept taught. For example, if the teacher is presenting a unit on the solar system, some of the information is verbally presented, some is visually presented, and some is addressed in tactile/kinesthetic formats. Similarly, SLPs are encouraged to consider auditory, visual, and tactile/kinesthetic aspects of information and stimulus presentation when working with clients in therapy.

Cultural Diversity and Learning Styles

The parameters related to learning styles addressed earlier in this chapter have implications for clients from varying cultural orientations and experiences in that these clients may view different aspects of learning styles differently. For example, Cheng (1991) reported that Asian parents hold different expectations for their children in the educational setting than American teachers might hold for Asian children. Cheng noted that teachers often expect children to participate in classroom activities and discussions, whereas Asian parents expect their children to be quiet and obedient. Brice (2002) reported differences in learning styles as well for Hispanic children. Brice indicated that time is viewed differently by the Hispanic family in that the family takes precedence over professional appointments. Brice added that appointments with SLPs and teachers need to be flexible in that regard. Delpit (1995) similarly reported differences in African-American children across several areas for perceptions and preferences related to learning styles. Delpit noted, for example, that large numbers of African-American children prefer a global or synergetic learning style and that these children value learning in groups. Pewewardy (2008) noted that Native American children often are taught humility and harmony at home and tend to operate as field-dependent, whereby they may look to the teacher or authority figure for guidance rather than taking an independent lead in learning. This information suggests that Native American children may tend to prefer group participation more so than individual competition as a function of remaining consistent with their cultural views.

Hegde (2008), drawing from the work of several professionals (Kayser, 1995; Payne, 1997; Peña-Brooks & Hegde, 2000; Roseberry-McKibbin, 1995), offered valuable suggestions for the SLP professional working with clients from cultures other than his or her own. SLPs are encouraged to become familiar with Hegde's (2008) suggestions as well as the work of others addressing differences in learning styles for culturally diverse populations and to make appropriate adaptations in the therapeutic process to accommodate the varying needs of clients from diverse cultural backgrounds and cultural orientations.

Basic Concepts from Learning Theory Applied to Speech-Language Pathology

As SLPs prepare to work with clients in various areas of therapy, it is important for the clinician to keep in mind the basic concepts related to learning theory that impact the client's abilities to achieve his or her therapeutic successes. SLPs are encouraged to help build client successes by properly constructing the therapeutic learning event. Client successes for achieving goals in therapy are significantly decreased if the SLP inappropriately constructs the progressions, expectations, or other important parameters of the therapeutic session. For example, clients will find it difficult to maintain satisfactory progress in the later stages of therapy if the proper foundations for sustained progress are neglected in the early stages of therapy.

The SLP should become comfortable with constructing therapy sessions that appropriately address several basic concepts related to *attention and focus, connections to prior learning, relevance, stages of acquisition of the skill, proficiency, maintenance,* and *generalizations of skills* (Siegler, 1991). The following brief guidelines are designed to help the SLP properly address client needs for orderly and sensible learning.

1. *Learning proceeds from the concrete to the abstract* (Siegler, 1991). Actual objects (books, cars, shoes) are more concrete than photographs; photographs are more concrete than line drawings; line drawings are more concrete than words; and words are the least concrete, the most abstract of all. When we are trying to teach the word *book*, or the concept of a book, it is easier for the client to learn "book" if we actually show the client a book as we teach the concept. In time, of course, the client will be expected to understand and use the word *book* in its abstract verbal expressive form.

2. *Learning proceeds from the general to the specific* (Siegler, 1991). For example, the developing child will learn the concept of "dog" as an animal characterized by four legs and a furry coat. Once learned, any animal with four legs and a furry coat becomes "dog" (generalized) until words for specific animals such as horse, cow, and lion are learned.

3. *Learning proceeds from simple to complex* (Siegler, 1991). For example, the developing child will learn simple singleton consonants before consonant blends. Within the concept of transportation, the child will likely learn *car* before *helium balloon* unless an experiential base powerfully impacts learning, such as the child accompanying a parent daily as mother or father works with helium balloons. In this case, the child may well learn *helium balloon* before he or she learns *car.*

4. *Attention and focus are necessary for learning to take place* (Perry, 2002). New signals are necessary to stimulate the client's attention; focus is stimulated by sustained interest in persons, objects, words, events, and so forth.

5. *The duration of attention, in minutes, is expected for the developing child roughly equivalent to the child's age in years.* For example, a 3-year-old child's attention span is expected to equal approximately 3 minutes; a 4-year-old child's attention span is expected to equal approximately 4 minutes, and so forth. SLPs should plan therapy sessions based on the client's probable attention span. For the older adolescent and adult, the attention expectation occurs in "curves or waves" of high attention and engagement for the first few minutes of presentation, with declining engagement, attention, and focus thereafter, significantly over the next few minutes. However, the cycle, or wave, repeats itself, with refocusing, but the initial peak for learning does not reach as high as it was at the beginning of the learning activity. Because of the nature of attending and focus over time, *SLPs are encouraged to plan several activities designed to accomplish the same objective for use within any given therapy session.*

6. *Processing and remembering new information occurs best when the information is personalized, organized, and developed around prior knowledge* (Mann & Sabatino, 1985). "These are *your* cards for today; let's see how many of *your* words we can say correctly." Expressions such as these help the client personalize the therapy experiences. ***Cognitive*** or ***graphic organizers***, pictorial, or physical presentations of a concept designed to give the learner a visual organizer of information to be addressed are effective ways to organize information (Sloan, Daane, & Giesen, 2004). A classic graphic organizer familiar to adults is the United States Department of Agriculture's Food Pyramid. A typical graphic or cognitive organizer for young children needing to remember three parts of any new learning task is a train: (1) the engine, (2) the middle car, and (3) the caboose.

7. *Most educators and researchers rely on repetitions for learning. Although there is no clear indication of how many repetitions are required for new speech and language learning, SLPs are encouraged to offer clients opportunities for as many repetitions as possible during elicitations in the session.*

8. *Rapport is an important part of learning and is an essential element for effective teaching.* Showing genuine concern, positive caring, and interest in the client helps establish rapport with the client. Several researchers indicated that rapport impacts learning (Marzano, 1992). SLPs are encouraged to practice rapport-building as the initial segment of all therapy sessions.

These items are not exhaustive of the concepts from learning theory that impact speech-language therapy. It is safe to say that dozens of other ideals associated with learning theory have direct application to the client's progress in therapy. SLPs are encouraged to seek greater understanding of how clients learn and to incorporate that information into therapy designed individually for clients in order to positively impact progress in therapy.

Summary

The impact of learning theories is present throughout the therapeutic process. Regardless of whether the clinician is stimulating for therapy through use of models, prompts, or cues, or whether the client is working to understand how much pressure must be exerted to change pitch to a more acceptable range, learning theory impacts speech-language therapy in profound ways. SLPs are encouraged to study several learning theories for their value in helping increase client progress. Similarly, an understanding of how clients are impacted in therapy by individual differences relates to both learning modality preferences and cultural communication-related preferences. Finally, SLPs are encouraged to become familiar with basic concepts from learning as they apply to therapeutic progress.

Learning Tool

1. Partner with a peer to develop a brief speech or language activity based on one of the four learning theories presented in this chapter. Write the name of the theory, and your idea for exemplifying it in the space below.

   _____

   _____

   _____

   _____

2. Develop an activity to address each of the major learning modalities (auditory, visual, and tactile/kinesthetic) for teaching the concept *ball*. Write your ideas here.

   _____

   _____

   _____

   _____

3. List considerations that need to be made to address at least five culturally diverse populations: the four groups mentioned in the discussion, plus an additional culturally diverse group of your choice.

   _____

   _____

   _____

   _____

References

Atkinson, G. (1989). Kolb's learning style inventory—1985: Test-retest deju vu. *Psychological Reports, 3*(64), 991–995.

Ayers, J. (1972). *Sensory integration and learning disorders.* Los Angeles, CA: Western Psychological Services.

Backus, O., & Beasley, J. (1951). *Speech therapy with children.* Cambridge, MA: Riverside Press.

Barbe, W. B., & Milone, M. N. (1981). What we know about modality strengths. *Educational Leadership, 38*, 378–380.

Brice, A. E. (2002). *The Hispanic child: Speech, language, culture and education.* Boston, MA: Allyn & Bacon.

Bruner, J. (1960). *The process of education.* Cambridge, MA: Harvard University Press.

Cheng, L. L. (1991). *Assessing Asian language performance: Guidelines for evaluating limited English-proficient students.* Oceanside, CA: Academic Communication Associates.

Combs, A. W. (1982). Affective education or none at all. *Educational Leadership, 39*(7), 494–497.

Crawford, K. (1996). Vygotskian approaches to human development in the information era. *Educational Studies in Mathematics, 31,* 43–62.

Delpit, L. (1995). *Other people's children: Cultural conflict in the classroom.* New York, NY: The New Press.

Dewey, J. (1910). *How we think.* Boston, MA: D. C. Heath.

Dunn, R. (1981). A learning styles primer. *Principal, 60*(5), 31–34.

Dunn, R. (2000). Learning styles: Theory, research, and practice. *National Forum of Applied Educational Research, 13*(1), 3–22.

Dunn, R., & Dunn, K. (1978). *Teaching students through their individual learning styles: A practical approach.* Reston, VA: Reston.

Good, T. L., & Brophy, J. E. (1990). *Educational psychology: A realistic approach* (4th ed.). White Plains, NY: Longman.

Hausfather, S. J. (1996). Vygotsky and schooling: Creating a social contest for learning. *Action in Teacher Education, 18,* 1–10.

Hegde, M. N. (2008). *Hegde's pockeguide to treatment in speech-language pathology* (3rd ed.). Clifton Park, NY: Delmar.

Johnson, D. W., & Johnson, R. T. (1989). *Cooperation and competition: Theory and research.* Edina, MN: Interaction Book.

Johnson, D. W., & Johnson, R. T. (1999). Making cooperative learning work. *Theory into Practice, 38*(2), 67–73.

Johnson, J. A., Musial, D., Hall, G. E., Gollnick, D. M., & Dupuis, V. L. (2005). *Introduction to the foundations of American education* (13th ed.). Boston, MA: Allyn & Bacon.

Jones, K. A., Jones, J. L., & Vermette, P. J. (2013). Exploring the complexity of classroom management: 8 components of managing a highly productive, safe, and respectful urban environment. *American Secondary Education, 41*(3), 21–33.

Kayser, H. (1995). *Bilingual speech-language pathology: An Hispanic focus.* San Diego, CA: Singular.

Keefe, J. W. (1979). *Student learning styles.* Reston, VA: National Association of Secondary School Principals.

Knowles, M. S. (1978). *The adult learner: A neglected species* (2nd ed.). Houston, TX: Gulf Publishing.

Kolb, D. (1983). *Experiential learning: Experiences as the source of learning and development.* Englewood Cliffs, NJ: Prentice Hall.

Lefrançois, G. R. (1994). *Psychology for teaching* (8th ed.). Belmont, CA: Wadsworth.

Low, H. M., & Lee, L. W. (2011). Teaching of speech, language and communication skills for young children with severe autism spectrum disorders: What do educators need to know? *New Horizons in Education, 59*(3), 16–27.

Lemire, D. (2001). Brief report: An introduction to learning styles for college teachers. *Journal of College Reading and Learning, 32,* 86–92.

Mann, L., & Sabatino, D. A. (1985). *Foundations of cognitive process in remedial and special education.* Rockville, MD: Aspen Systems.

Marzano, R. (1992). *A different kind of classroom.* Alexandria, VA: ASCD.

Maslow, A. H. (1954). *Motivation and personality* (2nd ed.). New York, NY: Harper & Row.

McCarthy, B. (1987). *The 4MAT system: Teaching to learning styles with right/left mode techniques.* Barrington, IL: EXCEL.

Merriam, S. B., & Caffarella, R. S. (1991). *Learning in adulthood: A comprehensive guide.* San Francisco, CA: Jossey-Bass.

Mickler, M. L., & Zippert, C. P. (1987). Teaching strategies based on learning styles of adult students. *Community and Junior College Quarterly of Research and Practice, 1*(11), 33–37.

Nicolosi, L., Harryman, E., & Kresheck, J. (2004). *Terminology of communication disorders: Speech-language-hearing* (5th ed.). Baltimore, MD: Lippincott Williams & Wilkins.

Oakes, J., & Lipton, M. (2003). *Teaching to change the world* (2nd ed.). Boston, MA: McGraw-Hill.

Patterson, C. H. (1973). *Humanistic education.* Englewood Cliffs, NJ: Prentice Hall.

Pavlov, I. (1926). *Conditioned reflexes: An investigation of the physiological activity of the cerebral cortex.* Oxford, UK: Oxford University Press.

Payne, J. C. (1997). *Adult neurogenic language disorders: Assessment and treatment.* San Diego, CA: Singular.

Pewewardy, C. (2008). Learning styles of American Indian/Alaska Native students. In J. Noel (Ed.), *Classic edition sources: Multicultural education* (pp. 116–121). New York, NY: McGraw-Hill.

Peña-Brooks, A., & Hegde, M. N. (2000). *Assessment and treatment of articulation and phonological disorders in children.* Austin, TX: Pro-Ed.

Perry, B. D. (2002). Starting school: Why it can be overwhelming. *Scholastic Early Childhood Today, 17*(1), 30–32.

Piaget, J. (1954). *Construction of reality in the child.* New York, NY: Basic Books.

Rogers, C. (1951). *Client-centered therapy.* Boston, MA: Houghton Mifflin.

Rogers, C., & Freiberg, H. J. (1993). *Freedom to learn* (3rd ed.). New York, NY: Merrill.

Roseberry-McKibbin, C. (1995). *Multicultural students with special needs.* Oceanside, CA: Academic Communication Associates.

Siegler, R. S. (1991). *Children's thinking* (2nd ed.). Englewood Cliffs, NJ: Prentice Hall.

Skinner, B. F. (1953). *Science and human behavior.* New York, NY: Macmillan.

Sloan, T., Daane, C. J., & Giesen, J. (2004). Learning styles of elementary pre-service teachers. *College Student Journal, 3*(38), 494–501.

Smith, R. M. (1982). *Learning how to learn: Applied theory for adults.* Chicago, IL: Follett.

Thompson, D. E., Orr, B., & Thompson, C. (2002). Preferred learning styles of postsecondary technical institute instructors. *Journal of Industrial Teacher Education, 39*(4), 1–13. Retrieved from http://scholar.lib.vt.edu/ejournals/JITEv39n4/thompson.html

Vygotsky, L. (1962). *Thought and language* (E. Hamsman & G. Vankan, Eds. & Trans.). Cambridge, MA: MIT Press.

Vygotsky, L. (1978). *Mind in society.* Cambridge, MA: Harvard University Press.

Wallace, J. (1995). When teachers' learning styles differ from those of their students. *Journal of Instructional Psychology, 22,* 99.

Watson, J. (1913). Psychology as the behaviorist views it. *Psychological Review, 20,* 158–177.

Exercise 4–1.

Answers.

Answer Pool: A. Maslow B. Pavlov C. Piaget D. Rogers E. Skinner F. Vygotsky G. Watson

(Several answers per question may be correct based on rationales. Be sure you are clear about the rationales that you offer if your answers are different from those given.)

1.	F	6.	C
2.	E	7.	C
3.	G	8.	A
4.	E	9.	D
5.	B	10.	F

Exercise 4–2.

Answers.

Answer Pool: A. Behavioral B. Cognitive C. Humanistic/Experiential D. Social

(Several answers per question may be correct based on rationales. Be sure you are clear about the rationales that you offer if your answers are different from those given.)

1.	A	6.	B
2.	D	7.	C
3.	A	8.	B
4.	D	9.	C
5.	A/D	10.	C

5

Developmental Domains and Special Classifications Related to the Therapeutic Process: An Overview

Introduction

Speech-language pathologists (SLPs) are nationally certified, autonomous professionals (ASHA, 2001). However, autonomy does not mean that SLPs work in a vacuum separate from other professions. In fact, it is believed that because of the autonomous nature of the speech-language pathology profession, greater care must be taken to ensure that SLPs remain cognizant of and closely aligned with both the practices of the speech-language pathology profession, and also the practices of other professions as we work to serve clients with communication disorders. This chapter is devoted to helping the speech-language pathology professional focus on developmental expectations and special classifications of clients who may present with other difficulties along with existing communication disorders.

Clients seen for speech-language therapy may present in one of two broad categories or profiles for patient management: (a) speech-only, or (b) speech as secondary to another disability, or difficulty. Speech-only clients generally have of a diagnosis in one or more areas of communication or swallowing disorders *with no other difficulties* identified or suspected. In these situations, the SLP is typically the case manager of record, with the requirements of client or patient management seen as more routine for the SLP in terms of patient profiles and areas of patient need. However, clients categorized as speech disordered secondary to another disability typically present with issues that may compound speech services, sometimes in every aspect of services across evaluation, diagnosis, treatment, and necessary follow-ups. The purpose of this chapter is to offer rudimentary information that may help increase awareness of the varying needs that clients have when presenting with suspected or diagnosed difficulties in other areas of functioning—in addition to communication disorders. Concepts related to broad-based typical development, recognized disability categories, and their impacts on speech-language therapy are addressed in this chapter.

Typical Developmental Expectations (Overview)

Development is the process of natural progression from a previous, lower stage of functioning to a more complex or adult-like stage (Nicolosi, Harryman, & Kresheck, 2004). The SLP should be aware of several areas of developmental expectations that may have an impact on expected speech-language progress in therapy. For example, motor difficulty throughout the body might also impact articulation due to difficulty with executing the exact fine motor movements of the tongue, lips, and palate in a coordinated fashion to correctly produce phonemes. Similarly, a client with reduced cognitive functioning may also experience difficulty grasping and retaining various concepts related to semantics, syntax, morphology, phonology, and pragmatics skills. For these reasons, information across five *developmental domains* (Gerken, Eliason, & Arthur, 1994; Newborg, Stock, Wnek, Guidubaldi, & Svinicki, 1988; Perry, 2001) is judged to be important in relation to impacts on speech-language therapy for the developing child, with most domains also having an impact for adult functioning as well. These domains include the *communication, cognitive, motor, self-help/adaptive,* and *social-emotional* domains.

It is believed that clients benefit when the SLP has a working knowledge of developmental expectations across various areas of functioning. However, rather than suggesting that the SLP learns every aspect of various areas of development, it is recommended that the SLP becomes familiar with *developmental milestones* associated with various developmental domains. **Developmental milestones** are those "markers" or skills that serve to indicate the client's functioning level compared to age expected levels across various areas of functioning. Developmental milestones are typical for motor, communication, adaptive/self-help, social-emotional, and cognitive skills. For example, if a client is expected to babble by age 6 months, but instead begins babbling at 2 months, the SLP has a "marker," a skill (babbling) that can be viewed in relation to its expected age of development to determine that the child in this scenario is performing the babbling skill 4 months earlier than expected; this scenario is an example of a child with skills *above age-level expectation* in this area of functioning. Above age-level expectation means that the child reached the developmental milestone sooner, or *before expected*, suggesting that the child is *above* average functioning in this area.

In another example, if a client is expected to sit independently by age 6 months and reaches age 12 months before sitting independently, the SLP has a marker, a skill (sitting) that can be viewed in relation to its expected age of development to arrive at the conclusion that the child in this scenario is performing the sitting skill 6 months later than expected; the child, in this case, is performing *below age-level expectation* in this area of functioning. Below age-level expectation means that the child reached the developmental milestone later, or *after expected*, suggesting that the child is *below* average functioning in this area. It is important to note that precocious skills in one area, for example, the child's early babbling in the previous scenario, do not necessarily indicate advanced skills in other areas of functioning. Similarly, skills below age-level expectation in one area of functioning for a client do not necessarily indicate that other skills are also below age-level expectations. For example, the child who sits later than expected may develop speech-language skills at age-appropriate times.

The SLP is the professional responsible for assessment and diagnosis of speech-language skills; therefore, inherent expertise in the communication developmental milestones is expected. However, SLPs are *not* expected to serve as an expert in other developmental domains (cognitive, motor, self-help/adaptive, and social-emotional). In fact, SLPs may need to consider making appropriate referrals for clients to be seen by professionals outside of speech-language pathology when client skills appear to be below age-level expectations in areas other than speech-language; referrals also may need to be made for clients who appear gifted (or significantly above age-level expectations) in various domains.

Interestingly, often case history forms tap into a young child's developmental milestones by asking parents to recall ages at which their child sat, crawled, walked, spoke first word, and so forth—all as a function of gathering information related to developmental milestones—markers for helping to determine whether the child exhibited expected developmental skills at age-expected times. Even though expertise in all developmental areas is not expected, in efforts to increase effectiveness in providing speech-language services to clients, SLPs are encouraged to obtain general knowledge regarding expected functioning for cognitive, motor, self-help/adaptive, and social-emotional skills, in addition to established expertise in speech-language expectations. Each of these five developmental domains (*communication, cognitive, motor, self-help/adaptive*, and *social-emotional*) is discussed briefly in the following sections.

Communication Domain

The following overview on the communication domain is likely to be redundant because of information obtained in various courses in communication disorders, particularly language and articulation/phonological acquisition courses. However, to facilitate ease in comparisons of client behaviors across all developmental areas discussed in this chapter, the communication domain overview is presented along with the four other developmental domains.

Receptive Language

Receptive language is defined as the spoken or visual (signed or written) words one understands (Nicolosi et al., 2004). Language reception involves competence for the user's underlying knowledge of the systems of rules that dictate language (Anderson & Shames, 2010). The primary learning modalities for language reception—visual, auditory, and tactile/kinesthetic—are intact and available for use by the infant immediately following birth (Brazelton, Scholl, & Robey, 1966). In fact, these authors indicated that the infant's abilities for fixation and pursuit (visual tracking) of a visual stimulus signifies intact functioning of the central nervous system, the sensory reception and motor expressive system needed for speech. Infants begin at birth absorbing information from the environment that is used for receptive communication, and they continue this development, ideally, throughout adulthood. Through use of receptive communication skills, the child develops understanding for ideas, thoughts, concepts, grammar, meanings of sounds, and appropriate uses of language in context (Bloom & Lahey, 1978).

Expressive Language

Expressive language is the use of conventional symbols (words, signs, etc.) to communicate one's ideas, thoughts, or intentions toward others (Nicolosi et al., 2004). Spoken words are, perhaps, the most convenient way to engage in expressive communication, but of course, signs, symbols, and printed words qualify as expressive communication as well. Speech is often referred to as an expressive motor act of communication (Nicolosi et al., 2004). Even though we typically use more spoken, or *verbal*, communication than signed or written, the infant and young child actually engage in *nonverbal* expressions through crying, laughter, pointing, and audible vocal behaviors (squeals, grunts, etc.) long before first words are spoken. Once expressive speech begins, however, nonverbal communication minimizes as the primary mode of communication, but, nonetheless, remains an important part of overall expressive communicative effectiveness. Ages at which the child coos and gurgles, babbles, reduplicates, shows intent to communicate, says first words, uses jargon, uses joint attending, and uses two-word utterances are a few examples of early speech and language developmental milestones. SLPs are encouraged to revisit speech-language milestones often in relation to the other four developmental domains: *cognitive, motor, self-help/adaptive,* and *social-emotional.*

Cognitive Domain

Cognitive skills address abilities in broad areas of perception, memory, imagination, conceptualization, and reasoning (Nicolosi et al., 2004). Although there are numerous contemporary researchers in the area of cognitive development, Jean Piaget remains one of the names best recognized for investigations into the cognitive area of learning (Siegler, 1991). Piaget's cognitive orientation theory was presented in Chapter 4, with detailed indicators of the *Sensorimotor Period* (birth–2 years), *Preoperational Period* (2–7 years), *Concrete*

Operations Period (7–12 years), and *Formal Operations Period* (12 years and beyond). Cognitive development is important to a number of parameters affecting the SLP's intervention program, including appropriateness of goals, stimulus presentation, materials selection, and much more. SLPs are encouraged to increase awareness of clients' skills in all aspects of development, particularly in areas of cognitive skills. Ages at which the child visually tracks, attends, focuses, exhibits object permanence, and exhibits cause–effect behavior are a few examples of the early cognitive developmental milestones.

Motor Domain

Motor skills are typically addressed across two broad functioning areas: *gross motor* and *fine motor* skills.

Gross Motor Skills

Gross motor skills are the large muscles and torso skills associated with kicking, rolling, sitting, crawling, standing, walking, running, climbing, throwing, and so forth. In fact, ages at which children are able to perform these skills serve as indicators of the child's gross motor developmental milestones. The muscle systems involved in gross motor skills are in the arms, legs, and torso and are generally responsible for large muscle control, body coordination, and locomotion (Newborg et al., 1988). The muscles associated with gross motor skills do not necessarily develop at the same rate, so often when describing clients' gross motor skills, it is important to distinguish whether the gross motor skills under discussion relate to the upper body, lower body, right or left sides of the body, and so forth, with the lateral difficulties holding particular interest for SLPs working with clients who have had strokes or are diagnosed with other medically or neurologically based difficulties. For example, clients with right-side motor difficulties often present with insult to the left side of the brain, possibly within the major speech, language, or hearing centers of the brain (Chapey, 2001; Davis, 2000).

Fine Motor Skills

Fine motor skills are the smaller muscle skills of the body and often impact hands, fingers, feet, and toes. Grasping, releasing, hand manipulations, and writing all qualify as fine motor skills. Because of the discrete movements of small muscles required for **articulation**, a series of overlapping ballistic movements, articulation is often likened to a fine motor skill in that very small and specific muscle movements are required to produce phonemes (Bauman-Wangler, 2012). In fact, Bernthal, Bankson, and Flipsen, (2009) noted that "speech requires rapid changes in the activation of about 100 muscles" (p. 9).

An awareness of developmental milestones and consideration for the client's motor functioning is important for SLPs during the therapeutic process. For example, in more severe articulation cases, such as a client with dysarthria of speech, the client's progress in speech therapy is often linked to his or her overall motor status.

Self-Help/Adaptive Domain

Self-help/adaptive skills are skills that demonstrate effectiveness in personal independence, social responsibilities, and environmental demands (Grossman, 1983). Specifically, self-help/adaptive skills relate to the client's abilities in dressing, feeding, toileting, negotiating safety, interacting appropriately within various settings, negotiating leisure, and other self-initiated tasks. Self-help/adaptive skills usually do not appear in the child's functioning until later due to the nature of the skills, themselves. For example, a 14-month-old child would not be expected to have full functioning in safety, dressing, or toileting skills at that age. However, there are some self-help/adaptive skills that may have earlier developmental expectations and increased significance for the SLP. For example, observing the client's appropriateness of interactions with others for possible connections to pragmatic language disorders is valuable when considering self-help/adaptive skills for the client. Although not all self-help/adaptive skills directly impact the client's performances in speech-language therapy, SLPs should note feeding skills for impacts on swallowing or possible oral defensiveness (difficulty accepting different textures, tastes, or temperatures in the mouth). Mouth breathing or other oral habits that might negatively impact progress in therapy should also be noted. For example, mouth breathing may suggest difficulties with adenoids or difficulty with other physical structures in ways that may negatively impact resonance or articulation skills related to muscle tone for the jaw and lips. Additionally, SLPs should note the presence of drooling during intervention in efforts to determine whether the client might require referral to medical or other professions. SLPs should note toileting skills for client comfort during therapy. Finally, attending and focus skills are sometimes viewed as being part of self-help/adaptive (as well as cognitive) skills and are important to SLPs for impacts associated with general learning during therapy.

Social-Emotional Domain

Social-emotional skills address the client's levels of maturation for expressions of affect (feelings), control of emotions, basic self-concept, and social roles (Grossman, 1983). SLPs typically note these areas of functioning, but, as expected, rarely take the lead in addressing these skills. However, difficulty in any of the social-emotional areas, if manifested during speech-language therapy, might negatively impact client progress in therapy. Appropriate referrals, in efforts to obtain additional insight for client management during speech-language therapy, are suggested. Additionally, SLPs are encouraged to practice effective behavioral management techniques during speech-language therapy sessions to help manage possible negative behaviors that impact effectiveness of speech-language intervention.

Conclusion Regarding Developmental Domains

SLPs who possess a good working knowledge of developmental domains and their implications for client functioning add significantly to the repertoire of clinical abilities for both assessment and intervention. SLPs are, therefore, encouraged to develop a grasp of the client's overall development in relation to speech and language developmental expectations. Nicolosi et al. (2004) presented *Developmental Sequences of Language, Developmental Sequences of Motor Skills, Developmental Sequences of Social Skills,* and *Normal Development of Feeding* in several appendixes of their text on terminology for communication disorders. Additionally, Bauman and Fishman (1991) published an inventory of child language and development that was viewed as helpful to professionals interested in increasing knowledge of developmental milestones across several areas of childhood development. Shipley and McAfee (2005) included developmental information across speech-language and motor skills as well. Finally, Gard, Gillman, and Gorman (1993) produced a speech and language development chart that includes a segment on developmental expectations for play in the young child. These publications serve as examples of the type of resources SLPs may find valuable in the search for information to increase knowledge and skills in developmental expectations for clients as applied to intervention successes in speech-language therapy.

Disability Categories and Their Impact on Speech-Language Therapy Progress

An overview of federal laws impacting speech-language pathology services was presented in Chapter 3 as support for helping clients develop trust in the therapeutic process. The intent in that chapter was to give SLPs information that might be shared with clients in times when client trust needed to be built on legal foundations. As concepts regarding disability categories are addressed in this current chapter, federal law will be revisited; however, this discussion is for purposes of helping the SLP increase understanding of the students served in speech-language therapy services under special education law.

Students may be eligible for special education and related services under 13 different disability categories under federal law, most recently, Individuals with Disabilities Education Act (IDEA) 2004. Based on various federal laws, and appropriate amendments to them (see Chapter 3), children from birth to 21 years may be served under categorical services. Additionally, noncategorical services are also available for children from birth to 9 years at the state's discretion. The disability categories under which most children will be served by the SLP in schools, or school-related settings, follow:

- Autism
- Deaf-blind
- Deafness
- Emotional Disturbance
- Hearing Impairment
- Mental Retardation
- Multiple Disabilities

- Orthopedic Impairment
- Other Health Impaired
- Specific Learning Disability
- Speech or Language Impairment
- Traumatic Brain Injury
- Visual Impairment including Blindness

Each of the above special education categories are discussed briefly across three dimensions: (1) definitions, (2) characteristics, and (3) implications for speech-language therapy. All definitions for these categories of special education were taken from the federal law (PL 105-17), Individuals with Disabilities Education Act, 1997 Amendment, Part B (*Federal Register*, online source).

Note to the Reader: The following information is meant as a general point of information for SLPs providing services to clients with an official diagnosis of specific disabilities other than Speech Impaired. This information is subject to changes as a result of future reauthorizations of federal law pertaining to the provisions of services to children and adults with diagnoses of disabilities. The SLP professional is advised to remain abreast of reauthorizations that may change, in some way, the information presented herein.

Autism

Autism is a developmental disability significantly affecting verbal and nonverbal communication and social interaction, generally evident before age three years, which adversely affects a child's educational performance. (*Federal Register*, online source)

Characteristics associated with autism include difficulties across broad areas of functioning including social-emotional difficulties, difficulties with daily living skills, and communication difficulties: Note the following characteristics associated with autism.

Social-Emotional Difficulties Characteristic of Autism

- lack of appropriate eye contact, or strange social gazes
- quick mood swings: becomes out of control easily and often; inappropriate outbursts of laughter
- short, but often, intense attention span
- may cling to one person, but often prefers little or no physical touching
- resistant to change of routines

- guarded personal space, with lack of interest in others
- highly interested in inanimate objects
- engagement in repetitive activities and stereotyped movements
- resistance to environmental change or change in daily routines
- unusual responses to sensory experiences
- low or no concept of emotions

Difficulties with Daily Living Skills Characteristic of Autism

- self-stimulation activities including rocking, spinning/twirling in full circles, hand-flapping, finger manipulations in front of face, sucking finger, biting parts of the body, scratching and self-mutilating activities, humming, singing, closing eyes tightly
- poor sleep habits
- fixation with eating only certain foods
- sensory issues: either *seeking* or *rejecting* stimulation for auditory, visual, tactile, kinesthetic, or vestibular systems
- occasional savant (giftedness or precociousness) for limited skills or behaviors

Communication Difficulties Characteristic of Autism

- absence of speech
- telegraphic speech
- echolalia or mimicked speech
- preservative speech
- use of very few pronouns; "I" often absent
- poor pragmatics
- low expressive semantics and syntax

Implications for Speech-Language Therapy and Autism

Moyes (2002) indicated that autism spectrum disorders range from milder cases, often classified as Asperger's syndrome, to more severely involved cases. SLPs often work as part of a team to serve clients with autism, with speech-language services for the child with autism often provided as a related service under federal law guidelines. As such, the classroom teacher may serve as the primary case manager for the child's intervention program; however, in more and more situations, schools appear to be moving toward management structures that place children with autism in language classrooms managed by SLPs, and as a result, "speech-language pathologists are often among the first professionals to work with young children with autism" (Rollins, 1999, p. 1).

Heflin and Simpson (1998) discussed a number of options for working with children with autism, including programs specific to autism intervention. In addition to commanding the expected skills in speech-language therapy when working with the child with autism, SLPs are encouraged to investigate programs specific to autism intervention in conjunction with team decisions regarding most appropriate intervention for the child. Agreement and consistency among professionals regarding intervention strategies for working with the child with autism should be practiced by all persons involved in the intervention program.

Hegde (2008) offered several suggestions for intervention with the child with autism that appeared applicable regardless of the implementation of specific programs for autism. Among these intervention strategies were suggestions such as using concrete objects rather than pictures for stimulus objects, teaching eye contact as part of interaction, and teaching turn-taking skills. Of particular interest was the finding by Mundy, Sigman, and Kasari (1990) that development of joint attention (use of eye gaze or gestures by two people to share attention) preceded advances in expressive language development, suggesting that working on the child's skills in pointing, showing, and eye gaze for objects with another was valuable for the child with autism (Rollins, 1999). Low and Lee (2011) noted that, "in general, the teaching of speech, language and communication skills to children with ASD [Autism Spectrum Disorders] is based on the behaviorism perspective that teachers can shape the learning directions and behaviors of these children by manipulating the external stimuli to elicit the desired learning outcomes" (p. 20). Although the behavioral perspective has been shown to be a powerful format for working with children with autism, SLPs are encouraged to refer to a variety of resources for further suggestions when working with the child with autism. Finally, SLPs should be aware of counseling strategies (Shames, 2000) associated with parent and family needs when working with a child with autism.

Deaf-Blindness

Deaf-blindness refers to concomitant hearing and visual impairments, the combination of which causes such severe communication and other developmental and educational needs that they cannot be accommodated in special education programs solely for children with deafness or children with blindness. (*Federal Register*, online source)

Characteristics for deaf-blindness impact communication, education, and social and mobility difficulties. Following are the characteristics associated with deaf-blindness.

Communication Difficulties Characteristic of Deaf-Blindness

- need for alternative forms of communication including tactile/kinesthetic
- high degree of pragmatic difficulty
- most will maintain a slight degree of either auditory or visual channel learning, but communication must be directed appropriately to that channel

Educational Difficulties Characteristic of Deaf-Blindness

- cognitive skills are strong determiners for educational management
- cognitive skills vary from gifted to profound intellectual disability

Social and Mobility Difficulties Characteristic of Deaf-Blindness

- often unsure of surroundings, so mobility is limited
- orientation in space is often unclear
- occasional self-stimulation or self-mutilation to create sensory input

Implications for Speech-Language Therapy and Deaf-Blindness

Although federal laws regarding disability classifications maintain the term *deaf-blindness*, Marchant (1992) reported best practices in the field to be the terms *multiple sensory impairment* or *dual sensory impairment*. However, because the term deaf-blind is currently used for IDEA and work in schools, deaf-blind is used for this discussion.

The National Technical Assistance Consortium for Children and Young Adults Who Are Deaf-Blind (NTAC) estimated that, in 2004, more than 10,000 children (ages birth to 22 years) qualified as deaf-blind, or dual sensory impaired, in the United States. Because of the inability to see or hear, the young child who is deaf-blind lives in world limited to touch. Miles (2005) noted that "such children are effectively alone if no one is touching them" (p. 1). The SLP is likely not the professional primarily responsible for the education of the child who is deaf-blind. However, because the challenge of learning to communicate is among the greatest difficulties that children who are deaf-blind face, the SLP may be a member of the team helping to develop communication skills for the child. Fryauf-Bertschy, Kirk, and Weiss (1993) reported that children who are blind experience difficulty with taking the perspectives of others, and experience difficulty with referents, deictic terms (here/there), relative pronouns (me, you, I), and mobility concepts. Children who are deaf-blind experience these difficulties as well (Miles, 2005). SLPs working with children who are deaf-blind are encouraged to (a) consider the child's cognitive skills; (b) use a variety of prompts, cues, and reinforcement strategies in a systematic instructional pattern; and (c) include environmental orientation and mobility skills as part of instruction (Downing & Chen, 2003; Miles, 2005; Smith, Polloway, Patton, & Dowdy, 1998).

Deafness

Deafness is a hearing impairment that is so severe that the child is impaired in processing linguistic information through hearing, with or without amplification, which adversely affects a child's educational performance. (*Federal Register*, online source)

Characteristic of deafness is absence of enough measurable hearing (usually pure tone average of 66–90+ decibels, American National Standards Institute, without amplification) such that the primary sensory input for communication may be other than the auditory channel. Communication may be accomplished through the following modes:

- sign language (often American Sign Language, referred to as ASL or Ameslan)
- finger spelling
- speech reading
- total communication

Implications for Speech-Language Therapy and Deafness

Implications for SLPs working with children who are deaf are somewhat different than might be expected compared to other disability categories in that deafness is viewed as not a disorder, but as a biological and cultural characteristic by the Deaf culture (Paul & Quigley, 1990). SLPs must, therefore, work closely with educational professionals and family members to determine how to best offer services to the deaf. Tyler (1990) indicated that the most important attribute of the Deaf culture is its language, ASL. Although SLPs are generally exposed to sign language in training programs, SLPs do not generally acquire enough experience in academic manual communication coursework alone to become proficient with sign language for teaching purposes. Teachers of the hearing impaired or educators of the deaf (depending on specific state certification requirements) are usually the professionals assigned as classroom teachers for children who are deaf. However, SLPs are encouraged to provide services to children who are deaf in accordance with agreed upon goals and best practice standards for each child individually and always in conjunction with parent inputs. Raimondo (2010) reported that approximately 39% of children who are deaf were found to also have other issues that impacted education; these additional issues may also have impact for SLPs providing services to clients who are deaf. Finally, SLPs are encouraged to review *Guidelines of the American Speech-Language Hearing Association (ASHA) on Roles of Speech-Language Pathologists and Teachers of Children Who Are Deaf and Hard of Hearing in the Development of Communicative and Linguistic Competence* (ASHA, 2004) as an additional resource when working with children who are deaf.

Emotional Disturbance

Emotional disturbance is a condition exhibiting one or more of the following characteristics over a long period and to a marked degree that adversely affects a child's educational performance:

1. an inability to learn that cannot be explained by intellectual, sensory, or health factors
2. an inability to build or maintain satisfactory interpersonal relationships with peers and teachers

3. inappropriate types of behavior or feelings under normal circumstances

4. a general pervasive mood of unhappiness or depression

5. a tendency to develop physical symptoms or fears associated with personal or school problems

The term includes schizophrenia. The term does not apply to children who are socially maladjusted, unless it is determined that they have an emotional disturbance. (*Federal Register*, online source)

Characteristics of emotional disturbance should be evaluated across three broad parameters: *duration, frequency,* and *intensity* of occurrences of specific defining components of the disability.

Duration Issues Characteristic of Emotional Disturbance

• no established sustained time for the behavior

• professionals judge impact of time on the behavior in relation to circumstances that might be transitory, such as illness or death in the family

Frequency Issues Characteristic of Emotional Disturbance

• no established frequency for the behavior

• professionals judge impact of frequency on the behavior in relation to circumstances that might be transitory, such as parental separations or divorce

Intensity Issues Characteristic of Emotional Disturbance

• no established intensity for the behavior

• professionals judge impact of intensity of the behavior in relation to circumstances that might be transitory, such as lack of housing or frequent relocations of the family

Students may be placed in crisis support services prior to completion of full due process procedures whenever duration, frequency, or intensity issues become an issue according to the judgment of appropriate professionals.

Implications for Speech-Language Therapy and Emotional Disturbance

The child with emotional disturbance is different from other children with disabilities in that he or she is likely to act out, causing disruptions in the classroom setting, especially in the general education setting (Smith et al., 1998). SLPs must become proficient at managing behavior in order to successfully implement a speech-language intervention program for the child who has emotional disturbance. Rules for order and behavior in the therapy session are helpful as both general and specific rules (Walker & Shea, 1995). The ultimate goal is for the SLP to facilitate behavior management in order to support therapy. Part of the consideration for maintaining appropriate behavior was addressed by Zabel and Zabel (1996) who discussed the importance of the physical environment in helping maintain discipline. For example, these researchers suggested considering appropriate seating arrangements as one way to help facilitate appropriate behavior. Additionally, preventive measures related to establishing high expectations, following rules, positive reinforcers, and structure in the curriculum were reported to be important for maintaining appropriate behavior in the classroom (Sabatino, 1987). SLPs are encouraged to incorporate the use of classroom rules, appropriate arrangements of the physical environment, and preventive behavior management strategies to help maintain appropriate behaviors for children with emotional disturbance. The SLP must work with the classroom teacher so that consistency and support are achieved to promote the behavioral plans applicable for the child within the classroom setting as well as within the speech-language therapy setting. Finally, SLPs should remain focused on the goals and objectives of the therapy session when working with children with emotional disturbance in the following manner:

- Remind the child often of the goals or objectives of the session.
- Reiterate often how well the child is doing in focusing on the goals or objectives of the session.
- Offer corrective feedback when the child is having difficulty with not only the goals or objective of speech-language therapy, but also offer corrective feedback related to behavior difficulties noted in the therapy session. However, rely on team members and experts in behavior management to assist with guidance in this arena, based on the child's needs.

Hearing Impairment

Hearing impairment is an impairment in hearing, whether permanent or fluctuating, that adversely affects a child's educational performance but that is not included under the definition of Deafness in this section. (*Federal Register*, online source)

Characteristic of hearing impairment is absence of enough measurable hearing (usually pure tone average of 30 to 65 decibels, American National Standards Institute, without amplification) such that the ability to communicate is adversely affected; however, the student who is hearing impaired relies on the auditory channel as the primary sensory input for communication. The child may require educational support or environmental adaptations (preferential seating, visual aids, etc.). Smith et al. (1998) noted several characteristics typical of children who are hearing impaired across psychological, communication, social-emotional, and academic parameters. These include:

- intellectual abilities similar to hearing peers
- problems with certain conceptualizations
- poor speech production (unintelligibility)

- possible voice quality problems
- less socially mature
- may resent having to wear aides
- may become overly dependent on the teacher
- spelling problems. (p. 216)

Implications for Speech-Language Therapy and Hearing Impairment

Hearing impairment, even milder forms, greatly impacts language abilities (Smith et al., 1998). SLPs are encouraged to review guidelines of the American Speech-Language Hearing Association (ASHA) on *Roles of Speech-Language Pathologists and Teachers of Children Who Are Deaf and Hard of Hearing in the Development of Communicative and Linguistic Competence* (ASHA, 2004) when working with children who have hearing impairments. Additionally, Smith et al. (1998) suggested several strategies applicable to services to children with hearing impairments:

- make sure adequate lighting is available for lip or speech reading

- make sure students are attending

- provide short, clear instructions

- teacher's face should be visible to students during all communicative interactions

- use gestures and facial animation/expressions

- if the student has an interpreter, maintain eye contact with the student, not the interpreter

- repeat comments of others who speak in the setting with the student who is hearing impaired

Intellectual Disability

Intellectual disability is significantly subaverage general intellectual functioning, existing concurrently with deficits in adaptive behavior, and manifested during the developmental period, that adversely affects the child's educational performance. (*Federal Register*, online source)

Characteristics of intellectual disability encompass four categories:

1. Mild Intellectual Disability (MID)
   - 55 to 70 IQ
   - deficits in adaptive behavior that significantly limit effectiveness in meeting the standards of maturation, learning, personal independence or social responsibility, and especially school performance, that is expected of the individual's age level and cultural group, as determined by clinical judgment.

2. Moderate Intellectual Disability (MoID)

    - 40 to 55 IQ

    - deficits in adaptive behavior that significantly limit effectiveness in meeting the standards of maturation, learning, personal independence or social responsibility, and especially school performance, that is expected of the individual's age level and cultural group, as determined by clinical judgment.

3. Severe Intellectual Disability (SID)

    - 25 to 40 IQ

    - deficits in adaptive behavior that significantly limit effectiveness in meeting the standards of maturation, learning, personal independence or social responsibility, and especially school performance, that is expected of the individual's age level and cultural group, as determined by clinical judgment.

4. Profound Intellectual Disability (PID)

    - below 25 IQ

    - deficits in adaptive behavior that significantly limit effectiveness in meeting the standards of maturation, learning, personal independence or social responsibility, and especially school performance, that is expected of the individual's age level and cultural group, as determined by clinical judgment.

Each level of reduction in intelligence quotient (IQ) score yields progressively more difficulty for the child to negotiate his or her environment for several parameters including attention, memory, motivational, academic, social, communication, generalized learning, and adaptive needs (Smith et al., 1998).

Implications for Speech-Language Therapy and Intellectual Disability

The SLP's work with children with intellectual disability is dictated, of course, by existing goals on the Individualized Education Plan (IEP) and may be offered collaboratively within the classroom. However, Smith et al. (1998) indicated that several broad accommodations should be made when working with children with intellectual disabilities.

1. Ensure attention to relevant task demands.

2. Teach ways to learn content while teaching content itself.

3. Focus on content that is meaningful to the student, to promote learning and to facilitate application.

4. Provide training that crosses multiple contexts.

5. Offer opportunities for active involvement in the learning process (p. 202).

Additionally, SLPs must work to understand that the greater the reduction in intellectual functioning, often the greater the difficulty in acquiring speech and language, particularly communication skills that require higher order cognitive tasks (memory, processing, inferring, synthesizing, and evaluating tasks). In instances of significantly reduced intellectual functioning, the SLP should adjust goals and objectives as well as presentation methods, materials, and evaluations to meet the needs of the client.

Multiple Disabilities

Multiple disabilities are concomitant impairments (such as intellectual disability-blindness, intellectual disability-orthopedic impairments, etc.), the combination of which causes such severe educational needs that they cannot be accommodated in special education programs solely for one of the impairments. The term does not include deaf-blind. (*Federal Register*, online source)

Characteristics of multiple disabilities are broad-based. Many students with intensive, multiple disabilities present challenging characteristics and need highly individualized strategies for coping with their disabilities. Any number of challenges within numerous contexts and configurations may characterize the child with multiple disabilities. For example, communication skills may be characterized by individual variations that include personalized expression methods or communication modes, such as mixing expressive words with gestures, symbols, objects, lights, pictures, and so forth for communication (Downing & Chen, 2003; Olson & Platt, 2000). Other areas of functioning may require similar, unique management strategies across the child's constellation of presenting characteristics.

Implications for Speech-Language Therapy and Multiple Disabilities

The SLP working with the child with multiple disabilities will be guided, of course, by requirements of the IEP. However, overall intervention in this area will be guided by (a) cognitive skills, (b) sensory modalities that provide the best avenue for learning, and (c) expressive outputs that are in place for use by the child. Intervention may include needs for alternative/augmentative modes of communication. Hegde (2008) discussed several basic principles that SLPs should consider when selecting an augmentative communication mode or system.

• Assess the client's speech as well as nonspeech communication potential.

• Consider the client's strengths and limitations for cognitive, sensory, motor and language comprehension skills.

- Select a mode of communication that gives the maximum advantage to the client.

- Consider cost.

- Consider the client's acceptance of the mode or system.

- Consider the communicative demands the client faces.

- Consider the amount of training required.

- Consider how the client and family will use the mode or system. (p. 85)

Orthopedic Impairment

Orthopedic impairment is a severe difficulty with the skeletal systems (bones, joints, limbs, and associated muscles) to a degree that adversely affects a child's educational performance. The term includes impairments caused by congenital anomaly (e.g., clubfoot, absence of some member, etc.), impairments caused by disease (e.g., poliomyelitis, bone tuberculosis, etc.), and impairments from other causes (e.g., cerebral palsy, amputations, and fractures or burns) that cause contractures. (*Federal Register*, online source)

Characteristics of orthopedic impairment most often involve "muscular and skeletal problems in the legs, arms, joints, or spine, making it difficult or impossible for the child to walk, stand, sit, or use his or her hands" (Hallahan & Kauffman, 2000, p. 437). Common difficulties include muscular dystrophy, juvenile rheumatoid arthritis, and scoliosis. Although technically a result of neurological damage, cerebral palsy often manifests itself in limb involvement and motor disability.

Implications for Speech-Language Therapy and Orthopedic Impairments

Typically, the child's intelligence is unaffected in orthopedic impairments unless there are associated difficulties manifesting that result in reduced intelligence. However, due to limitations in mobility, the child with orthopedic impairments often has reduced concepts related to action verbs and other language concepts associated with physical activity. For example, words associated with participation sports and physical games may be limited for the child with orthopedic impairments because of limited mobility and participation in such activities. In degenerative impairments such as muscular dystrophy, musculature motor articulation control is eventually affected as the difficulty progresses and muscle fibers degenerate (Batshaw & Perret, 1986). Speech-language services generally are not indicated for children with degenerative muscular disorders in later stages of progression. However, the SLP will need to be guided by the dictates of the IEP for children with orthopedic impairments, particularly degenerative disorders over time.

Cerebral palsy, on the other hand, is a static-state disorder in terms of progression; it is not a disorder that is expected to get worse over time for the child's overall functioning for muscular skills, unless, of course, left untreated. With appropriate treatment from medical and support services such as physical therapy and occupational therapy, symptoms of cerebral palsy may decrease over time. Because of the relationship between the child's general motor state and progress in speech-language therapy, the SLP working with the child with cerebral palsy is encouraged to work closely with other professionals serving the child in order to monitor overall general motor skills. Therapy techniques addressing dysarthria of speech are often appropriate for children diagnosed with dysarthria of speech as a result of cerebral palsy.

Other Health Impairment

Other health impairment is having limited strength, vitality or alertness, including a heightened alertness to environmental stimuli, that results in limited alertness with respect to the educational environment that:

(a) is due to chronic or acute health problems such as asthma, attention deficit disorder or attention deficit hyperactivity disorder, diabetes, epilepsy, a heart condition, hemophilia, lead poisoning, leukemia, nephritis, rheumatic fever, and sickle cell anemia; and

(b) adversely affects a child's educational performance. (*Federal Register*, online source)

Characteristics of other health impairments vary widely due to the number of disabilities included in the category. Children with health impairments of the nature mentioned previously in the definition often have difficulty completing tasks, making transitions between tasks, interacting with others, following directions, producing work consistently, and organizing multistep tasks. Children who are medically fragile may require oxygen support, medications several times daily, and often are enrolled in school with nursing assistance (Hallahan & Kauffman, 2000). Children with communicable diseases also are served in schools under the other health impairment category. For the protection of both clients and the SLP, SLPs are encouraged to take universal health precautions when working with all clients, particularly both children and the elderly with diagnoses of other health impairment.

Implications for Speech-Language Therapy and Other Health Impairments

Speech-language therapy often takes a back seat to medical difficulties that threaten health and life. Children who are medically fragile often have health needs that demand immediate attention to preserve life or to prevent further medical deterioration (Hallahan & Kauffman, 2000). During times of medical crisis, children may not be seen for speech-language therapy because of difficulties related to breathing or feeding that are counter-indicated for working on speech. However, as soon as the child's health permits, and he or she returns to speech therapy, the SLP resumes work in speech-language therapy related to the goals of the child's IEP.

Specific Learning Disability

Specific learning disability is defined as follows:

(a) *General:* The term means a disorder in one or more of the basic psychological processes involved in understanding or in using language, spoken or written, that may manifest itself in an imperfect ability to listen, think, speak, read, write, spell, or to do mathematical calculations, including conditions such as perceptual disabilities, brain injury, minimal brain dysfunction, dyslexia, and developmental aphasia.

(b) *Disorders not included:* The term does not include learning problems that are primarily the result of visual, hearing, or motor disabilities, of mental retardation, of emotional disturbance, or of environmental, cultural, or economic disadvantage. (*Federal Register*, online source)

Characteristics of specific learning disabilities are relatively broad. Children diagnosed with specific learning disabilities have a measured IQ in the average or above average ranges, with a discrepancy noted between achievement and intellectual ability; the child does not perform to expected levels when performances are compared to intellectual ability in one or more of the abilities listed in item (a) of the definition for understanding or using language, listening, thinking, speaking, reading, spelling, writing, or doing math.

Implications for Speech-Language Therapy and Specific Learning Disability

Specific learning disabilities and speech-language therapy are closely aligned at several points along the possible diagnostic indicators for specific learning disabilities. For example, understanding and using language, listening, thinking, and speaking are skills often addressed by the SLP regardless of the client's age or disability area; therefore, clients with specific learning disabilities in areas that interface with speech-language often also qualify for speech-language therapy. However, based on tenets of federal laws regarding serving children in least restrictive environments, students with difficulties in specific learning disabilities that parallel the skills addressed in speech-language therapy often are adequately served for those language deficits within the specific learning disabilities program, with no additional services from the SLP required. Ultimately, the committee of professionals and parents responsible for developing the child's IEP determines the programs suited to meet the child's individual needs. Once the SLP finds that the child with specific learning disabilities is recommended for receiving speech-language services, the SLP, of course, provides services in accordance with the prescribed IEP goals for the child.

Speech or Language Impairment

Speech or language impairment under federal law is a communication disorder, such as stuttering, impaired articulation, a language impairment, or a voice or resonance impairment, that adversely affects a child's educational performance. (*Federal Register*, online source)

Characteristics of children who are speech-language impaired include difficulty with reception and expression of language skills in areas of semantics, phonology, morphology, syntax, or pragmatics, and may also include difficulty with speech areas such as stuttering, voice, resonance, or articulation/phonology skills.

Implications for Speech-Language Therapy and Speech Impaired

As indicated earlier in this chapter, SLPs may serve children in schools under two management structures: (a) as the *primary service provider*, as in the case of a child whose only special needs classification is speech or language impaired, or (b) as *a related service* when the primary special needs classification is any category other than speech or language impaired, but with the child also requiring speech-language services. The child's placement committee determines the structure under which the child is seen for speech-language services (as a primary service, or as a related service). Therapy is provided based on the IEP and in collaboration with other professionals serving the child.

Traumatic Brain Injury

> *Traumatic brain injury* is an acquired injury to the brain caused by an external physical force, resulting in total or partial functional disability or psychosocial impairment, or both, that adversely affects a child's educational performance. The term applies to open or closed head injuries resulting in impairments in one or more areas, such as cognition; language; memory; attention; reasoning; abstract thinking; judgment; problem-solving; sensory, perceptual, and motor abilities; psychosocial behavior; physical functions; information processing; and speech. The term does not apply to brain injuries that are congenital or degenerative, or to brain injuries induced by birth trauma. (*Federal Register*, online source)

Characteristics of traumatic brain injury (TBI) vary greatly depending on the degree of insult to the brain, location of the insult, general status and functioning prior to insult, and degree of recovery following insult. Currently, placement of a child classified as having TBI indicates that the child is served by appropriate certified teachers who address identified needs; however, there is no TBI certified teacher, per se. Mira, Tucker, and Tyler (1992) discussed characteristics of TBI injury across several areas of functioning: physical, sensory, cognitive, language, and behavioral/emotional, with a child needing services typically placed with the teacher best qualified to address the specific areas of deficit presented by the individual child. Mira et al. (1992) noted that children with TBI experience numerous difficulties that included reduced stamina and fatigue, vision/hearing problems, memory and attention deficits, reasoning and problem-solving difficulties, socially inappropriate verbal behavior, problems in planning and organizing, over activity, impulsivity, and lack of self-direction. Additionally, children with TBI may experience difficulty with sleep disorders, evaluating executive functions, and altered diet preferences.

Implications for Speech-Language Therapy and Traumatic Brain Injury

Children with TBI range broadly across difficulties, with TBI manifesting differently in each child's individual profile. Mira et al. (1992) offered the following suggestions for working with the child with TBI that are applicable for use by the SLP.

- Limit amount of information presented at one time.
- Provide simple instructions for only one activity at a time.
- Teach rehearsal skills to use before speaking.
- Teach self-regulating skills for attending; that is, "Am I paying attention?"
- Reduce distractions.
- Provide both visual and auditory directions.
- Allow the child to complete a project rather than written assignments.
- Allow extra time for fine motor activities.
- Help students understand the nature of their injuries. (p. 254)

As with any other special category of functioning, the child with TBI will be served by the SLP in accordance with individual goals on the IEP. SLPs should work closely with other professions for consistency in managing the needs of the child with TBI.

Visual Impairment Including Blindness

> ***Vision impairment including blindness*** is impairment in vision that, even with correction, adversely affects a child's educational performance. The term includes both partial sight and blindness. (*Federal Register*, online source)

Characteristics of vision impairment including blindness manifest in numerous ways. Most often, federal law interpretation of vision impairment considers the method of reading that must be addressed as a result of the child's vision difficulty (Hallahan & Kauffman, 2000). Based on this rationale for classifying vision impairments in children, the classifications, by the degree of visual acuity, include functionally blind, legally blind, and partially sighted. The child with functional blindness is legally blind and unable to use print material as the reading medium; consideration of instruction in Braille is essential to this student's education. The child classified as legally blind has a visual acuity of 20/200 or less in the better eye after correction or has a limitation in the field of vision that subtends an angle of 20 degrees. Some students who are legally blind have useful vision and may read print. In fact, Willis (1976) found that only 18% of students classified as legally blind were totally blind. Partially sighted acuity falls within the range of 20/70 in the better eye after correction or when reading 18-point print at any distance. Some students with a visual acuity greater than 20/70 will need specialized help for a limited time. Regardless of the acuity, the educational team has to decide if the child's vision loss constitutes an educational disability.

Implications for Speech-Language Therapy and Visual Impairment Including Blindness

The impact of vision difficulty on speech-language therapy is determined by the level of vision disability. Hallahan and Kauffman (2000) reported that some researchers believe that the lack of vision does not have a significant effect on the ability to understand and use language. However, based on findings related to early onset total blindness, it was determined that communication difficulties existed for children who were deaf-blind, with several parameters related more to blindness. Fryauf-Bertchy et al. (1993) indicated the following for children who are visually impaired, including blindness.

- They have a need for alternative/expanded forms of receptive communication including tactile/kinesthetic.
- They experience a high degree of pragmatic difficulty due to lack of vision.

As with other areas of categorical disabilities, SLPs are encouraged to work from the requirements of the IEP to address the needs of the child in the area of speech-language skills.

Summary

SLPs working with children and adults may better service clients if the difficulties observed in speech-language skills are viewed in relation to the totality of the overall developmental status of the client. Consideration for developmental domains (cognitive, motor, self-help/adaptive, social-emotional) along with speech-language development often allows the SLP professional to more clearly determine specifics of intervention that are best suited for the client's overall progress in therapy. Similarly, knowledge of characteristics of various disabilities, in conjunction with implications for speech-language therapy, serves to strengthen the SLP's skills in providing therapy to clients who present with varying difficulties as accompaniments to speech-language disorders.

Learning Tool

1. *Mini Child Develop Chart*. Choose a developmental domain (cognitive, motor, self-help/ adaptive, or social-emotional) and compare the expected development in that domain with expected development in speech-language skills for a child birth through age 5 years. Choose two major milestones per year for both the selected domain and speech-language development, and develop a chart of the development for ease in comparing across ages. For example, beginning at age 4 or 5 months, determine what the child should be doing in the area of speech-language skills; then, determine what the child should be doing in the selected domain (motor, for example) at 4 or 5 months. Place both skill areas on a chart so that the reader easily sees what skills in both areas are expected of the child at age 4 or 5 months. Then choose another age from the first year

of life and make the same comparison and charting. Select two ages per year through age 5 years, 11 months for your comparison. *Use sources suggested in the text for this chapter, along with other available resources, to support this learning effort.*

2. *Program Modifications.* Select a disability from those presented in the chapter. List five modifications that the SLP might be expected to make for a client who is diagnosed as having the disability. (For example, several modifications are likely needed if the SLP works with a client who has multiple disabilities, not including deaf-blindness; the SLP needs to be aware of what those modifications might include.) Once selected, indicate the disability you've chosen, and list the likely modifications in the spaces provided.

Disability: _____

Modifications:

a. _____

_____

b. _____

_____

c. _____

_____

d. _____

_____

e. _____

_____

References

American Speech-Language-Hearing Association. (2001). *Scope of practice in speech-language pathology.* Rockville, MD: Author.

American Speech-Language-Hearing Association. (2004). *Roles of speech-language pathologists and teachers of children who are Deaf and hard of hearing in the development of communicative and linguistic competence.* Rockville, MD: Author.

Anderson, N., & Shames, G. H. (2010). *Human communication disorders: An introduction* (8th ed.). Boston, MA: Allyn & Bacon.

Batshaw, M. L., & Perret, Y. M. (1986). *Children with handicaps: A medical primer*. Baltimore, MD: Paul H. Brookes.

Bauman, C., & Fishman, S. E. (1991). *The child chart*. Vero Beach, FL: The Speech Bin.

Bauman-Wangler, J. (2012). *Articulatory and phonological impairments: A clinical focus* (4th ed.). Boston, MA: Allyn & Bacon.

Bernthal, J. E., Bankson, N. W., & Flipsen, Jr., P. (2009). *Articulation and phonological disorders: Speech sound disorders in children* (6th ed.). Boston, MA: Allyn & Bacon.

Bloom, L., & Lahey, M. (1978). *Language development and language disorders*. New York, NY: John Wiley & Sons.

Brazelton, T. B., Scholl, M. L., & Robey, J. S. (1966). Visual responses in the newborn. *Pediatrics, 37*(2), 284–290.

Chapey, R. (Ed.). (2001). *Language intervention strategies in aphasia and related neurogenic communication disorders* (4th ed.). Baltimore, MD: Lippincott Williams & Wilkins.

Davis, G. A. (2000). *Aphasiology: Disorders and clinical practice*. Boston, MA: Allyn & Bacon.

Downing, J. E., & Chen, D. (2003). Using tactile strategies with students who are blind and have severe disabilities. *Teaching Exceptional Children, 36*(2), 56–61.

Federal Register. IDEA '97 Final Regulations, 34 CFR Part 300, Assistance to States for the Education of Children with Disabilities (Part B of the Individuals with Disabilities Education Act). (n.d.). Retrieved May 28, 2005, from http://www.ed.gov/legislation/FedRegister/proprule/1998-3/081498a.html

Fryauf-Bertschy, H., Kirk, K. I., & Weiss, A. L. (1993). Cochlear implant use by a child who is Deaf and blind: A case study. *American Journal of Audiology, 2*(1), 38–47.

Gard, A., Gilman, L., & Gorman, J. (1993). *Speech and language development chart* (2nd ed.). Austin, TX: Pro-Ed.

Gerken, K. C., Eliason, M. J., & Arthur, C. R. (1994). The assessment of at-risk infants and toddlers with the Bayley Mental Scale and the Battelle Developmental Inventory: Beyond the data. *Psychology in the Schools, 31*, 181–187.

Grossman, H. J. (1983). *Classification in mental retardation*. Washington, DC: American Association on Mental Deficiency.

Hallahan, D. P., & Kauffman, J. M. (2000). *Exceptional learners: Introduction to special education* (8th ed.). Boston, MA: Allyn & Bacon.

Heflin, L. J., & Simpson, R. (1998). Interventions for children and youth with autism: Prudent choices in a world of exaggerated claims and empty promises. Part II: Legal/policy analysis and recommendations for selecting interventions and treatments. *Focus on Autism and Other Developmental Disabilities, 13*, 212–220.

Hegde, M. N. (2008). *Hegde's pocketguide to treatment in speech-language pathology* (3rd ed.). Clifton Park, NY: Delmar.

Low, H. M., & Lee, L. W. (2011). Teaching of speech, language and communication skills for young children with severe autism spectrum disorders: What do educators need to know? *New Horizons in Education, 59*(3), 16–27.

Marchant, J. M. (1992). Deaf-blind handicapping conditions. In P. J. McLaughlin & P. Wehman (Eds.), *Developmental disabilities* (pp. 113–123). Boston, MA: Andover Press.

Miles, B. (2005). *Overview on Deaf-blindness*. Monmouth, OR: The National Clearinghouse on Children Who Are Deaf-Blind.

Mira, M. P., Tucker, B. F., & Tyler, J. S. (1992). *Traumatic brain injury in children and adolescents: A sourcebook for teachers and other school personnel*. Austin, TX: Pro-Ed.

Moyes, R. A. (2002). *Addressing the challenging behaviors of children with high-functioning autism/Asperger's syndrome in the classroom: A guide for teachers*. Philadelphia, PA: Jessica Kingsley.

Mundy, P., Sigman, M., & Kasari, C. (1990). A longitudinal study of joint attention and language development in autistic children. *Journal of Autism and Developmental Disorders, 22*, 115–127.

Newborg, J., Stock, J., Wnek, L., Guidubaldi, J., & Svinicki, J. (1988). *Diagnostic Battelle Developmental Inventory*. Allen, TX: DLM Teaching Resources.

Nicolosi, L., Harryman, E., & Kresheck, J. (2004). *Terminology of communication disorders: Speech-language-hearing* (5th ed.). Baltimore, MD: Lippincott Williams & Wilkins.

Olson, J., & Platt, J. (2000). *Teaching children and adolescents with special needs* (3rd ed.). Upper Saddle River, NJ: Merrill Prentice-Hall.

Paul, P. V., & Quigley, S. P. (1990). *Education and deafness.* New York, NY: Longman.

Perry, B. D. (2001). The importance of pleasure in play. *Scholastic Early Childhood Today, 15*(7), 24–26.

Raimondo, B. (2010, Spring/Summer). Deaf children with disabilities: Rights under IDEA. *Odyssey: New Directions in Deaf Education, 11*(1), 10–14.

Rollins, P. R. (1999). Early pragmatic accomplishments and vocabulary development in preschool children with autism. *American Journal of Speech-Language Pathology, 8*(2), 181–190.

Sabatino, D. A. (1987). Preventable discipline as a practice in special education. *Teaching Exceptional Children, 19*, 8–11.

Shames, G. H. (2006). *Counseling the communicatively disabled and their families: A manual for clinicians.* (2nd ed.). New York, NY: Psychology Press.

Shipley, K. G., & McAfee, J. G. (2005). *Assessment in speech-language pathology: A resource manual* (3rd ed.). New York, NY: Thomson Delmar Learning.

Siegler, R. S. (1991). *Children's thinking* (2nd ed.). Englewood Cliffs, NJ: Prentice Hall.

Smith, T. E. C., Polloway, E. A., Patton, J. R., & Dowdy, C. A. (1998). *Teaching students with special needs in inclusive settings* (2nd ed.). Boston, MA: Allyn & Bacon.

Tyler, R. S. (1990). Speech perception with the nucleus cochlear implant in children trained with the auditory/verbal approach. *American Journal of Otology, 11*, 99–107.

Walker, J. E., & Shea, T. M. (1995). *Behavior management* (6th ed.). Columbus, OH: Merrill.

Willis, D. H. (1976). *A study of the relationship between visual acuity, reading mode, and school systems for blind students.* Louisville, KY: American Printing House for the Blind.

Zabel, R. H., & Zabel, M. K. (1996). *Classroom management in context.* Boston, MA: Houghton Mifflin.

6

Hands-On Core Skills: The Speech-Language Pathologist as Facilitator of Positive Communication Change

Introduction

A brief discussion in Chapter 2 of this text addressed words used for characterizing the role of the speech-language pathologist (SLP) in the therapeutic process, words used to describe the *facilitative role* of the SLP in the therapeutic process. The role of the SLP in therapy is to *facilitate*, or *promote*, increased communication skills in clients. SLPs accomplish this by blending a thorough knowledge of the profession with the skillful, even artful, implementation of core skills in the therapeutic process. These core skills, called *therapeutic-specific skills*, are fundamental skills that the SLP employs as an ongoing, underlying, and integral part of therapy. Therapeutic-specific skills constitute the underlying fiber, the essence of what SLPs do, fundamentally, to facilitate increased communication skills in clients; ***therapeutic-specific skills*** are what the term implies: skills that are specific to the act of providing speech-language therapy in a manner conducive to effecting communicative improvement in clients. As an illustration, consider the architectural profession and the task of building a home.

Though, perhaps, unable to cite the specifics of design, materials quantity, safety, or durability codes, and so forth, the lay public probably has some understanding that, in order to build a home, there needs to be some place to locate the structure, something from which to build it, and some way of ensuring that it holds together over time. Architects know these things, as well. In fact, architects know that no matter how great, or small, the job, there are some underlying basic considerations that must be made in the daily task of operating as an architectural professional; factoring gravitational pull is probably one of those considerations. The architect may also consider the impact of natural elements such as rain, heat, cold, wind, and so forth when working through a project. Regardless of the size, or cost, of the project, it is inconceivable that an architect would design, or oversee, the construction of even a small storage building without considering the basic, underlying principles that serve, so powerfully, to impact activities of that profession. SLPs should view therapeutic-specific skills in the same manner: no matter how easy, or difficult, a case, no matter how old or new the clinical techniques employed, there are some basic considerations that are required as a function of operating as a clinician in the speech-language pathology profession; basic hands-on therapeutic-specific skills are among those considerations. Certainly, therapeutic-specific skills are not all particular to the speech-language pathology profession, for many of these same skills are used by educators, psychologists, and others. However, if used well by the SLP, in conjunction with a good knowledge base of the profession, these skills may well separate the SLP who is adequate from one who is excellent.

By design, therapeutic-specific skills are basic and global skills; they remain the underlying skills that SLPs bring to the implementation of most, if not all, speech-language therapy intervention programs and techniques. For example, when designing a specific fluency program aimed at reducing repetitions, blocks, and prolongations, authors of the program typically outline specific components for intervention, specifying how, when, and why the SLP should implement various aspects of the program. Rarely does the author of a fluency intervention program take the time, however, to teach or remind the SLP of the importance of *pace, volume, proximity, enthusiasm, antecedents, direct teaching*, and so forth, unless one or more of these therapeutic-specific skills is viewed as an integral part of the fluency intervention program itself; in this case, pace, for example, may be discussed as an integral part of some fluency intervention programs. Yet, it is believed that the authors of any intervention program expect SLPs to inherently know that, in addition to learning the specifics of the intervention program, the SLP must also exhibit good clinical use of the core skills mentioned: pace, volume, proximity, enthusiasm, antecedents, direct teaching, and so forth. However, as mentioned, rarely does the author of a specific intervention program build in instruction in the core skills of therapy. How, then, is the SLP expected to acquire these core skills? Other than random occurrences of therapeutic-specific skills dispersed among various intervention programs, clinical supervisors are left to teach therapeutic-specific skills on an "as needed" basis as situations arise during clinical training for SLP students. Fortunately, most clinical supervisors have done good jobs of teaching these core skills, perhaps, using "teachable moments" as a major factor in instruction design. However, it is believed that information presented in this text, particularly in this chapter, serves to systematically help SLPs learn and implement underlying basic core skills that are integral to speech-language therapy.

Therapeutic-Specific Skills

There are, in all likelihood, a number of skills that professionals might suggest for inclusion as therapeutic-specific core skills. However, based on approximately 20 years of classroom instruction designed to teach core therapeutic-specific skills to beginning SLP students, it became apparent that the skills discussed in this chapter constitute more than an adequate start for developing the underlying skills needed by SLPs to effect communication improvements in clients. The following 28 selected therapeutic-specific core skills are highlighted in this chapter, with 21 of these skills specifically addressed in a DVD accompaniment to the chapter. The skills highlighted on the DVD are indicated by a media symbol to the left of the topics, and appear in **bold**.

1. Motivation
2. ☉ **Communicating Expectations**
3. ☉ **Enthusiasm**, **Animation**, and **Volume** in the Therapeutic Process
4. ☉ **Seating Arrangements**, **Proximity**, and **Touch** in the Therapeutic Process
5. ☉ **Preparation**, **Pacing**, and **Fluency** for Therapeutic Momentum
6. ☉ Antecedents: **Alerting Stimuli**, **Cueing**, **Modeling**, and **Prompting**
7. ☉ Direct Teaching: **Learning Modalities**, Describing/Demonstrating, **Questioning**, and **Wait-Time**
8. ☉ Stimulus Presentation: **Shaping (Successive Approximations)**
9. ☉ Positive Reinforcers: **Verbal Praise**, **Tokens**, and **Primary Reinforcers**
10. ☉ **Corrective Feedback** in the Therapeutic Process
11. ☉ **Data Collection** in the Therapeutic Process
12. Probing in the Therapeutic Process
13. Behavioral Management in the Therapeutic Process
14. Troubleshooting in the Therapeutic Process

Overview of Workshop Tutorials: How to Use This Chapter

Twenty-eight core therapeutic-specific skills are discussed in this chapter. Considerable time will be devoted to presenting definitions, rationales, and relevant points of application to the speech-language pathology profession for each therapeutic-specific skill addressed in the chapter. The presentation format for the therapeutic-specific skills is a series of *mini-workshops*, opportunities to receive tutorials in individual therapeutic-specific skills in concise sequences of activities contained on a Therapeutic-Specific Workshop Form (Figure 6–1 and Figure 6–2).

Example: Workshops Forms Without a DVD Vignette
Therapeutic-Specific Workshop (TSW) Form: _____

Name: _____ Date *Post Organizer* Completed _____

Section A		
(Read this section *before* proceeding to Section B.)		
Definitions	Rationale	Relevance to SLP Profession

Section B
(Read this section *before* proceeding to Section C.)

Advance Organizer

Topic:

Purpose:

SLP Action:

Background:

Links to Prior Learning:

Objective and Clarification of Skill to be Learned:

Rationale:

New Vocabulary:

Individualized SLP Outcomes/Performance Objectives:

_____

_____

Figure 6–1. Therapeutic-Specific Workshop (TSW) Form. This example is for workshops *without* the DVD vignettes. Workshops 1, 12, 13, and 14 *do not* have DVD vignette accompaniments. *continues*

Section C
(Read this section *before* proceeding to Section D.)

Description/Demonstration

Example 1:

Example 2:

Section D
(Complete this section *before* proceeding to Section E.)

Think-Out-Loud Questions

☑ Read questions aloud.

☑ Verbalize answers to help with cognitive processing and the practice effect.

☑ Write short answers in spaces provided.

1. What is the first thing that I must do in order to _____?

   _____

2. What are the next step(s) that I must take in order to _____?

   _____

3. What vocabulary must I use in order to _____?

   _____

4. What should I say or do in interactions with the client to _____?

   (To help with authenticity, give your client an imaginary name!)

   _____

   _____

   _____

5. How will I know that I am appropriately _____?

   _____

Figure 6–1. *continues*

Section E

(Complete this section *before* proceeding to Section F.)

Prompts for Practice Opportunity

Practice the skills discussed in Sections A–D above. Revisit Sections A–D as needed to increase comfort with this section. *Use SLP peers, friends, parents, other relatives, large dolls positioned in a chair in front of you to pose as the "client(s)," etc., for your practices. If no one is available to serve as your client(s), use yourself as the client(s) by standing or sitting in front of a large mirror as you practice; the effect of "using yourself as client(s)" is the same, and sometimes more powerful, than having another pose as client(s).* Repeat practices until therapeutic features 1–3 below are accomplished. (You may require more or less than the practice check boxes provided.) Check one box each time a skill is practiced. Enter date each skill is accomplished to your satisfaction in the date spaces provided. (Dates may/may not be the same for each skill accomplishment.)

1. ❑ ❑ ❑ ❑   Accuracy in the skill sequence accomplished.   Date: _____

2. ❑ ❑ ❑ ❑   Personal comfort in the skill sequence accomplished.   Date: _____

3. ❑ ❑ ❑ ❑   Adequate speed/fluency in the skill sequence accomplished. Date: _____

Section F

(Complete this section *before* entering the date for *Date Post Organizer Completed,* upper right, page 1.)

Post Organizer

What I Accomplished in this Workshop: _____

_____

_____

Importance of My Accomplishment(s) to My Therapy: _____

_____

_____

My Assessment of My Performance of the Skill(s) Presented in this Workshop:

   The Easiest Parts for Me: _____

   The Most Difficult Parts for Me: _____

Thought Processes/Emotions I Experienced Learning the Skill(s) Presented in this Workshop Compared to What I Ultimately Learned from this Effort (Reflection Exercise):

_____

_____

_____

Date Post Organizer Completed: (Enter date here and in upper right corner, page 1): _____

Figure 6–1. *continued*

Example Workshops Forms With *the DVD Vignette* Therapeutic-Specific Workshop Form: _____

Name: _____ Date *Post Organizer* Completed _____

Section A

(Read this section *before* viewing the vignette on . . .)

Definitions	Rationale	Relevance to SLP Profession

Section B

(Read this section *before* viewing the vignette on . . .)

Advance Organizer

Topic:

Purpose:

SLP Action:

Background:

Links to Prior Learning:

Objective and Clarification of Skill to be Learned:

Rationale:

New Vocabulary:

Individualized SLP Outcomes/Performance Objectives:

_____

_____

Figure 6–2. Therapeutic-Specific Workshop (TSW) Form: (DVD Format). *continues*

Section C
(Read this section *before* viewing the vignette on . . .)

Description/Demonstration

Example 1:

Example 2:

Section D
(Complete this section *before* viewing the vignette on . . .)

Think-Out-Loud Questions

☑ Read questions aloud.

☑ Verbalize answers to help with cognitive processing and the practice effect.

☑ Write short answers in spaces provided.

1. What is the first thing that I must do in order to _____?

   _____

2. What are the next step(s) that I must take in order to _____?

   _____

3. What vocabulary must I use in order to _____?

   _____

4. What should I say or do in interactions with the client to _____?

   (To help with authenticity, give your client an imaginary name!)

   _____

   _____

   _____

5. How will I know that I am appropriately implementing _____?

   _____

Figure 6–2. *continues*

Section E

(Complete this section *after* viewing the vignette on . . .)

Prompts for Practice Opportunity

Practice the skills discussed in Sections A–D above and demonstrated in the DVD vignette on . . . Revisit the DVD demonstration and Sections A–D as needed to increase comfort with this section. *Use SLP peers, friends, parents, other relatives, large dolls positioned in a chair in front of you to pose as the "client(s)," etc., for your practices. If no one is available to serve as your client(s), use yourself as the client(s) by standing or sitting in front of a large mirror as you practice; the effect of "using yourself as client(s)" is the same, and sometimes more powerful, than having another pose as client(s).* Repeat practices until therapeutic features 1–3 below are accomplished. (You may require more or less than the practice check boxes provided.) Check one box each time a skill is practiced. Enter date each skill is accomplished to your satisfaction in the date spaces provided. (Dates may/may not be the same for each skill accomplishment.)

1. ☐ ☐ ☐ ☐ Accuracy in the skill sequence accomplished.   Date: _____

2. ☐ ☐ ☐ ☐ Personal comfort in the skill sequence accomplished.   Date: _____

3. ☐ ☐ ☐ ☐ Adequate speed/fluency in the skill sequence accomplished. Date: _____

Section F

(Complete this section *after* viewing the vignette on . . .)

Post Organizer

What I Accomplished in this Workshop: _____

_____

_____

Importance of My Accomplishment(s) to My Therapy: _____

_____

_____

My Assessment of My Performance of the Skill(s) Presented in this Workshop:

   The Easiest Parts for Me: _____

   The Most Difficult Parts for Me: _____

Thought Processes/Emotions I Experienced Learning the Skill(s) Presented in this Workshop Compared to What I Ultimately Learned from this Effort (Reflection Exercise):

_____

_____

_____

Date Post Organizer Completed: (Enter date here and in upper right corner, page 1): _____

Figure 6–2. *continued*

The **Therapeutic-Specific Workshop Form** (TSW Form) serves as a *learning tool* to guide students through the activities associated with learning new therapy skills; this form accompanies each skill to be learned. Additionally, 21 therapeutic-specific skills are highlighted on an accompanying DVD (found within the covers of this text) as demonstrations of how each respective therapeutic-specific skill might be represented within a therapeutic context. As a culminating experience for students learning therapy, two mini-therapy sessions (one approximately 11 minutes, the other approximately 20 minutes in length) are provided for a synthesized view of several therapeutic-specific skills when used within the context of a therapy session. The completion of each TSW Form serves as an indicator that the SLP has both worked through the skills addressed in the selected workshop and has attained an adequate self-assessed level of comfort with the materials presented in the workshop.

The basic foundation for the tutorials SLPs receive in this chapter is the **Explicit Instruction Model** of teaching, an instruction model that is both highly organized and task-oriented (Miller, 2002). Using an adaptation of this model, SLPs will be provided five cognitive aids designed to help focus content, attention, and learning: *advance organizers, descriptions/demonstrations, think-out-loud questions, practice opportunities,* and *post organizers.* These cognitive aids help the SLP process the components and requirements of each skill addressed in this chapter.

Before going further, it is important that students obtain a basic understanding of what is required in the workshops for each therapeutic-specific skill. A TSW Form (see Figure 6–1 or Figure 6–2) is provided for each skill to be studied and contains specific procedures students are to follow in learning the selected therapeutic-specific skill. As an example, the *Workshop Forms* list sections for advance organizers, descriptions/demonstrations, think-out-loud questions, practice opportunities, and post organizers. An **advance organizer** is information introduced in advance of the new skill to be learned and is designed to bridge the gap between current knowledge and knowledge to be acquired (Williams & Butterfield, 1992). *Advance organizers* are presented before students proceed in acquiring a new therapeutic-specific skill. Advance organizers are an important part of understanding and gaining comfort in acquiring the therapeutic-specific skills presented in this chapter. **Descriptions**, well-organized explanations of the skills to be learned and the steps taken in learning the new therapy skill, along with **demonstrations**, written or visual presentations of skills implemented by the SLP, also serve to help students acquire the skills presented. **Think-out-loud questions,** which the learner verbalizes to him- or herself, help processing of new information by combining two modalities, auditory and visual, to reinforce retention of new concepts. **Prompts for practice opportunities** are designated points in learning to practice new skills with help from prompts in the vignettes or on the TSW Form. Prompts for practice opportunities provide the essence of the workshop opportunity; for it is the practice opportunities that ultimately lead to the desired comfort level that students achieve in the learning experience. *Prompts for Practice Opportunities* offer practice at three levels: (a) practice for accuracy in accomplishing the skill, (b) practice for personal comfort in accomplishing the skill—needed because students often report "feeling strange" practicing the skills, and (c) practice for speed/fluency in accomplishing the skill. Finally, a ***post organizer***, a concluding activity that helps students further conceptualize new material, is used at the end of each workshop experience. Working through the workshop experiences, using the TSW Forms, the DVD, and information from this text, students gain both understanding and practice in numerous therapeutic-specific skills.

SLPs are encouraged to work through this chapter in the following manner for maximal benefit.

1. Select a therapeutic-specific skill to be studied and read the introductory information from this chapter that accompanies the selected skill. For example, if selecting the therapeutic-specific skills for Enthusiasm, Animation, and Volume, read the information from this chapter related to those skills.

2. Select the *Therapeutic-Specific Workshop (TSW) Form* that accompanies the skill selected. For example, the skills Enthusiasm, Animation, and Volume have an accompanying TSW Form, TSW Form 3, which you will need when studying the skills on Enthusiasm, Animation, and Volume.

3. Fill in your name in the space provided on the TSW Form.

4. Read the definitions, rationales, and relevant statements located in Section A of the TSW Form.

5. Complete the *Advance Organizer* portion of the TSW Form located in Section B for the skill selected.

6. Read the *Description/Demonstration* information located in Section C on the TSW Form.

7. Locate the *Think-Out-Loud* questions located in Section D on the TSW Form and answer the questions before viewing the vignette on the topic selected.

8. (If no DVD accompanies the selected therapeutic-specific skills, proceed to item 10 below.) If there is a DVD accompaniment to the selected therapeutic-specific workshop, view the DVD accompaniment to the skill selected as often as needed to become comfortable that the demonstrated skill(s) are clear. Each skill on DVD is demonstrated in a short vignette segment designed to provide the viewer a visual representation of possible way(s) the skill may be represented; the DVD also prepares the viewer for *Prompts for Practice Opportunities* related to the skill(s) selected.

9. Stop the DVD at the end of the vignette on the selected skill.

10. Read the *Prompts for Practice Opportunity* section located in Section E on the TSW Form. Practice the skills demonstrated in the vignette, if applicable, and in Sections A–D of the TSW Form. Repeat practices until (a) accuracy in the skill sequence is accomplished, (b) personal comfort for the skill sequence is accomplished, and (c) appropriate speed/fluency in the skill sequence is accomplished.

11. Fill in the dates skills for *accuracy, personal comfort,* and *speed/fluency* were accomplished in the *Prompts for Practice Opportunities* section of the TSW Form,

Section E. (Note: For some skills, it is likely that all three levels of practice, *accuracy*, *personal comfort*, and *speed*, will be accomplished within one or two practice sessions. For others, however, it is not uncommon for students to require only one or two practices to accomplish *accuracy* for the skill, but to still need several more practice sessions before *personal comfort* is achieved; most often even more practice is required to achieve the *speed/fluency* deemed appropriate for therapeutic intervention.)

12. Once all three of the skill levels in *Prompts for Practice Opportunities* (accuracy, comfort, speed) are accomplished, complete the *Post Organizer* activities in Section F. Fill in the date the Post Organizer was completed in the lower right-hand corner of Section F and in the upper right-hand corner of page 1 of the TSW Form. This date in the upper right-hand corner indicates the date this particular therapeutic-specific skill was accomplished.

Workshop Tutorials

Therapeutic-specific skills are most often learned independently of other skills without a hierarchical order. Therefore, skills may be selected in the order presented in this text, as preassigned in class, or as otherwise selected by the individual SLP.

Motivation *(Therapeutic-Specific Workshop: Form 1; No DVD Vignette)*

Motivation is defined as a stimulus or force that causes a person to act (*Webster's*, 1996). In speech-language therapy, this stimulus or force might be any number of things including the client's desire to improve communication skills, or for the clinician, the commitment to optimize the client's communication skills. Sometimes motivating stimuli are considered to be *extrinsic*, caused by something external to the client, or clinician; sometimes the motivating force is *intrinsic*, caused by an internal force or stimulus. Most researchers agree that intrinsic motivation is stronger for impacting learning because intrinsic motivators teach on their own; in this way, children and adults want to learn for the sake of learning (Brandt, 1995; Chance, 1992; White, 1959). For example, White (1959) believed that one of the most important intrinsic motivators was the need to feel competent. White thought that the motivation to achieve competence explained the practice behavior seen in learning and further discussed the feeling of pride in personal effectiveness as an intrinsic motivator. SLPs are encouraged to help clients find intrinsic motivators to keep in the forefront as therapy proceeds. However, when intrinsic motivators appear to have little or no impact on client motivation, systems of extrinsic motivators (token rewards, performance contracts, etc.) may prove helpful. Work through various concepts associated with motivation using *Therapeutic-Specific Workshop: Form 1, Motivation. (There is no DVD vignette for this skill.)*

⚙ Communicating Expectations *(Therapeutic-Specific Workshop: Form 2; DVD Vignette 1)*

The concept of communicating expectations is based on research regarding teacher expectations (Learman, Avorn, Everitt, & Rosenthal, 1990; Rosenthal & Jacobson, 1968; Smith, 1980). Rosenthal and Jacobson (1968) found that gains in children's IQs were related directly to the classroom teacher's expectations for IQs to increase. Replications of Rosenthal and Jacobson's (1968) work, often referred to as the "Pygmalion in the Classroom Study," were performed within numerous contexts over several decades (Brophy, 1983; Eden, 1990; Edmonds, 1979), with results indicating that children will perform to the levels expected and communicated, even when such communications are inadvertent nonverbal behaviors (Ambady & Rosenthal, 1992). In fact, Feldman and Theiss (1982) found that teacher expectations influenced student achievement and that preconceptions influenced both student and teacher attitudes. The effects of communicated expectations have broadened to wider circles over the past 20 years in that researchers found relationships between communicating expectations and performance indicators in courtrooms (Blanck, Rosenthal, Hart, & Bernieri, 1990), in management (Eden, 1990), and in skilled nursing facilities (Brophy, 1983; Learman et al., 1990).

Good and Brophy (1984) suggested ways in which educators may reduce communicating expectations that have negative impacts on students. Among these suggestions were recommendations for:

- setting goals for individuals in terms of minimally accepted standards and indicating to students that they have the ability to meet those standards,

- stressing progress relative to previous levels of mastery by the individual student, rather than comparing the student's performances to performances of others, and

- encouraging students to achieve as much as possible by stretching and stimulating students' minds to achieve.

SLPs are encouraged to communicate positive expectations to clients at all times and to practice communicating positive expectations during therapy, particularly at the beginning of the body of therapy, and at other advantageous times as well. Activities associated with *Therapeutic-Specific Workshop: Form 2, including DVD Vignette 1*, are designed to help with increasing these skills.

⚙ Enthusiasm, Animation, and Volume in the Therapeutic Process *(Therapeutic-Specific Workshop: Form 3; DVD Vignette 2)*

The personality traits found among SLPs tend to be representative of the basic personalities found in the general population: some of us are "bubbly," energetic, and enthusiastic, whereas others are sedate, serene, and low-key in affect. *Affect* was discussed in Chapter 2 and was defined as the feelings, emotion, mood, and temperament associated with a thought (Nicolosi, Harryman, & Kresheck, 2004). Although some SLPs naturally possess an enthusiastic personality, there is no consistent way to tell beforehand whether that enthusiasm will translate into the interpersonal interactions needed for conducting speech-language therapy. **Enthusiasm** is defined as a strong excitement or feeling for something; a zest or zeal for a subject (*Webster's*, 1996). Often enthusiasm is portrayed in body movements, changes in vocal pitch and volume, or general attributes of animation. *Webster's* (1996) defined **animation** as relating to spirit, movement, zest, and vigor. Some SLPs admit that they are not interested in portraying the animation suggested for working with very young clients, even though some of the same SLPs describe themselves as being enthusiastic. Clinical supervisors must, therefore, survey student SLPs for expressions of enthusiasm and animation sufficient for effective speech-language therapy. When that level of enthusiasm is not present, it must be taught. This is where the concept of *Showtime* becomes important.

Showtime, as discussed in Chapter 2, is used as a concept to help SLPs understand the significance of the therapy provided to clients. The significance of therapy takes precedence over the SLP's personal preferences for expressions of emotions, affect, and enthusiasm. Although not characteristic of—or even preferred as a personal personality trait—animation, role-playing, or otherwise displaying pitch and volume ranges beyond normal may be necessary for SLPs to demonstrate a level of enthusiasm sufficient to keep the client interested in therapy and motivated to perform well in all aspects of therapeutic intervention. Several researchers found that students responded with increased attention and on-task behavior to dynamic, energetic speech, and speech that was perceived as extroverted, displaying expanded pitch ranges, and increased volume and pitch (Bettencourt, Gillett, Gall, & Hull, 1983; Nass & Lee, 2000). These vocal traits—dynamic, energetic speech, expanded pitch ranges, and increased volume and pitch—were characterized as the vocal styles used by master teachers for whom children answered 16% more science questions than for teachers with decreased emotional affect. Reissland and Shepherd (2002) found that mother's use of a higher pitch increased the infant's eye gaze toward the mother. Coulston, Oviatt, and Darves (n.d., online resource) found that 77% of children ages 7 to 10 years adapted the volume of their responses to match the volume of animated speakers; the children increased volume as the animated speaker's volume increased, and they decreased volume in response to speakers using a decreased volume. These studies suggested that enthusiasm, indicated by vocal manipulations for both pitch and volume, has a positive impact on a young child's attending, academic engagement, and focus on the speaker. However, it was unclear as to the age limits of generalizations of these impacts. For example, most studies involving the impact of pitch, perceived animation, and volume manipulations in the voice were conducted on children age 10 years and younger. It was uncertain whether the enthusiastic voice had an impact on older children and adults. The SLP, therefore, must make a clinical judgment as to how much animation is needed for each client, depending on age, functioning level, and therapeutic objectives.

Nonverbal affect was found to be important for infants reading social signals of their mothers. In fact, several researchers found that infants perceived stimuli as pleasant or unpleasant, depending on adult facial expressions (Klinnert, Campos, Sorce, Emde, & Svejda, 1983; Mumme, Fernald, & Herrera, 1996). Similarly, nonverbal communication for the SLP such as eye contact, facial expression, body language, and even proximity are important communicators of enthusiasm and animation during speech-language therapy. For example, a common nonverbal expression of excitement and enthusiasm is the "high five."

SLPs are encouraged to work toward manipulations and controls of both verbal (vocal pitch and volume range manipulations) and nonverbal (facial expressions) stimuli in the provision of speech-language services. Activities associated with *Therapeutic-Specific Workshop: Form 3, including DVD Vignette 2*, are designed to help with increasing these skills.

⊛ Seating Arrangements, Proximity, and Touch in the Therapeutic Process *(Therapeutic-Specific Workshop: Form 4; DVD Vignette 3)*

Numerous researchers addressed the impact of seating arrangement on learning and behavior (Cegelka & Berdine, 1995; Miller, 2002; Reith & Polsgrove, 1994). Miller (2002) indicated that design and arrangement of the physical dimensions of a classroom are very important because they affect student learning and behavior. SLPs often work in small physical spaces regardless of whether employed in clinics, hospitals, or schools, and typically, we use a variety of seating arrangements. Among the seating arrangements used by SLPs are (a) diagonal-table seating, (b) across-the-table seating, (c) side-by-side table seating, and (d) kidney-shaped table seating. (See Figure 6–3 for schematics of these seating designs.)

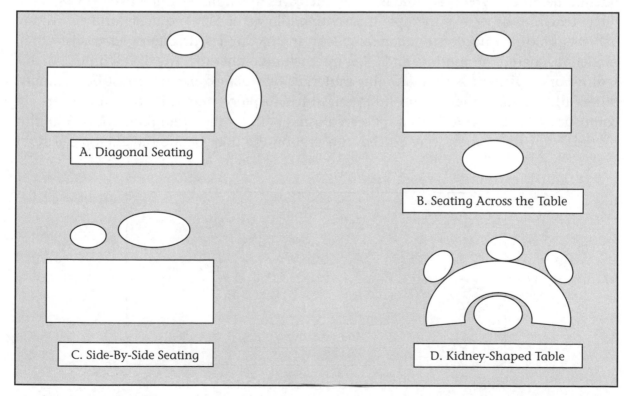

Figure 6–3. Four seating arrangements typical of speech-language therapy settings: **A.** Diagonal Seating; **B.** Seating Across the Table; **C.** Side-By-Side Seating; **D.** Kidney-Shaped Table.

No research was available to suggest the better seating model for learning during speech-language therapy, but most SLPs can be observed using one or more of the mentioned arrangements, depending on the work setting, number of clients in the session, and nature of the goals of the client. Wengel (1992) especially urged teachers to think about instructional goals and to select a seating arrangement that best supports those goals. Additionally, Miller (2002) listed both cultural diversity of the learner and specific needs dictated by the disability of the client as considerations for choosing seating arrangements. For example, Wortham, Contreras, and Davis (1997) found that persons from Latino families tended to prefer seating arrangements that allowed group interaction, such as semicircle seating as offered in the kidney-shaped table arrangement. Native Americans and African-Americans tended to prefer group interaction for learning as well (Lewis & Doorlag, 1991; Sadker & Sadker, 2005). However, the size of some kidney-shaped tables must be monitored, if this type of table is used, to help increase interaction among clients. Often the tables are so large that clients are not seated near enough to each other to foster the type of interaction desired.

Another type of semicircle arrangement is presented in Figure 6–4. This type of seating is an interactive arrangement for groups of clients focusing on communication skills that can be enhanced by peer or group interactions and models. In this seating arrangement, *cluster seating*, the SLP chooses a semicircle for interactive purposes, but removes the table to achieve better proximity and increased ease in creating opportunities to facilitate interaction among clients.

Both cluster seating in chairs and cluster seating on the floor are possible. The advantage of this type of seating is that it increases the intimacy and effectiveness of the direct teaching aspects of therapy; this seating allows the SLP to quickly and effortlessly achieve proximity needed for addressing learning modalities, describing, demonstrating, modeling, cueing, prompting, and other interactions of therapy. The disadvantage of this seating arrangement is that stimulus materials and data collection must be managed differently because there is no table on which to place materials or data sheets. To compensate for this, one SLP was observed using pails for managing materials. Stimulus materials for the session were placed in a pail on the floor beside the SLP on her right

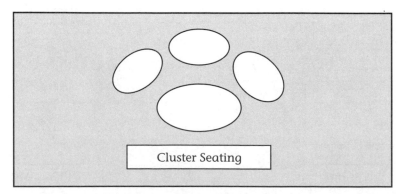

Figure 6–4. A schematic of cluster seating, a table-less grouping for sitting in chairs or on the floor.

side. As the SLP finished with an item, it was placed in another pail on the floor to her left. The SLP used a small clipboard for support during writing for data collection. Considerations for the management of therapy materials and data collection in relation to the space available to the clinician once acceptable seating arrangements are established are important. In particular, SLPs need to consider space requirements for both the material being used in therapy and the amount of space required in taking data during the session. Data collection is addressed later in this chapter, and materials management is addressed in Chapter 8.

Another effective, but not as often used, seating arrangement is *wall-mounted mirror seating*. In this arrangement, the SLP seats clients facing a large mirror that is mounted on the wall. The SLP then sits behind the clients. This type of seating works well for clients who require a lot of visual feedback for placement of the articulators, such as in the initial phases of placements for phonemes, or for clients who may need visual feedback for facial muscular movements or head or torso posture following stroke or traumatic brain injury. (See Figure 6–5 for a schematic of this seating arrangement.)

Proximity, the degree of closeness in physical distance between persons, as related to increased learning was addressed by a number of researchers involved in both teacher expectation and nonverbal communication investigations (Burgoon, Stern, & Dillman, 1995; Miller, 1988; Ridling, 1994; Sills-Briegel, 1996). In a study investigating the impact of five nonverbal cues—eye contact, proximity, body positioning, smiling, and touch—Burgoon et al. (1995) found that when the power of the cues were considered, relative to one another, proximity carried the greatest weight. In a study addressing the impact of proximity, Miller (2002) listed four categories of informal space that were established for the United States: *intimate space* (up to 1.5 feet), the zone reserved for close relationships, sharing, protecting, and comforting; *personal space* (1.5 to 4 feet), informal conversations between friends; *social space* (4 to 12 feet), generally accepted for interactions among strangers, business acquaintances, and teachers and students; and *public space* (12 to 25 feet), one-way communication as exhibited by lecturers. The distance between SLP and client is extremely important for therapeutic success. Therefore, the recommended

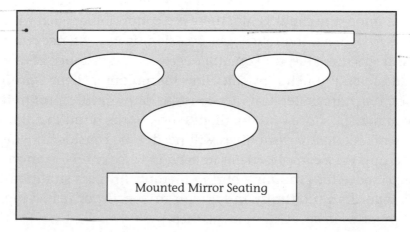

Figure 6–5. Mounted mirror seating.

distance for SLP to client interaction is the lower limits of personal space, or no more than 2 feet distance between the SLP's and client's faces for typical interactions. Of course, there are times when the SLP may need to move closer than 2 feet to the client for therapeutic interaction, and times when the distance between the SLP's face and the client's face will be greater than 2 feet, depending, of course, on therapeutic objectives.

SLPs should respect the client's cultural and personal dictates for personal space preferences and comfort levels with ***nonthreatening therapeutic touch***, touching the client's shoulder, upper arm, neck, torso, and facial areas in order to support clinical instruction. For example, the SLP may need to touch the client's thorax or diaphragm areas for instruction regarding proper breathing for speech. In other instances, portions of the head may need to be touched to help make a point during instruction regarding impacts of stroke or dementias. However, some Southeast Asians may feel it to be spiritually inappropriate to be touched on the head, whereas African-Americans may feel a touch on the head to be demeaning rather than kind (Sadker & Sadker, 2005). Sadker and Sadker further noted variability in perceptions of "getting in someone's face" as clinicians may need to do to be effective in therapy, in that such closeness may either be perceived as threatening or kind. One way to eliminate or lessen the negative perceptions that clients may form regarding proximity and therapeutic touch is to simply discuss the steps or actions the clinician will take in providing services. For example, telling a client that the chin will be touched to help establish proper swallowing posture and discussing any reservations clients might express (verbally or nonverbally) helps lessen client feelings of violation of any kind. However, SLPs are cautioned that Asian-Americans and Native-American children are likely to avoid asking for help, even in resolving a discomfort related to interaction (Sadker & Sadker, 2005). In these instances, the SLP will need to be sensitive to both the client's discomfort with therapeutic touch and the discussion of that discomfort. SLPs will need to take the lead in ensuring the client's comfort by initiating appropriate discussion of the client's needs in these areas.

In addition to consideration of the distance between the SLP's face and the client's face for determining appropriate proximity for therapy, SLPs are urged to use an informal rule for determining appropriate therapeutic proximity. This rule, referred to as the ***hand-to-chin rule***, dictates a proximity span whereby when the clinician's upturned palm is extended to touch under the client's chin, there is a comfortable reach without overextension of the elbow to achieve the touch. On occasion, it may be necessary to lessen this space for teaching specific skills, and on other occasions, a distance of a few more inches more than a hand-to-chin touch may still allow for maximal client learning.

Regardless of the parameter used to consider appropriate proximity for therapy (distance between the SLP's face and the client's face, or the hand-to-chin rule), the physical needs for clients related to disabilities will need to be considered when determining proximity for therapy. For example, clients in beds, in wheelchairs, or in casts may require more than typical space for proximity during therapy. In these situations, the SLP must make decisions regarding proximity in relation to best fit for achieving proximity for maximal client progress in speech-language therapy.

In summary, in all instances of establishing seating arrangements and proximity for therapeutic touch and intervention, the clinician should remember (a) the established goals for the client, (b) needs of the client related to cultural diversity, and (c) needs of the client dictated by the presenting disability. Activities associated with *Therapeutic-Specific Workshop: Form 4, including DVD Vignette 3* are designed to help with increasing these skills.

⊛ Preparation, Pacing, and Fluency for Therapeutic Momentum *(Therapeutic-Specific Workshop: Form 5; DVD Vignette 4)*

Therapeutic momentum is defined as the speed, thrust, or force of moving between sections of the session. For example, in Chapter 7, three major sections of a therapy session are addressed, the *Introduction, Body,* and *Closing.* Regardless of techniques used, SLPs must promote therapeutic momentum through proper preparation, pacing, and fluency as therapy proceeds through the major sections of the session. Being properly prepared for each segment of therapy, monitoring the pace of progressions for stimulus presentation and client responses, and monitoring the flow (fluency) of therapy help support therapeutic momentum.

Miller (2002) noted that it is important to maintain momentum during teaching so that lessons progress without lulls that result in **nonproductive time**, time that is wasted during therapy. Toward the end of Chapter 2, SLPs were encouraged to adopt a *minutes matter attitude* to avoid wasting time during therapy and to increase time-on-task. Time-on-task is increased when the SLP is well prepared and organized for progressions between and within various sections of therapy. When the clinician is *organized,* understands the order of segments of therapy to be addressed, and has all needed materials properly placed at hand, time-on-task and instructional momentum are enhanced. In fact, Miller (2002) reported that the best way to maintain instructional momentum is to be *prepared* and *organized.* Imagine the loss of momentum, the lull in time, and the nonproductive therapeutic time that occurs when the SLP has to stop therapy to go to a cabinet, shelf, or desk to find an item of material needed for the session.

A number of researchers (Good & Brophy, 1984; Miller, 2002) found that quick-paced lessons facilitated student involvement in learning and helped maintain momentum. Miller (2002) indicated that **quick-paced lessons** refer to the *presentation rate* used in teaching, not the number of minutes or total amount of time spent in teaching a skill. For example, the customary amount of time that a client is scheduled for therapy per session is not shorted by quick-paced presentations of information. Rather, quick-paced lessons refer to the SLP's skilled practice of moving effectively and efficiently through the task of presenting stimuli and eliciting responses from the client and moving smoothly from one segment of therapy to the next. Occasionally, however, the SLP may choose to purposely slow the pace, just for a few moments, to (a) allow a little more time for the client to process more challenging information or (b) change the impetus for a moment to reorient the client's attending and focus skills.

The smooth movement or transition between various parts of therapy is referred to as *fluency* within the therapeutic session. Fluency is promoted by quick-paced lessons and good preparation and organization for the session; fluency ensures the absence of "fumbling around" during the session, and it helps the SLP avoid repeated uses of *nonsemantic fillers,* the "ahs," "ums," "okays," and "let me sees" often characteristic of those unsure of what should happen next in therapy. Another way to increase fluency within the flow of the therapeutic session is to use a guide (physical or mental) to help ensure that the SLP is aware of both the scope and sequence of the session.

Scope refers to the range or depth of activities of the session; *sequence* refers to the order in which the activities occur within the session. For example, when teaching a session on following one-step directions using a scope and sequence guide to help the session remain fluent, or flow well, the SLP might establish a scope (range of activities) of three one-step commands given to the client to assess skills in this area. A scope that includes asking the client to follow a one-step command just once during therapy is not enough range or depth of the activity to assess client skills, whereas asking the client to follow a one-step command 50 times during the session is far more than the range or depth needed to assess this skill. In this same scenario, the SLP establishes a *sequence,* or order, for not only which of the three questions used should be asked first, second, and third, but which sequence helps the SLP determine where to go or what to do next in the session, depending on client responses. Other guides to help increase fluency in the session are visuals such as graphic organizers (discussed in Chapter 4), charts, posters, computerized projections, and so forth. Some SLPs use note cards, lesson plans, color-coded files, or other media aids to serve as props or reminders of progression of therapy so that both momentum and fluency are maintained.

In summary, therapeutic momentum is enhanced by the SLP who is well prepared and organized for therapy, uses a quick pace for presenting stimuli and eliciting responses, and maintains fluent movement between sections of therapy throughout the session. Activities associated with *Therapeutic-Specific Workshop: Form 5, including DVD Vignette 4* are designed to help increase these skills.

⊛ Antecedents: Alerting Stimuli, Cueing, Modeling, and Prompting
(Therapeutic-Specific Workshop: Form 6; DVD Vignette 5)

Hegde (2008) noted the following regarding *antecedents*: "Events that occur before responses; stimuli or events the clinician presents in treatment. Antecedents may be objects, pictures, re-created or enacted events, instructions, demonstrations, modeling, prompting, manual guidance, and other special stimuli" (p. 9). For purposes of this discussion, the events that will be highlighted as antecedents are *alerting stimuli, cueing, modeling,* and *prompting.*

Alerting Stimuli

Alerting stimuli are the various means of drawing the client's attention to the coming treatment stimuli (Hegde, 2008); alerting stimuli serve, essentially, as a "heads-up" alert to help the client prepare for the stimuli to which a response is required. Alerting stimuli may be verbal such as, "Watch my face," or nonverbal, such as holding up a hand to alert the client that the stimulus is about to be presented.

Cueing

Cueing is an aid to promote correct responses (Nicolosi et al., 2004). Cues may be (a) auditory such as verbal expressions that may include stress, pitch, quality, intonation, and duration markers; (b) visual such as gesture, posture, or facial expression; and (c) tactile-kinesthetic such as touch to the speech mechanisms.

Modeling

Hegde (2008) defined *modeling* as the clinician's production of a target behavior for the client to imitate and listed the following suggestions for using modeling.

- Provide live or mechanically delivered model (audio or videotaped or computer presented)
- Use the client's own correct response as a model (presented mechanically)
- Model frequently in the beginning stage of treatment
- Ask the client to imitate as closely as possible
- Reinforce the client for correct imitations or approximations
- Withdraw or fade modeling in gradual steps as the client's imitative responses stabilize. (p. 334)

A typical model is the clinician's correct production of the /s/ phoneme for the client to imitate during traditional articulation therapy. Additionally, clients may serve as the models for peers during group therapy. Meyer (2004) noted several possible problems that SLPs may face in modeling: (a) *unnatural productions*, (b) *ungrammatical utterances*, and (c) the *"OK" syndrome*. Meyer referred to **unnatural productions** as pronunciations presented to the client in which unnatural stress, syllabification, or other abnormalities in modeled presentation occur. An example includes *"but ton"* for *"but on."* **Ungrammatical utterances**, the use of grammatically incorrect language during therapy, was also discussed by Meyer (2004). A typical example often seen in SLPs in the beginning stages of therapy includes the use of feedback to the client in the form of the grammatical incorrect, "You did good!" rather than the grammatically correct, "You did well!" Meyer (2004) described the **"OK" syndrome** as the overuse of "OK," including five possible reasons why SLPs use "OK." Meyer noted that "OK" is used (a) as a conversational, or nonsemantic filler, (b) as a tag question, (c) to provide feedback, (d) as a positive reinforcer, and (e) as an answer to a question. Based on observations of SLPs throughout training, two aspects of the "OK" syndrome were noted.

1. It appeared that the "OK" syndrome diminished over time, particularly its use as a nonsemantic filler and as a tag question, as the SLP gained experience and confidence in therapy. Often as skills in preparation, pace, and fluency increased, unnecessary uses of "OK" appeared to decrease.

2. SLPs whose primary service delivery was individual therapy appeared to maintain the unnecessary uses of "OK" longer than SLPs conducting mostly group therapy. A speculation for this perceived phenomenon is that SLPs engaged in group therapy are responsible for more semantic content due to the requirements of interactive therapy; perhaps, there simply are less noncommunicative "spaces to fill" with nonsemantic verbalizations. In other words, because of the interactive nature of group therapy, there simply may be less time for nonsemantic units.

SLPs should record themselves periodically during therapy and count the number of inappropriate uses of "OK" during therapy. Increased skills in therapy should result in decreases in unintentional uses of "OK."

Prompting

Prompting is using special stimuli, verbal or nonverbal, to increase the probability that the client will respond in a desired manner. For example, if prompting a client to respond with the word *nose*, the clinician may say, "I smell with my" while either pointing to his or her nose, at the same time verbally prompting with the /n/ phoneme. Hegde (2008) recommended the following regarding prompting.

*   Prompt promptly, as the client hesitates (e.g., in treating naming in a client with aphasia: "What is this?" "The word starts with a /t/.")
*   Prompt more frequently in the beginning to reduce errors
*   Prefer a subtle or short prompt to ones that are loud or long (e.g., in training a person who stutters to speak slowly: "Slower" instead of "Speak at a slower rate."). Prefer a gesture to a verbal prompt (e.g., in training a person who stutters to speak slowly: make a hand gesture to suggest a slower rate.)
*   Use Partial Modeling as a prompt
*   Fade prompts as the responses become more consistent. (pp. 358–359)

In summary, antecedents such as alerting stimuli, cueing, modeling, and prompting hold valuable places in therapeutic intervention. The SLP should practice these skills and become comfortable using them in the therapeutic process. Activities associated with *Therapeutic-Specific Workshop: Form 6, including DVD Vignette 5* are designed to help with increasing these skills.

⊛ Direct Teaching: Learning Modalities, Describing/ Demonstrating, Questioning, and Wait-Time in the Therapeutic Process *(Therapeutic-Specific Workshop: Form 7; DVD Vignette 6)*

Direct teaching for speech-language therapy refers to instances when the SLP's task is to *teach, instruct, or train* the client in a new skill. Although SLPs are not certified as teachers, there are times when best teaching practices are beneficial in helping SLPs accomplish therapeutic objectives. During those segments of therapy, the SLP is encouraged to consider several concepts from teaching and learning literature, namely, information regarding *learning modalities, describing, demonstrating, questioning skills,* and application of appropriate *wait-time* during instruction.

Learning Modalities

Typically, SLPs rely on visual, auditory, and tactile (expanded to include tactile/kinesthetic) modalities for teaching clients new information. This means that stimuli are presented (a) visually to address the visual modality, (b) verbally to address the auditory modality, and (c) through touch to address the tactile/kinesthetic modality. However, other modalities such as taste and smell are used by SLPs as well, if client goals determine the need for these stimulations. Although most typical learners are capable of learning through all modalities, learners most often have a **preferred learning modality**, the sensory modality through which information appears easiest to learn (e.g., auditory, visual, or tactile/ kinesthetic). (See Chapter 4.) As professionals responsible for establishing goals for clients, and planning successful activities designed to address those goals, it is important for SLPs to be aware of the various modality preferences presented by clients.

Describing and Demonstrating

Major components of teaching are describing and demonstrating. **Describing** refers to telling or detailing the major features, functions, characteristics, or aspects of an item or concept deemed important. For example, when describing a ball, the SLP might say the following: "It's round and it bounces. We can throw it, catch it, roll it, or kick it." Descriptions may include the following **attributes**, the primary characteristics or features of the item being described: *size, shape, color, function,* and *remote associations*. **Remote associations** are defined as distal times, locations, or activities when the client may have encountered the item being described. For example, a remote association for a ball might be, *"There are three balls in your classroom."*

   Demonstrating refers to using well organized, step-by-step explanations in language that is easily understood to give examples. Teacher demonstrations of materials and concepts to be learned were found to be helpful teaching tools (Rivera & Smith, 1987). The use of visuals, models, actions, gestures, and so forth may also help in making demonstrations more powerful for clients. Demonstrations paired with feedback (Rose, Koorland,

& Epstein, 1982) and demonstrations paired with modeling (Rivera & Smith, 1987) were found to be helpful to children in generalizing learning. Demonstrating using short, repetitive units such as sentences or actions are recommended. For example, in demonstrating how to turn on overhead lights, the SLP might go over to the light switch and turn on the light while saying, "I flip the switch up, and the light comes on; I flip the switch down, and the light goes off. Watch again, flip up, the light goes on; flip down, the light goes off. Up, goes on; down, goes off. Up, on; down; off." SLPs should become comfortable in designing demonstrations for clients that are systematic and effective teaching tools. The tendency to "talk too much," *loquaciousness,* as described by Meyer (2004) should be avoided during demonstrations and at other times during therapy when possible. However, due to the nature of describing and demonstrating, therapy during these times is likely to require more talking from the SLP than might be necessary at other times.

Questioning

Questioning is a technique of direct teaching designed to assess learning and facilitate further learning (Miller, 2002). Questions help focus attention on important information and keep students actively involved in the session (Gall, 1984). Hegde (2008) listed the following four types of questions:

1. Intonation questions: Essentially declarative statements (not syntactically correct questions) that serve as questions because of their unique intonation

2. Tag questions: Declarative expressions with an interrogative tag added at the end (e.g., "You can do it, can't you?")

3. Wh-questions: Question forms that begin with *who, what, which, when, where, whose, why,* and *how*

4. Yes–No Questions: Question forms that require either a Yes or a No as the response. (p. 372)

Questioning is a valuable part of direct teaching, but SLPs are encouraged to use questions for intended purposes under the concept of *"taking it to the bank,"* a term used to help SLPs understand that answers to questions should not be assumed present in the client's repertoire of skills, unless the SLP has exposed the client to instruction designed to *deposit* the information in the client's *skills bank.* Remember the purpose of questions (assessing learning and fortifying additional learning) and use questions thoughtfully and appropriately.

Wait-Time

Wait-time is the amount of time the SLP waits for a response from a client after asking a question or giving a command. Cotton (1995) supported the use of longer wait-time during questioning. A wait-time of between 3 to 5 seconds used by classroom teachers following questioning was generally reported in the literature (Rowe, 1986; Tobin, 1980). However, SLPs are encouraged to consider wait-time in reference to goals of the client and his or her communication skills. For example, a high-functioning client with goals for increasing semantic, syntactic, or pragmatic skills within challenging contexts may be given more wait-time than a client with moderate intellectual disability who needs immediate interactions for best learning. Based on prior discussion regarding loquaciousness, waiting 3 to 5 seconds for clients to respond following questions or commands may be difficult. Fortunately, interactions not involving questions or commands do not require the 3 to 5 seconds wait time.

In summary, direct teaching is often required during the therapeutic process. SLPs are encouraged to develop skills in using various learning modalities, describing, demonstrating, questioning, and appropriate use of wait-time to enhance clinical skills. Activities associated with *Therapeutic-Specific Workshop: Form 7, including DVD Vignette 6* are designed to help with increasing these skills.

⊛ Stimulus Presentations: Shaping (Successive Approximations) *(Therapeutic-Specific Workshop: Form 8; DVD Vignette 7)*

Stimulus presentations, the methods used for presenting stimuli during therapy, vary according to the stage of therapy being addressed. Stimulus presentations may be as simple as a verbal model given to help the client understand how the /s/ phoneme should sound. However, some stimulus presentations are considerably more involved. For example, when trying to determine the best method of presenting a stimulus to a client experiencing difficulty understanding the concept for "over," the SLP may need to consider several parameters before proceeding. Aspects of direct teaching (presented in the prior section) will need to be considered, along with the concept of consistency in method of presentation. One commonly occurring aspect of therapy that requires consistency in presentation is the bridging of client skills between the time when the client is unable to produce the desired response and the eventual acceptable production of the response. This bridging concept is *shaping* or *successive approximations* and SLPs are encouraged to develop skills in effectively shaping client responses in therapy.

Shaping (successive approximations) is a technique used for obtaining responses that are not in the client's repertoire (Nicolosi, Harryman, & Kresheck, 2004). These researchers indicated several steps for *shaping* a client's response:

> First, the desired response is specified, and then responses which resemble that response (even remotely) are reinforced. Once the frequency of these responses has been increased, the subject must emit a response even more like the desired one; at this point, the technique is a special form of differential reinforcement. The criterion for reinforcement is continuously shifted in the direction of the desired response until that response is emitted, reinforced, and acquired. (p. 279)

Hegde (2008) reported that shaping, or successive approximations, was supported by experimental evidence and was viewed as highly useful in teaching a variety of skills. Hegde listed the following steps to take in using successive approximations.

1. Select a terminal target response (e.g., the production of /m/ in word initial positions)

2. Identify an initial component of that target response the client can imitate (e.g., putting the two lips together)

3. Identify intermediate responses (e.g., humming or other kinds of vocalizations, opening the mouth as humming is continued)

4. Teach the initial response by modeling an immediate positive reinforcement (e.g., putting the lips together on several trials)

5. In successive stages, teach the intermediate responses (e.g., adding humming when the lips are closed; opening the mouth when the humming is continued; adding other sounds to form words)

6. Continue until the terminal response is taught. (pp. 391–392)

To continue Hegde's example, if the terminal response is /m/ in the word *man,* the SLP should model and elicit the target word *man.* Once the client makes an error in producing /m/, the clinician immediately responds to the error by reinforcing the client's effort (attempt) to make /m/, telling the client what was correct about the /m/ sound, what aspects were incorrect about the /m/ sound, then modeling the correct /m/. The SLP then directs the client through a systematic sequence of shaping or successive approximations to elicit a correct /m/ in the word *man.* Four parts of the sequence are required at all phases of successive approximations to achieve correct production of /m/ in *man:* (a) telling the client what is about to be elicited, (b) modeling the structure to be elicited, (c) eliciting client's production of the modeled unit, and (d) reinforcing the client's effort. Note this progression in the sequence in Figure 6–6.

SLPs are encouraged to practice shaping, or successive approximations, for enhanced therapeutic skills. Activities associated with *Therapeutic-Specific Workshop: Form 8, including DVD Vignette 7* are designed to help with increasing these skills.

Positive Reinforcers: Verbal Praise, Tokens, and Primary Reinforcers *(Therapeutic-Specific Workshop: Form 9; DVD Vignette 8)*

Nicolosi et al. (2004) defined **positive reinforcers** as "anything, following a response, which increases the frequency of that response; may be extrinsic, such as a token, edible item, or money, or social, in the form of praise" (p. 263). *Positive reinforcers,* then, might take the form of the clinician's exclamation, "Great job!" or "Easy for you!" Gestures such as the high five, or other gestures of excitement such as handclapping, may serve as a positive reinforcer for some clients. For others, a statement in conversational tones such

Clinician	Client
Tell me *man.*	-an.
I saw you trying, and your lips almost touched together, but you left off the /m/. Tell me /m/.	/m/
Wonderful. Your lips touched together, and you made a strong "humming" sound. Now, let's put that sound back into your word. Let's break your word into two parts: /m/ an.	/m/ an
Perfect! Good /m/ sound; good "an." Now, let's put them a little closer together: /m/ an	/m/ an
Very good on both parts. Now, let's blend the sounds together: "man"	"man"
Great job! You made a good /m/ with your lips touching together, and you put that /m/ back into the word *man.*	

Figure 6–6. Shaping/successive approximations for eliciting /m/ in *man.*

as, "That was exactly correct; your tongue was in exactly the right place" is sufficient. SLPs are encouraged to become proficient in using verbal praise as a positive reinforcer and to *avoid the use of edibles as positive reinforcers if at all possible during therapy.*

Verbal Praise

Hegde (2008) described **verbal praise** as a type of reinforcement in which the client is praised for giving correct responses or for imitating modeled responses. Hegde offered the following suggestions regarding the use of verbal praise as a positive reinforcer.

- Praise the client promptly for producing or imitating a correct response
- Use such phrases as "Good Job!" "I like that!" "That was correct!" "Excellent!" and so forth; select the phrases and words that are appropriate for the client's age, education, and cultural background
- Deliver verbal praise in a natural manner, with appropriate emotion and facial expression

- Keep an accurate record of response frequency to make sure that the verbal consequences are indeed functioning as reinforcers (i.e., the response rate is increasing)
- Use other forms of reinforcers if verbal praise does not work (e.g., tokens or primary reinforcement). (p. 428)

SLPs are encouraged to become proficient in using verbal praise as a reinforcer. However, when verbal praise proves ineffective, additional reinforcers may be explored.

Tokens

Tokens are items that have little inherent value (chips, tickets, stars, marks on a tally sheet, etc.), but which may be given as a temporary reinforcer to be later exchanged for a **backup reinforcer**, something that the client does value (markers, book or video checkouts, etc.). A system of behavior management under the concept of *token economy* will be discussed later in this chapter. However, for purposes of this section, Hegde (2008) indicated that SLPs should set a low ratio in the beginning stages of using tokens as a reinforcer (e.g., a one-to-one [1:1] ratio in which one token may be exchanged for one backup item), then gradually increase the number of tokens needed to obtain the desired backup reinforcer. Backup reinforcers may be *tangible reinforcers* or *nontangible reinforcers*. **Tangible reinforcers**, nonedible items that are reinforcing, are used as rewards on occasion to provide variety in reward routines so that the effectiveness of a verbal (social) reinforcer is not diminished (Kerr & Nelson, 2002). For example, clinicians often use stickers as tangible rewards. **Nontangible reinforcers**, reinforcers that often constitute actions or activities as a reward, may also serve to provide variety in reinforcement routines. For example, a teenage female client with moderate intellectual disability was intrigued with fashion and makeup. She worked diligently in the clinic in exchange for the opportunity to pose for a photograph in the campus photo lab. Of course, this nontangible backup reinforcer of *posing for the photograph* eventually became a tangible backup reinforcer when the client was allowed to work toward the reward of obtaining the photograph to take home. Backup reinforcers should be items that are readily available, chosen by the client, and given in exchange on a predetermined ratio (Hegde, 2008).

Primary Reinforcers

Primary reinforcers are reinforcers that do not depend on prior learning and typically satisfy a biological need (e.g., hunger or thirst). Hegde (2008) suggested using primary reinforcers with clients who do not respond well to social reinforcers such as verbal praise. Hegde further suggested pairing the primary reinforcer with a social reinforcer and gradually withdrawing the primary reinforcer. Primary reinforcers for SLPs often take the form of **edible reinforcers**, food given as a *positive reinforcer* to increase the frequency of a desired response. Although there are clients for whom primary reinforcers seem most appropriate (young, nonverbal, low-functioning clients), Kerr and Nelson (2002) identified four difficulties with the use of edible reinforcers with students not responding well to *social reinforcers.*

1. The student must be hungry for food to be effective.
2. Food preferences negate the value of some foods as reinforcers.
3. Health factors such as food allergies and parental preferences must be taken into account.
4. Many schools have policies restricting the use of edible items in classrooms.

Additionally, because of possible undiagnosed swallowing disorders, SLPs are cautioned about the use of food as a reinforcer and should *avoid food as a reinforcer* whenever possible; the liability for mishaps related to giving a client food is simply too great, in many cases. Kerr and Nelson (2002) added that "fortunately, behavior analysis technology has advanced to the point where teachers seldom have to rely exclusively on edible reinforcement" (p. 140).

Regardless of whether positive reinforcers are tangible or nontangible, a *schedule of reinforcement,* how often the clinician reinforces following client responses, should be taken into consideration during therapeutic intervention. Two specific reinforcement schedules appear to have strong applicability to the speech-language pathology profession: a *continuous schedule of reinforcement* and an *intermittent schedule of reinforcement.* In a **continuous schedule of reinforcement**, the client receives a reinforcer following each response. In an **intermittent schedule of reinforcement**, the client receives a reinforcer only after a certain predetermined number of responses, for example, after 3, 5, or even 10 responses. A continuous schedule of reinforcement is often more powerful in the beginning stages of therapy, whereas the intermittent schedule of reinforcement is typically reserved for intermediate and advanced stages of therapy (Hegde, 2008).

In summary, SLPs are urged to take advantage of recent technology to avoid using food as a primary reinforcer when possible and to become proficient in using verbal praise, tokens, and primary reinforcers. Activities associated with *Therapeutic-Specific Workshop: Form 9, including DVD Vignette 8* are designed to help with increasing these skills.

⊛ Corrective Feedback in the Therapeutic Process *(Therapeutic-Specific Workshop: Form 10; DVD Vignette 9)*

Beginning SLPs often experience difficulty giving corrective feedback because of lack of confidence in pinpointing (a) whether a response was correct, or (b) what exactly about the response was correct or incorrect. **Corrective feedback** is the information the clinician gives the client regarding the quality, feature, or correctness of a preceding response. When the beginning clinician is unclear about the nature of that response, it is difficult to adequately give corrective feedback. Nonetheless, beginning SLPs are encouraged to think critically, and systematically, about the nature of client responses in efforts to develop skills in corrective feedback.

Corrective feedback is most often *verbal* and is based on the SLP's skills in correctly determining the correctness of client responses and communicating these findings to the client immediately after a response. The following steps are recommended for increasing accuracy of assessment of client responses.

1. *Increase knowledge of the objective/target in the client's response.* For example, if the target of client's response is the /s/ phoneme, the clinician should become familiar with the *place and manner* for the production of /s/ and should become comfortable with his or her own ear training for recognition of correct /s/ sounds.

2. *Compare the client's response to the expected target.*

3. *Task-analyze the response to help pinpoint specific features of the response for correctness.* For example, are the structures and functions of the articulators adequate for the /s/ sound production? Did the posture of the client's body adequately support correct production of /s/? Was the client's tongue in the correct place? Did the airstream achieve the directionality needed to be emitted from the mouth properly?

4. *Explain to the client the aspects of the target /s/ that were correct, based on results of the task-analysis.*

5. *Address the feature/aspect of the /s/ revealed as incorrect.* This step is accomplished through use of any number of techniques designed to teach and demonstrate correct production of /s/ through clinician model or through other presentation avenues.

Additionally, Hegde (2008) recommended minimizing the negative connotations associated with corrective feedback by giving more positive than negative points during corrective feedback. As a rule, always communicate to the client the aspects of production that were correct, first, then add the aspects that were incorrect along with the analysis of why the production was incorrect. Activities associated with *Therapeutic-Specific Workshop: Form 10, including DVD Vignette 9* are designed to help with increasing skills in corrective feedback.

⊛ Data Collection in the Therapeutic Process *(Therapeutic-Specific Workshop: Form 11; DVD Vignette 10)*

Data collection is recording client responses during the therapeutic session. There are any number of formats for taking data, and SLPs are encouraged to select a method that is both simple to manage on a daily basis and effective for accuracy in recording client responses. Some SLPs prefer a simple (+) or (–) system of data collection, whereby (+) equals a correct client response, and a (–) equals an incorrect client response. Others prefer a (1) or (✓) system where (1) equals a correct client response and (✓) equals an incorrect client response. Simpler, still, may be a system of "tick marks" as used in counting where a (I) equals a correct client response and an (X) equals an incorrect client response. Additionally, "clickers" for data collection are commercially available. Generally, SLPs may use any desired system for marking and tallying client responses as long as consistency in data collection is maintained.

Data collection forms, the form used to note or write results of the responses of clients for tally and analysis, are useful for data collection. Some forms are simple base-10 formats allowing up to 10 client responses to be recorded on a line or in a block. Other data collection forms are more creative and represent artistic flair in design. These forms may allow data collection on various shapes or colors set in the context of familiar themes. For example, there may be 30 brightly colored apples on a tree, with the 30 apples serving as the spaces for data collection of client responses or *clinical trials*.

Clinical trials are defined as structured opportunities for the client to produce a response in therapy. Hegde (2008) discussed a number of different opportunities for the client to respond during therapy intervention, that is, during establishment of baseline data and during treatment. Clinical trials also occur as part of evaluation/assessment when the clinician uses repeated opportunities for the client to respond in an effort to determine amounts of progress made on a specific therapeutic goal. For example, the clinician determines the percentages of correct productions on a specific objective by asking the client to repeatedly produce the target of the goal a specified number of times (clinical trials); the clinician determines the amount of progress by comparing the number of correct trials to the number of opportunities to produce the target. For example, if the client achieves 90% correct production of /k/, this result means that the client correctly produced /k/ 9 times out of 10 clinical trials. Computing the percentages of correct productions of targets on clinical trials is a widely used format of *collecting data* during collection of baseline data, therapeutic interaction, and assessment/evaluation activities.

The primary issue in taking data is more focused on consistency in taking data than in the method used or the forms on which tallies are made. SLPs are encouraged to become comfortable in managing data collection throughout a therapeutic session. Activities associated with *Therapeutic-Specific Workshop: Form 11, including DVD Vignette 10* are designed to help with increasing these skills.

Probing in the Therapeutic Process
(Therapeutic-Specific Workshop: Form 12; No DVD Vignette)

Probing is investigating a client's skills in producing nontargeted responses on the basis of generalization. For example, after 4 weeks of working on word initial /t/ using *take, tie, tell, top,* and *tide* as *exemplars*, or example words for training /t/, the SLP probes /t/ to determine production on nontargeted or generalized words such as *tax, toe, tame, tip,* and *toad.* Probes may be conducted in all areas of therapy (voice, fluency, language, etc.) and are used to (a) determine whether the targeted skills may be advanced to higher levels and (b) make dismissal decisions. Hegde and Davis (2005) noted "you cannot decide that a behavior (e.g., the /s/, the present progressive, oral resonance, normal voice quality, naming) is tentatively trained because the responses on selected training words or phrases have been correct. Instead, you conduct a probe" (p. 315). Hegde (2008) provided steps for conducting both *pure probes* and *intermixed probes,* whereby only nontargeted words (pure probe) versus both nontargeted and targeted words are used for the probe (intermixed). Productions of targets for a probe do not count toward the client's productions of targets for that session; the probe is strictly a planning tool.

Modified probes for articulation indicate if nontargeted **homorganic phonemes**, phonemes made in the same anatomical area, but different by one feature, often the manner of production, are positively impacted by work on the target. For example, /s/ and /t/ are homorganic phonemes; they are made in the same anatomical place, but in a different manner. Often correction of one of these phonemes appears to positively impact correct production of the other. A probe addressing the nontargeted phoneme in this case may be helpful, particularly if the nontargeted phoneme is being considered for targeting in the near future.

SLPs are encouraged to become comfortable using probes to determine the client's level of skills for a target not yet addressed during the treatment period. Activities associated with *Therapeutic-Specific Workshop: Form 12* are designed to help with increasing these skills. *(There is no DVD vignette for these skills.)*

Behavioral Management in the Therapeutic Process *(Therapeutic-Specific Workshop: Form 13; No DVD Vignette)*

SLP students often possess both the interpersonal communication and the therapeutic-specific skills needed to conduct effective speech-language therapy. However, many beginning-level SLPs experience difficulty in properly managing client behavior, thereby negating therapeutic effectiveness. It is extremely difficult, or impossible, to conduct effective therapy when clients are noncompliant, defensive, antagonistic, or are otherwise behaving in ways that are not conducive to participation in speech-language therapy. **Behavior management** is a system that the SLP uses to establish and maintain appropriate client behavior for therapeutic intervention. Miller (2002) discussed student behavior and behavior management programs and noted the following.

> Most students display appropriate behavior when academic expectations are clear; lessons are engaging and motivating with clear rationales; lessons are challenging, but within the students' capability; lessons are delivered effectively; and a positive, supportive atmosphere is evident. It is possible, however, for students to display behavioral difficulties in spite of the presence of strong academic and social programs. Thus, teachers must organize behavioral programs to address these difficulties should they emerge. (p. 86)

Several concepts presented in Miller's (2002) quote are significant for SLPs. To properly manage clients' behavior, it is important for SLPs to take the following steps.

1. Communicate clear clinical expectations.

2. Conduct therapy sessions that are engaging and motivating with clear rationales.

3. Establish clinical objectives that are challenging, but within the client's capabilities.

4. Deliver lessons or activities of the session effectively.

5. Create a positive, supportive atmosphere within the therapeutic setting.

However, when further behavioral management is needed within the therapeutic setting, SLPs should consider the establishment of either low-intensity or medium-intensity techniques for managing student behavior (Miller, 2002).

Low-Intensity Behavioral Management Techniques

Low-intensity behavioral management techniques include *establishing class rules, using specific praise,* and *ignoring behaviors* (Miller, 2002). Several researchers discussed the concept of establishing rules for classroom behavior (Kerr & Nelson, 2002; Miller, 2002). Miller (2002) indicated that *class rules* (a) communicate teacher expectations, (b) communicate a sense of fairness, (c) help build a climate of trust, and (d) help teachers determine the type of praise statements to use with students (Miller, 2002). For example, if the class rule is, "We respect our neighbor by listening when he or she is talking," teachers are able to easily link praise with the rule. The SLP might announce, "Kenitra, I like the way you are following our class rule on respecting others by listening to Lydia when she talks." Because of the importance of class rules in managing behavior, Miller (2002) advised that "before deciding upon class rules, teachers must think about whether or not they will be comfortable using and enforcing the rules with every student in their class" (p. 87). SLPs are encouraged to think through parameters of establishing class rules in a similar manner. Miller (2002) noted that regardless of the constellation of rules established in a classroom, general guidelines for developing rules are widely accepted. These rules include (a) limiting the number of rules to no more than three to four, (b) stating the rules in positive language, (c) aligning class rules with activity goals, and (d) posting class rules in a prominent location.

SLPs are encouraged to use *specific praise* as a part of behavioral management techniques. **Specific praise** refers to verbalizing to the student the specific aspect of behavior the student is performing well. For example, when Tim puts away his materials, the teacher might use specific praise by telling Tim, "You did a wonderful job of putting away your materials."

Miller (2002) indicated that occasionally students will continue an undesirable behavior because of the attention it attracts. In these instances, ***ignoring undesirable behaviors,*** a behavior management skill that is *planned* and used to negate a disruptive behavior each time it occurs, is advised. However, ignoring behaviors should not be used when someone's safety is jeopardized. Once the SLP determines that ignoring the behavior is the appropriate management technique, the technique should be applied consistently because (a) the undesirable behavior is likely to increase as the client works harder to get the teacher's attention; and (b) if the planned ignoring is not consistently applied, the client learns that escalating the undesirable behavior results in the client getting what he or she wants.

Based on Miller's (2002) work, the use of the classroom rules, specific praise, and ignoring undesirable behaviors are powerful behavioral management techniques when used together as the SLP's behavioral management program. SLPs are encouraged to practice these low-intensity behavioral management techniques and to employ them as the first rules of behavioral management. However, when undesirable behaviors persist, Miller (2002) recommended escalating behavioral management techniques to include *medium-intensity behavioral management techniques.*

Medium-Intensity Behavioral Management Techniques

Medium-intensity behavioral management techniques include *contingency contracting, token economy systems,* and *self-management strategies.* These strategies, by their natures, represent increased intensity for application requirements on the part of the SLP in addressing behavioral difficulties seen in clients. For example, they require more time and effort to implement, but Miller (2002) reported these behavioral management techniques to be reasonable for diverse classroom settings.

Contingency contracting is based on an agreement (verbal or written) between the client and the SLP regarding expected client behavior within the therapeutic setting. The concept of contingency contracting was first introduced by David Premack in 1959. Premack encouraged participation in nonpreferred activities by using preferred activities as a reinforcer. Premack's (1959) work became known as the *Premack Principle,* also known as *Grandma's Law* because grandmothers typically tell children things such as "You can have dessert as soon as you finish your vegetables." The Premack Principle, or *Grandma's Law,* gradually became known as contingency contracting (Homme, 1970). The general procedure for contingency contracting is deceptively simple: the clinician arranges the conditions so that the client gets to do something he or she wants to do following some-thing the SLP wants the client to do (Homme, 1970). Miller (2002) noted that contingency contracts, written documents developed by the SLP, should include the following:

- a statement related to the desired student(s) behavior
- terms or conditions of the agreement (e.g., time frame for demonstrating the desired behavior, amount of behavior required, amount of reinforcers, when the reinforcer will be available);
- a statement related to the activity or reinforcer that will be rewarded contingent on fulfilling the conditions of the contract;
- signatures of the student(s) and teacher. (pp. 90–91)

Smith, Polloway, Patton, and Dowdy (1998) found that to be most effective, contracts should (a) make some attempt to reward imperfect *approximations* of the desired behavior;

(b) provide frequent rewards; (c) reward accomplishments rather than obedience; and (d) be fair, clear, and positive.

Smith et al. (1998) also discussed three types of *group contingency contracts*, contingencies for groups, and reported these to be excellent alternatives for managing behavior of special needs children in regular classroom placement.

- *Dependent contingencies:* All group members share in the reinforcement if one individual achieves a goal (e.g., all children participate in a video party because one child achieved 100% correct production of a goal 2 consecutive days in therapy).

- *Interdependent contingencies:* All group members are reinforced if all collectively (or all individually) achieve the stated goal (e.g., all children participate in a video party because all children achieved 70% correct production of their phonemes by the end of the week).

- *Independent contingencies:* Individuals within the group are reinforced for individual achievements toward a goal (e.g., Anthony and Joe received passes to the book room because they each achieved their goals for the week).

Smith et al. (1998) reported that independent contingencies are most often used in classrooms, but that each type of contingency has specific value; they noted that the "benefit of group contingencies (or peer-mediated strategies, as they are often called) include the involvement of peers, the ability of teachers to enhance motivation, and increased efficiency for the teacher" (p. 370).

Tokens were discussed briefly in the positive reinforcers section of this chapter and were described as items that have little inherent value (chips, tickets, stars, marks on a tally sheet, etc.), but which may be given as a temporary reinforcer to be later exchanged for something that the client does value. Tokens relate directly to the use of *token economy systems* of behavior management, another medium-intensity behavioral management technique often used by SLPs. **Token economy** is a system of behavioral management involving nonsocial conditioned reinforcers (e.g., chips, points, paper clips, etc.) earned for exhibiting desired academic or social behaviors that may be exchanged for back-up reinforcers of predetermined token value (Kerr & Nelson, 2002). Token economy systems have been proven effective for managing student behavior (Miller, 2002). Kerr and Nelson (2002) indicated that the essential ingredients of a token economy system are (a) the tokens (items for which client will work), (b) backup reinforcers (tangibles or activities) for which tokens may be exchanged, (c) contingencies specifying the conditions under which tokens may be obtained or lost, and (d) the exchange rate of tokens for back-up reinforcers. The SLP employing a token economy system must decide these parameters. Miller (2002) suggested considering the following steps before implementing a token economy system.

Step 1: Determine which behaviors will result in earning tokens (may want to focus on three or fewer behaviors per student)

Step 2: Decide what will be used as tokens taking into consideration durability, expense, safety, attractiveness, and ease of dispensing (e.g., plastic chips, play money, points on a point card). Plastic chips are usually colorful, durable, and reinforcing. Play money provides opportunities to combine behavior management with teaching money skills. Point cards are easy to manage and less apt to result in ownership debates since the student's name is written on the card.

Step 3: Identify reinforcers that students will be motivated to earn and determine how many tokens each reinforcer will cost (e.g., 100 tokens = 5 minutes of computer time or 1 baseball card or 1 pencil sharpener; 200 tokens = 10 minutes to play a game or 1 comic book or 2 arcade tokens to use after school; 300 tokens = pass to media center or 1 baseball cap or 1 poster). More valuable items cost more tokens. Thus, students have the opportunity to practice deferred gratification and the value of saving.

Step 4: Decide whether to display the reinforcers in a classroom "store" (e.g., special bookcase or cabinet) or whether to list the items on a poster board. In either case, the number of required tokens should be indicated so students know what they have to earn. The store and/or poster will serve as a visual reminder to demonstrate the behaviors that result in earning tokens.

Step 5: Decide when students will be permitted to trade in earned tokens (e.g., as soon as they have enough or at designated times throughout the day or at the end of the day/class period).

Step 6: Establish rules for the token economy system (e.g., students should not be given tokens if they ask for them; students should not be allowed to take tokens from other students or give tokens to other students).

Step 7: Explain the token system and accompanying rules to students to ensure they understand what behaviors will result in earning tokens, how many are needed for the various reinforcers, and when the trading may occur. (pp. 94–95)

It is important to remember that when using a token economy system, the emphasis is on positive student behaviors. Miller (2002) recommended pairing verbal praise with the use of tokens to help with the transition into the student's acceptance of positive social reinforcers. Similarly, when the student misbehaves, make sure the verbal pairing to redirect the student is appropriate. For example, "As soon as you sit quietly, tokens can be earned." Miller (2002) reported that verbal cues, paired with tokens tend to redirect inappropriate behaviors while still maintaining a positive classroom atmosphere, particularly when the verbal reinforcer is used at an increasing quantity over time and the token ratios become greater and greater.

Both contingency contracting and token economy systems are teacher-directed medium-intensity behavior management systems. *Self-management strategies* also qualify as a medium-intensity behavior management system. However, ***self-management strategies*** are behavioral techniques that are student-directed and typically are instituted once teacher-directed behavior management strategies are demonstrated consistently. These include *self-monitoring, self-evaluation,* and *self-reinforcement* techniques. ***Self-monitoring*** requires the student to record the frequency of a particular behavior, usually on a card or other form. ***Self-evaluation*** requires students to compare their behavior to a preset standard to determine whether the criterion is being accomplished. *Self-reinforcement* involves having students reward or reinforce themselves following appropriate behavior (Miller, 2002). It is possible to use all three self-management techniques concurrently for a given student, but teacher support and suggestions for students using self-management may be needed, particularly when students are determining rewards and reinforcers.

High-Intensity Behavioral Management Techniques

High-intensity behavioral management techniques, which are highly structured behavioral programs and classrooms involving multiple individuals, are available to the SLP. Typically, when low- and medium-intensity techniques are not successful for behavioral management, the SLP works with several other professions (teachers, parents, behavioral specialists, etc.) to help the client facilitate positive behavioral changes (Miller, 2002). Often the behavioral changes needed, once a child is placed on high-intensity behavioral techniques, require the student's enrollment in special programs, and occasionally, special classes for children with behavioral disorders. It is likely that children who require high-intensity behavioral techniques exhibit behavioral difficulties across several areas of functioning including classroom, home, and social settings, in addition to behavioral difficulties exhibited in speech-language therapy.

Behavioral management techniques and skills are very important to the therapeutic process. Often clinicians with otherwise adequate clinical skills are rendered ineffective because of inability to manage client behavior. It, therefore, is important that SLPs understand the rudiments of choosing and developing an appropriate behavior management plan for clients experiencing behavioral difficulty in therapy. Activities associated with *Therapeutic-Specific Workshop: Form 13* are designed to help with increasing these skills. (*There is no DVD vignette for these skills.*)

Troubleshooting in the Therapeutic Process *(Therapeutic-Specific Workshop: Form 14; No DVD Vignette)*

Troubleshooting refers to the concept of constant *mental scanning,* whereby the SLP constantly looks for indicators of difficulty when therapy is not proceeding well. Often, the SLP is unable to make adequate professional judgments regarding the level of acceptability of various aspects of therapy as the session proceeds. Most often, this inability to troubleshoot occurs across two broad areas: *clinician-focused difficulties* or *client-focused* difficulties. Regardless of the cause of difficulties in therapy, the result is the same: lack of appropriate client progress in therapy.

As a general rule, SLPs are encouraged to assess their own behaviors in therapy as a beginning point of troubleshooting. *Clinician-focused difficulties* are difficulties the SLP experiences in therapy that result in ineffective therapy and lack of client progress. Difficulty in therapy for the SLP often takes the form of (a) ineffective interpersonal communication skills, (b) ineffective therapeutic-specific skills, and (c) lack of knowledge and skills in specific intervention programs needed to address client goals/objectives. SLPs must constantly scan to determine if difficulty in therapy is related to insufficient command of one or more clinical skills during the therapeutic process. Troubleshooting, for example, helps the SLP recognize a problem with fluency in therapy caused by poor preparation and organization or helps the SLP recognize difficulties with modeling or cueing. **Scanning** refers to asking questions, the right questions, about clinical skills and performances. Examples of questions that help the SLP determine if difficulty in therapy is clinician-focused follow.

1. Are my personal and interpersonal communication skills appropriate for working with this client?

2. Am I establishing the correct goals and objectives for this client?

3. Are those goals/objectives established at the correct levels? For example, are the goals too high, or too low, for this client's current levels of functioning?

4. Do I properly communicate goals, objectives, and expectations to this client?

5. Do I exhibit the proper level of enthusiasm for encouraging progress for this client?

6. Do I understand the specific components of the therapy program I am implementing?

7. Am I properly implementing each segment of the therapy program for my client (stuttering program, voice program, language program, articulation program, swallowing program, etc.)?

8. Am I accurately keeping data regarding the performance of my client?

9. Am I making the correct analysis of client performances on a consistent basis?

10. Am I making the correct plans and modifications based on client performances in therapy?

A second set of questions must also be addressed when therapy is not proceeding as well as hoped. These questions relate to client-focused difficulties. **Client-focused difficulties** are defined as difficulties that arise in therapy as a result of client behaviors that negatively impact progress in therapy. For example, the client may not be properly motivated for putting forth adequate effort in therapy, thus causing lack of sufficient progress. Typically, client-focused behaviors generate a shorter list because there are some client behaviors for which the SLP must ultimately take responsibility. For example, if a client lacks proper motivation for therapy, of course, some of that difficulty rests with the client. However, as the clinician, the person ultimately responsible for client progress, the lack of client motivation must be shared by the clinician. Examples of questions the SLP should ask when attempting to determine client-focused difficulties in therapy follow.

1. Does the client exhibit adequate motivation and enthusiasm for success in therapy?

2. Are there any hidden, inherent reasons for the client to negate or sabotage therapy? For example, does the client like the attention associated with

therapy, thereby rendering the prospect of improved communication or swallowing skills unattractive?

3. Does the client have proper family or other support for therapy progress?

Regardless of whether results of troubleshooting yield clinician-focused difficulty or client-focused difficulty, the SLP must develop skills in troubleshooting and take appropriate corrective actions to ensure adequate client progress in therapy.

Activities associated with *Therapeutic-Specific Workshop: Form 14* are designed to help with increasing these skills. *(There is no DVD vignette for these skills.)*

Summary

The 28 therapeutic-specific skills presented in this chapter are not all-inclusive of the skills needed by SLPs for providing effective speech-language therapy. However, it is believed that successful implementation of these 28 skills has a significant positive impact on therapy. SLPs implementing these skills should refer often to the 28 skills highlighted in this chapter through use of text, the 14 accompanying TSW Forms, along with the 10 DVD vignettes provided as learning supports.

Learning Tool

1. Work through the 28 skills in this chapter at a moderate pace using the 14 TSW Forms and the DVD accompaniments to help process information related to the 28 skills.

2. Task-analyze skills (segment skills into component parts) and practice the parts as needed. Put the parts together to develop comfort with the entire skill sequence.

3. Use peers to serve as "clients" as needed for your practices.

References

Ambady, N., & Rosenthal, R. (1992). Thin slices of expressive behavior as predictors of interpersonal consequences: A meta-analysis. *Psychological Bulletin, 111,* 256–274.

Bettencourt, E., Gillett, M., Gall, M. D., & Hull, R. (1983). Effects of teacher enthusiasm training on student on-task behavior and achievement. *American Educational Research Journal, 20*(4), 435–450.

Blanck, P. D., Rosenthal, R., Hart, A, J., & Bernieri, F. (1990). The measure of the judge: An empirically-based framework for exploring trial judges' behaviors. *Iowa Law Review, 75,* 653–684.

Brandt, R. (1995). Punished by reward? A conversation with Alfie Kohn. *Educational Leadership, 53,* 13–16.

Brophy, J. E. (1983). Research on the self-fulfilling prophecy and teacher expectations. *Journal of Educational Psychology, 75,* 631–661.

Burgoon, J. K., Stern, L. A., & Dillman, L. (1995). *Interpersonal adaptations: Dyadic interaction patterns.* New York, NY: Cambridge University Press.

Cegelka, P. T., & Berdine, W. H. (1995). *Effective instruction for students with learning difficulties.* Needham Heights, MA: Allyn & Bacon.

Chance, P. (1992). The reward of learning. *Phi Delta Kappan, 73,* 13–16.

Cotton, K. (1995). *Effective schooling practices: A research synthesis 1995 update.* Portland, OR: Northwest Regional Educational Laboratory.

Coulston, R., Oviatt, S., & Darves, C. (n.d.). *Amplitude convergence in children's conversational speech with animated personas.* Retrieved March 25, 2005, from http://www.cse.ogi.edu/CHCC

Eden, D. (1990). *Pygmalion in management: Productivity as a self-fulfilling prophecy.* Lexington, MA: Lexington Books.

Edmonds, R. (1979). Effective schools for the urban poor. *Educational Leadership, 37,* 15–18.

Feldman, R. S., & Theiss, A. J. (1982). Teacher and student as Pygmalions: Joint effects of teacher and student expectations. *Journal of Educational Psychology, 74,* 217–223.

Gall, M. (1984). Synthesis of research on teachers' questioning. *Educational Leadership, 42,* 40–47.

Good, T. L., & Brophy, J. E. (1984). *Teacher expectations.* New York, NY: Harper & Row.

Hegde, M. N. (2008). *Hegde's pocketguide to treatment in speech-language pathology* (3rd ed.). Clifton Park, NY: Delmar.

Hegde, M. N., & Davis, D. (2005). *Clinical methods and practicum in speech-language pathology* (4th ed.). New York, NY: Thomson Delmar Learning.

Homme, L. (1970). *How to use contingency contracting in the classroom.* Champaign, IL: Research Press.

Kerr, M. M., & Nelson, C. M. (2002). *Strategies for addressing behavior problems in the classroom* (4th ed.). Columbus, OH: Merrill Prentice Hall.

Klinnert, M. D., Campos, J. J., Sorce, J. F., Emde, R. N., & Svejda, M. (1983). Social referencing: Emotional expressions as behavior regulators. In R. Plutchnik & H. Kellerman (Eds.). *Emotions: Theory, research and experience. Volume 2: Emotions in early development.* Orlando, FL: Academic Press.

Learman, L. A., Avon, J., Everitt, D. E., & Rosenthal, R. (1990). Pygmalion in the nursing home: The effect of caregiver expectations on patient outcomes. *Journal of the American Geriatrics Society, 38,* 797–803.

Lewis, R. B., & Doorlag, D. H. (1991). *Teaching special students in the mainstream* (3rd ed.). New York, NY: Merrill.

Meyer, S. M. (2004). *Survival guide for the beginning speech-language clinician* (2nd ed.). Austin, TX: Pro-Ed.

Miller, P. (1988). *Nonverbal communication* (3rd ed.). Washington, DC: National Education Association.

Miller, S. P. (2002). *Validated practices for teaching students with diverse needs and abilities.* Boston, MA: Allyn & Bacon.

Mumme, D. L., Fernald, A., & Herrera, C. (1996). Infants' responses to facial and vocal emotional signals in a social referencing paradigm. *Child Development, 67,* 3219–3237.

Nass, C., & Lee, K. L. (2000). Does computer generated speech manifest personality? An experimental test of similarity-attraction. *Proceedings on the Conference on Human Factors in Computer Systems.* Chicago, IL: ACM Press

Nicolosi, L., Harryman, E., & Kresheck, J. (2004). *Terminology of communication disorders: Speech-language-hearing* (5th ed.). Baltimore, MD: Lippincott Williams & Wilkins.

Premack, D. (1959). Toward empirical behavior laws: I. Positive reinforcement. *Psychological Review, 66,* 219–233.

Reissland, N., & Shepherd, J. (2002). Gaze direction and maternal pitch in surprise-eliciting situations. *Infant Behavior & Development, 24,* 408–417.

Reith, H. J., & Polsgrove, L. (1994). Curriculum and instructional issues in teaching secondary students with learning disabilities. *Learning Disabilities Research and Practice, 9,* 118–126.

Ridling, Z. (1994, April). *The effects of three seating arrangements on teachers' use of selective interactive verbal behaviors.* Paper presented at the annual meeting of the American Educational Research Association, New Orleans, LA.

Rivera, D. M., & Smith, D. D. (1987). Influence of modeling on acquisition and generalization of computational skills: A summary of research findings from three sites. *Learning Disability Quarterly, 10,* 69–80.

Rose, R. L., Koorland, M. A., & Epstein, M. H. (1982). A review of applied behavior analysis interventions with learning disabled children. *Education and Treatment of Children, 5,* 411–458.

Rosenthal, R., & Jacobson, L. (1968). *Pygmalion in the classroom: Teacher expectation and pupil's intellectual development.* New York, NY: Holt, Rinehart and Winston.

Rowe, M. B. (1986). Wait time: Slowing down may be a way of speeding up! *Journal of Teacher Education, 37,* 43–50.

Sadker, M., & Sadker, D. (2005). *Teachers, schools and society* (7th ed.). New York, NY: McGraw-Hill.

Sills-Briegel, T. M. (1996). Teacher-student proximity and interactions in a computer laboratory and classroom. *Clearing House, 1*(70), 21–24.

Smith, M. L. (1980). Teacher expectations. *Evaluation in Education, 4,* 53–55.

Smith, T. E. C., Polloway, E. A., Patton, J. R., & Dowdy, C. A. (1998). *Teaching students with special needs in inclusive settings* (2nd ed.). Boston, MA: Allyn & Bacon.

Tobin, K. G. (1980). The effect of an extended wait time on science achievement. *Journal of Research in Science Teaching, 17,* 469–475.

Webster's II New Riverside Dictionary (Revised ed.). (1996). Boston, MA: Houghton Mifflin.

Wengel, M. (1992). *Seating arrangements: Changing with the times.* (Rep. No. PS 020682). Washington, DC: U.S. Department of Education, Office of Educational Research and Improvement. (ERIC Document Reproduction Service No. 348 153).

White, R. W. (1959). Motivation reconsidered: The concept of competence. *Psychological Review, 66,* 297–333.

Williams, T. R., & Butterfield, E. C. (1992). Advance organizers: A review of the research, Part I. *Journal of Technical Writing and Communication, 22,* 259–272.

Wortham, S., Contreras, M., & Davis, L. (1997, April). *The organization of space and activities among Latinos: A strategy for making school more culturally familiar.* Paper presented at the annual meeting of the American Educational Research Association, Chicago, IL.

7

Basic Structure Within the Therapeutic Process

Introduction

This chapter focuses on *three management concepts* related to the speech-language therapy structure: *time frames for therapy, individual versus group therapy,* and *heterogeneous versus homogeneous groups.* Additionally, this chapter focuses on *three basic divisions,* or *components,* of a typical speech-language therapy session: *the Introduction, the Body,* and *the Closing.* These management and component structures help the speech-language pathologist (SLP) organize therapy, and they serve as the foundations for the daily logistics of therapy planning.

Management Concepts for Therapy

SLPs receive similar entry-level training and must go through the same credentialing process before being granted the Certificate of Clinical Competence (CCC), known as Cs of the American Speech-Language Hearing Association (ASHA). However, after completing the initial credentialing process and receiving the ASHA-Cs, SLPs may choose to work in a number of different settings, including hospitals, private and public clinics, and schools. Additionally, many SLPs also choose to develop specialties in one or more areas of practice. For example, SLPs often choose to become specialists in voice, fluency, swallowing, articulation/phonology, language, or resonance, and many specialize in related subset areas of interest, as well. Although each area of academic and clinical practice of the profession is supported with guidelines, policies, procedures, best practices statements, research, or other literature related to the specific area of practice, there are aspects of clinical practice that the SLP must determine for him or herself, regardless of the work setting. The SLP may be responsible for decisions regarding the *time frames* to schedule a client in therapy, whether to schedule the client for *individual or group sessions*, and if in a group, whether to schedule the client in *heterogeneous or homogeneous groups*.

Time Frames for Therapy

Two primary time frames for therapeutic intervention are important: (a) how often the client should be seen in therapy weekly, called **frequency of therapy,** and (b) how much time, typically, in minutes, the client should be seen in therapy during each session, called **duration of therapy**. Additionally, it is important to note time in therapy over a number of months. For example, clients enrolled in schools often are prescribed therapy that is designed to span a 12-month period. However, clients receiving speech-language therapy in medical settings often receive recommendations for therapy for significantly shorter lengths of time.

Frequency and duration of therapy are determined based on a number of indicators including (a) type and severity of the client's speech-language disorder; (b) customary practices in the service facility. For example, it is common for clients in a hospital setting to be served 5 to 7 days of the week, whereas children seen in schools are typically served 2 to 3 times per week; and (c) client's tolerance and stamina for frequency and duration of therapy. Hegde and Davis (2005) discussed in detail other parameters to consider in making frequency and duration decisions and summarized those details. Three of Hegde and Davis's suggestions are listed below and apply regardless of work setting.

1. Schedule sessions to optimize the effectiveness of treatment.
2. Coordinate speech-language pathology services with other services.
3. Allow time for indirect services (paperwork, evaluations, conferences, and breaks). (p. 139)

Several additional factors also must be considered when determining the amount of time to schedule for a client. These additional factors include (a) client's support system to help with therapy needs, (b) client's financial resources for paying for speech-language therapy services, and occasionally, (c) time requirements of the specific programs or techniques needed to accomplish the client's goals of objectives. For example, clients with more severe disorders may be scheduled for more time per session, but a client with a limited support system at home may not be able to attend more than short periods in therapy at a time. Similarly, clients with limited financial resources may choose fewer sessions over time. Finally, clients enrolled in specific therapy programs (e.g., stuttering camps) may need to be seen for specific times based on requirement of the training program. A final consideration that impacts frequency and duration of services is the *model of services* selected for delivering therapy to the client.

The **model of services** refers to the management strategies used in scheduling clients for therapy. The models of services typically utilized by SLPs include (a) the **pull-out model**, a model of services in which clients are taken from their typical setting (pulled-out) and served in a designated "speech room," (b) the classroom *collaborative model*, a model of services whereby the SLP serves clients in their respective classrooms as a collaborative effort with the classroom teacher, and (c) the *consultative model*, a model of services in which the SLP works with the client's teachers, parents, or other professionals to address the needs of the client on a limited direct contact basis (Hegde & Davis, 2005). Hegde and Davis referred to two additional service models used by the SLP, the *pull-in model* in which the SLP goes into the client's classroom and works with the student individually or in a small group, thereby "pulling-in" the student, and the *language and speech classroom*, a classroom established as one of the instructional periods of the day whereby students go to the language and speech classroom as part of a regular routine of courses, typically instituted in secondary school. Each of these management models will impact scheduling for the client, particularly in schools; SLPs should take into consideration the service model under which the client will be served when determining the client's therapy schedule.

Individual Versus Group Therapy

Clients may be served in therapy within the constructs of either individual or group therapy. An *individual therapy session* means that the SLP works with only one client or student at a time. Some of the same concepts used in determining the frequency and duration of services apply when considering whether a client should be seen in individual or group settings. For example, SLPs should consider type and severity of the client's speech-language disorder and customary practices in the service facility when determining whether to schedule the client for individual versus group therapy. For some clients group therapy is recommended, whereas individual therapy may be best for other clients (Eisenson & Ogilvie, 1977; Hegde & Davis, 2005). For example, some clients will need to be served individually for a number of factors, including type and severity of their communication difficulties, whereas clients with less severe difficulties may be seen for less intense services. Meyer (2004) noted that individual therapy seems to be the easiest for beginning SLPs to learn and added that often SLPs transfer the one-to-one interaction between client and SLP in individual therapy inappropriately to group therapy. The result of this inappropriate interaction is *individual therapy in a group* (Meyer, 2004), a phenomenon often seen when SLPs fail to facilitate the interaction needed within the structure of group therapy. Although Meyer believed that it is easier to teach new SLPs to do individual therapy, then, progress into group therapy, some clinicians and clinical researchers supported the view that, due to the interactive nature of communication, group therapy should be the foundation for speech-language therapy (Backus & Beasley, 1951).

As indicated in Chapter 1, Backus and Beasley (1951) believed that "group instruction should form the core of speech therapy" and that "group membership should be non-segregated in respect to kinds of speech symptoms" (p. 5). Backus and Beasley, therefore, supported not only group therapy as the foundation for therapeutic intervention, but promoted *heterogeneous groups* as well. Based on the teachings of Backus and Beasley

(1951), beginning SLPs often are introduced to therapeutic intervention within the context of group work first, then proceed to individual therapy as an additional or alternative form of providing services to clients. In this manner, beginning SLPs are taught the true concept of *group therapy* and, thus, do not become guilty of promoting *individual therapy in a group*. Instead, the interactive nature of group therapy is introduced to the new SLP from the beginning of training and is kept ever present as a major aspect of therapy. As support for group therapy, Hegde and Davis (2005) suggested that "although students receiving individual treatment receive more of your individual attention, group treatment also has advantages. The group setting may better reflect students' school environment than does a student's interaction with only the speech-language pathologist" (p. 138).

Homogeneous Versus Heterogeneous Groups

When the SLP makes a decision to provide group therapy, an ensuing decision must then focus on whether to provide group therapy within a *homogeneous* setting or within a *heterogeneous* setting. **Homogeneous groups** are therapy groups in which all clients are working on the same or similar objectives (e.g., /s/ or /k/). **Heterogeneous groups** are therapy groups in which clients are working on different objectives, often from different disability categories (e.g., /s/, semantics for body parts, fluency). Hegde and Davis (2005) noted that even though children with different disorders may comprise a heterogeneous group, another consideration for heterogeneous grouping should be age levels and basic functioning abilities of the children in the group. Hegde and Davis suggested that when making a decision between wide variability in ages versus variability in disorders, "it may be better to group according to age, so that the students share certain comprehension and attention levels" (p. 46). The advantage of heterogeneous grouping is that it provides the SLP with the ability to facilitate interaction among clients in roles as peer models and peer evaluators. SLPs are encouraged to develop heterogeneous groups as often as possible to better achieve a communication environment representative of the social environments in which clients must communicate and to achieve group interaction.

Interactive Group Therapy

SLPs are encouraged to implement elements of *interactive group therapy* at all times during group sessions, whether working with homogeneous or heterogeneous groups. **Interactive group therapy** is a therapy structure in which each member of the group serves as a peer model or evaluator for the productions of others in the group in a fashion similar to conversational exchanges, such that it is often difficult to determine whose turn it is at the moment.

During interactive group therapy, each group member listens, models, evaluates, or otherwise supports the productions of others' targets or objectives throughout the session. Ultimately, the SLP establishes this interaction through direct instruction. For example, when Robin experiences difficulty constructing a sentence using the word *fruit,* the SLP directs David to "Let Robin hear your sentence using *fruit*," after which David models the sentence, "I like fruit." The following scenario is typical of an interactive articulation group session.

SLP:	Adrienne, tell me *like*.
Adrienne:	*Like*.
SLP:	Good, tell me *long*.
Adrienne:	*Long*.
SLP:	Wonderful, *last*.
Adrienne:	*Last*.
SLP:	Good job. *Look*.
Adrienne:	*Wook*.
SLP:	Adrienne, you were really working to make a good /l/ sound, but instead of /l/, you gave me /w/ at the beginning of that word. I need a good strong /l/ with the tongue tip up behind your front top teeth, like this, /l/.
	Sherrie, show Adrienne your /l/ sound.
Sherrie:	/l/.
SLP:	Great job, Sherrie. Your tongue was up behind the front top teeth.
	Caleb, show Adrienne /l/.
Caleb:	/l/.
SLP:	Good work, Caleb; you made a nice strong /l/ and your tongue was in the right place.
	Now, Adrienne, you try. Get your tongue up behind your front top teeth and let the air go out the sides of your tongue, like this /l/.
Adrienne:	/l/.
SLP:	Perfect, Adrienne, great /l/ sound. Did you guys hear her /l/ sound? (surveying other clients)
Sherrie:	(gives a thumbs up)
Caleb:	(nods head, yes)
SLP:	The /l/ was exactly right, with the tongue up behind the front top teeth. Way to go, Adrienne. Now, let's put the /l/ back into your word, nice and slow.

In this scenario, all three clients worked by listening, modeling, or evaluating Adrienne's production of /l/. Clients remain actively involved in learning and communicating, with no time for coloring, cutting, pasting, or idle sitting.

It is possible to use the elements of interactive group therapy in homogeneous groups. However, the peer models may not be as accurate, particularly if everyone is working on the same concept and all are progressing at about the same pace. This decrease in peer modeling opportunities is one reason why homogeneous groups may not be the most desirable group configuration for therapy. SLPs are encouraged to institute elements of interactive group therapy at all possible opportunities.

Components of the Therapy Session

Regardless of the amount of time scheduled in therapy or the model of service delivery implemented for the client, each therapy session is divided into three basic components: *the introduction, the body,* and *the closing.* See Chart 7–1 for an outline of the therapy session at a glance.

Each of the components of therapy listed in Chart 7–1 is discussed in detail in an effort to help the SLP understand how to structure a basic therapy session. Although any number of time configurations may be used for therapy, most often clients are scheduled for either 30-minute, 45-minute, or 60-minute sessions one to two times weekly. However, for this discussion, the 30-minute session will be outlined. See Chart 7–2 for a detailed explanation of therapy progression.

Chart 7–1. The therapy session at a glance.

The Speech-Language Therapy Session at a Glance

Introduction

    Greeting and Rapport

    Review of Previous Session

    Collection of or Mentioning of Homework

Body

    Establishment Phase

    Eliciting and Recording Phase

    Teaching Phase

Closing

    Review the Session's Objectives

    Summarize Client's Performances

    Homework

    Rewards and Dismissal

Chart 7–2. Detailed therapy progression.

Here's How to Do Therapy
Sequence of Events Within the Typical Speech-Language Therapy Session

Component	Time	Definition	Procedures and Examples	TSW Skills Likely Needed
I. INTRODUCTION	2–3 Minutes	The opening or beginning of the speech-language therapy session.	Sets the stage for the work of therapy by orienting clients to the session and addressing preliminary tasks of the session.	
• Greeting and Rapport		The initial portion of the therapy session, designed to set an amicable, amenable, learning atmosphere for therapy.	• Hi, Karen. It's nice to see you today. Great shirt! • Welcome to therapy, Mr. Griffin. You look alert today. (Begin adjusting seating as needed.)	1, 3, 4
• Review of Previous Session		A brief questioning by the clinician of what the client worked on in the previous session.	• What have you been working on in therapy? • Tell me the sounds you are working on in therapy. (Remind clients as needed.)	1, 3, 9
• Collection of or mentioning of Homework.		A brief reminder of tasks related to therapy that clients were asked to complete outside of therapy.	• Dad was supposed to help you with /k/ at home. Did you have a chance to do that? • Did you remember to bring your homework? (Take homework from client and put it aside. Do not take time to evaluate homework at this time, but thank client for bringing it.)	1, 3, 9, 13

Component	Time	Definition	Procedures and Examples	TSW Skills Likely Needed
II. BODY	24–26 Minutes	The component of therapy in which the client is introduced to, practices, and masters the relevant aspects and skills for improving communication abilities.	The part of therapy in which the major concepts and progressions of therapy take place.	
• Establishment Phase – State intended objective of the session. – Model or prompt the target at the intended level of work.		The first phase within the body of the session used to determine whether planned or intended levels of work for the current session may be addressed.	• Juan, you're working on /k/ in all positions of words. Let me hear these words to see how well you are doing with /k/, one word at a time: *cake, rake, making*. (Juan correctly produces 3 of the 4 /k/ phonemes.) Wonderful, Juan, you got 3 of the 4 /k/ sounds; let's see if you can get 90% correct for your words today.	1, 2, 3, 5, 6, 11

continues

Chart 7-2. *continued*

Component	Time	Definition	Procedures and Examples	TSW
– Elicit the target 3 to 5 times to determine if client's skills match the intended objective. – State the actual level of work for the session, based on client's responses. – Set expectation for productivity or goal for the session			(No effort for teaching is made during this phase of work, and therefore, no feedback between production attempts is given.) • Lisa, you're working on full breaths for fluency. Tell me these three sentences using full breaths, one at a time: *The car is red; She is running; Where is Jared?* (Lisa correctly produces all three of the sentences.) Easy for you, Lisa! You used full breaths for all three sentences. Let's try for 100% correct production of full breaths.	
• Eliciting and Recording Phase – Model and elicit the target at the established level as previously stated in the establishment phase. – Record the responses. – Reinforce client efforts, verbally or nonverbally. – Provide corrective feedback regarding the nature or quality of the client's responses.		Bringing forth or drawing out responses from clients and writing down a tally of correct and incorrect client responses.	• Juan, let's start on /k/ in all positions of words. (Prepare to take data on correct and incorrect responses.) – Tell me, one word at a time, *cup, keep, can, cast, call* (Juan produces all /k/ phonemes correctly, one word at a time). Wonderful, Juan, tell me, one at a time, *make, rack, pick, sock, looking.* (Juan produces all /k/ phonemes correctly.) Excellent work, Juan, you got all /k/ sounds right. Your tongue was humped up in the back exactly right. • Lisa, use full breaths before these sentences, one at a time: (Prepare to take data on correct and incorrect responses.) – *Jake and Melvin went to the store to buy candy. They were late for the theatre last night. When did the airplane arrive?* (Lisa correctly produces the full breath before each sentence.) Great work, Lisa, you used full breaths for all sentences. Your rhythm and rate were smooth and your words were clear. Great job. (Continue modeling, eliciting, recording, and corrective feedback until an error occurs.)	1, 3, 5, 6, 7, 9, 10, 11, 13

174

Component	Time	Definition	Procedures and Examples	TSW

• Teaching Phase
  – Verbally reinforce the effort.
  – Give corrective feedback.
  – Demonstrate or model the target at lower or lowest tolerance level.
  – Use others in the session to add peer-modeling and interaction.
  – Elicit the target from the client being directly taught.
  – Use successive approximations.
  – Provide one additional slowly produced target to help reinforce correct productions.
  – Give corrective feedback.
  – Return to eliciting and recording phase of therapy.
		The segment of therapy in which the concepts associated with the target are taught.	(Note: The Teaching Phase begins immediately following an error production. **Dispense with recording during this phase.**)
			• Kevin, you're really trying to make that sound.
			  – But, instead of /k/, you made /t/. You put your tongue up behind the front top teeth and made /t/ instead of making /k/ in the back of the mouth.
			  – I need for you to make a good /k/, tongue down in the front, and humped-up in the back. Push the air over the hump, /k/.
			  – Maggie, let Kevin hear your /k/ sound.
			  – Great Maggie. Now, Kevin, you try /k/.
			  – Good /k/, Kevin. Now, let's put the /k/ back into your word. Let's break the word into two parts: /k/----an. Good. Now, let's make the sounds closer together: /k/---an. Good. Now, let's blend the sounds slowly, like this, *can*. Good work, Kevin.
			  – Now, tell me one final word, nice and slow: *keep*. Good /k/ in *keep*.
			  – Kevin. Excellent work, your tongue was humped up in the back exactly right.
			(Return to the eliciting and recording phase of therapy.)
				1, 3, 5, 6, 7, 8, 9, 10, 13

Component	Time	Definition	Procedures and Examples	TSW Skills Likely Needed

III. CLOSING
 	
• Review the session's objectives.
• Summarize each client's performances during the session.
• Give assignments and instructions or demonstrations of homework
• Give rewards, if desired, and dismiss the session.
	2–3 Minutes	The activities at the end of the session designed to review and reiterate objectives and end the session.	**Designed to give the client information regarding performances during the session.**
			• Tracy, you worked on /s/ today.
			  – You got 84% correct production on the /s/ sound. Way to go!
			  – No homework today, but tell mother how well you did in therapy.
			Everyone gets a sticker today. Great work everyone. Good-bye.
				1, 2, 3, 9, 10, 11, 12, 14

Therapeutic-Specific Skills and Components of the Therapy Session

As indicated in the introduction to Part I of the text, it is not necessary to proceed with learning all 28 therapeutic-specific skills discussed in Chapter 6 before proceeding to the detailed therapy progression presented in Chart 7–2. For those interested in correlating the TSW skills in Chapter 6 with the components of the therapy session addressed in the current chapter, a reference to TSW skills likely needed for each component of therapy and its subparts is indicated in the right-hand column of Chart 7–2. The numbers in the right-hand column of Chart 7–2 refer to the TSW skills addressed in Chapter 6, which are listed and numbered below for ease of reference when working with Chart 7–2.

1. Motivation
2. ☮ **Communicating Expectations**
3. ☮ **Enthusiasm**, **Animation**, and **Volume** in the Therapeutic Process
4. ☮ **Seating Arrangements**, **Proximity**, and **Touch** in the Therapeutic Process
5. ☮ **Preparation**, **Pacing**, and **Fluency** for Therapeutic Momentum
6. ☮ Antecedents: **Alerting Stimuli**, **Cueing**, **Modeling**, and **Prompting**
7. ☮ Direct Teaching: **Learning Modalities**, Describing/Demonstrating, **Questioning**, and **Wait-Time**
8. ☮ Stimulus Presentation: **Shaping (Successive Approximations)**
9. ☮ Positive Reinforcers: **Verbal Praise**, **Tokens**, and **Primary Reinforcers**
10. ☮ **Corrective Feedback** in the Therapeutic Process
11. ☮ **Data Collection** in the Therapeutic Process
12. Probing in the Therapeutic Process
13. Behavioral Management in the Therapeutic Process
14. Troubleshooting in the Therapeutic Process

Introduction of the Session

The *introduction of the session* is the opening or beginning of the speech-language therapy session. This part of therapy is designed to set the stage for the work of therapy by orienting clients to the session and addressing preliminary tasks of the session. Typically, the introduction is comprised of (a) *greeting and rapport*, (b) *review of the previous session*, and (c) *collection of or mentioning of homework*; **the introduction should take no more than 2 to 3 minutes of the session**, depending on the number of clients in the session, whether there was a previous session to review, and whether there is homework to collect. The ***greeting and rapport*** is designed to set an amicable, amenable, learning atmosphere for therapy. It is established using conversational interactions with the client that include a simple greeting ("Hi"; "Hello") and an acknowledgment of the client in a brief exchange designed to put the client at ease. Whittler and Martin (2004) noted that "when a teacher shows he or she genuinely cares about a student it tends to set students apart from academic work and helps gain their cooperation, keeping them motivated and on task. Generally, this might be viewed as teachers having positive rapport with students" (p. 16). Often a compliment works well for putting the client at ease for positive rapport. The *review of the previous session* during the introduction is a brief questioning by the clinician of what the client worked on in the previous session. However, if the client does not readily respond with the correct answer, the SLP provides the answer and encourages the client to try to remember the next time because this is *not* a teaching phase of therapy, nor is it an assessment that requires a correct response; questioning regarding previous session's work during the introduction is merely a quick way to get the client's attention and serves as a focus for the session. The last component of the introduction of the session is *collection of or mentioning of homework*, a brief reminder of tasks related to therapy that clients were asked to complete outside of therapy. Clients are asked if they remembered to do homework or to bring homework if a tangible product is expected from the client. However, any homework brought in by the client is collected, but not assessed at this time. Verbal praise and encouragements are used to help clients focus on remembering to do or return homework, but only a brief mention of homework is made during the introduction. Figure 7–1 details an example of a typical introduction of the session for a small group. The SLP is mindful of time and works to get through the introduction as quickly as possible (within 2–3 minutes) so that as much time as possible remains for the actual work to be done in the session.

Working at a moderate pace, the entire introduction scenario of Figure 7–1 takes approximately 1 minute and 45 seconds, allowing for the responses of the clients to be slower because spontaneous communication interactions for the clients are generally a little slower than are elicited utterances. One additional activity that sometimes adds a few seconds to the time spent in the introduction is the adjustments of seating, proper establishment of proximity using the "hand-to-chin" rule (discussed in Chapter 6), or other ways to ensure that proper proximity is in place for best therapeutic interaction.

Body of the Session

The body of the session is where the actual "work" of the SLP takes place. Often students are told, in jest, that this is "the place where the SLP actually earns his or her pay" because the progression of the body of therapy is what separates SLPs from other professionals who also work with speech-language clients (parents, teachers, and others). Of course, such a jest is an oversimplification of roles and responsibilities for the SLP professional. The point, however, is that the body of the session is the part of therapy in which the major concepts and progressions of therapy take place. The *body of the session* is the component of therapy in which the client is introduced to, practices, and masters the relevant aspects and skills for improving communication abilities. There are several parts, or stages, of the body of the therapy session: (a) *establishment*, (b) *eliciting and recording data*, and (c) *teaching*.

Introduction of the Session	
Clinician	**Client**
Hi, Jacob. That's a great shirt.	Jacob: Hi.
Good morning, Megan. You look focused and ready to work today.	Megan: Good morning.
Hi, Reginal. You have a new hair cut; it looks great.	Reginal: Hi. My dad took me to get it cut.
He did? Wonderful. Reginal, what have you been working on in here?	Reginal: Words.
That's right. You've been working on new vocabulary words. Good remembering. Jacob, what have you been working on in here?	Jacob: The /s/ sound.
Perfect, Jacob, the /s/ was perfect. Megan, What have you been working on in here?	Megan: The, ah, ah, the, the.
Megan, you're working on /k/; let me hear /k/.	Megan: /k/.
Excellent, Megan! You are working on /k/. Way to go. Reginal, did you remember to bring your homework?	Reginal: No, I forgot.
Did you get to do your homework with dad?	Reginal: Yes, we did it.
Good; try to remember to bring it the next time. Jacob, did you bring your homework?	Jacob: Yes, here it is (hands paper to the clinician).
(Takes the homework and puts it aside for later evaluation.) Good job of remembering your homework, Jacob. Megan, you didn't have homework this time, right?	Megan: Right.

Figure 7–1. Example of script for introduction of the therapy session.

Approximately 24 to 26 minutes of a 30-minute therapy session are devoted to the body of the session, depending on number of minutes required for the introduction and closing segments of the session.

Establishment Phase of the Body

The primary task in the **establishment phase**, the first phase within the body of the session, is to determine whether planned or intended levels of work for the current session may be addressed. The SLP needs to perform the following four tasks for each client (whether group or individual therapy) in order to execute the requirements of the *establishment phase of the body of therapy*.

1. State the intended objective of the session for each client.
2. Model or prompt the target of the objective at the intended level of work for each client.
3. Elicit the target three to five times to determine if client's skills match the intended objective.
4. State the actual established level of work for the session for each client, depending on client responses at item 3.

The primary reason establishment is required is because of **regression-recoupment**, a phenomena whereby clients gain a certain level of success in therapy by the end of a given session, but due to the time between therapy sessions, the level of accomplishment in the prior therapy session may no longer exist. Regression-recoupment most often occurs during notable time spans between therapy sessions. For example, SLPs are often aware that the level of accomplishment of therapy objectives may be reduced for the client who has a holiday, or takes vacation, thereby missing up to 2 weeks of therapy (e.g., winter holidays, summer holidays, etc.). However, regression-recoupment occurs for some clients during normally scheduled therapy time, even when the client misses no sessions. For example, clients who are scheduled for therapy on Tuesdays and Thursdays may accomplish a desired level of skills production by the end of the therapy session on Thursday. However, by the time the client returns to therapy the following Tuesday, 4 days have passed, and the client often experiences regression of skills. The client often reaches acceptable levels in skills by the end of therapy on Thursday, again, only to have another 4 days pass before returning to therapy the following Tuesday. The SLP must compare data from week to week to determine the impact of regression on the client's progress in relation to how much effort is needed for the client to recoup the drop in skill levels due to lack of therapy between sessions. Establishment is important for all clients, but especially so for clients for whom regression-recoupment is notable. SLPs must, therefore, determine whether the planned or intended therapeutic activities may be implemented, based on the levels of current functioning, compared to levels last achieved in therapy. If possible, the session proceeds as planned; if not, the SLP must adjust plans and provide therapy at an appropriate level, most often at a lower level of accomplishment than intended.

Establishment is accomplished through assessment of correct production of an *imitative verbal task*. An **imitative verbal task** is verbal response following a modeled verbal stimulus that takes the same form as the stimulus (Hegde, 2008). For example, when assessing the imitative verbal task for the production of /s/ in initial positions of words, the clinician gives a verbal model stimulus, one word at a time, "soup," "sip," "safe." The client is then expected to imitate, or repeat back to the clinician, "soup," "sip," "safe," one word at a time, imitating the verbal model. The SLP's assessment of how well /s/ was produced in the stimulus words *soup, sip, safe* helps determine whether the client should work at the planned level for the current session, or whether the client should be moved back to easier or prior levels of production, for the first portion of the session. There are no hard and fast rules about the number of imitative verbal tasks the clinician must model for the client during the establishment phase of the body of therapy or during any other phase of therapy. Typically, during the establishment phase of therapy, the stimuli items associated with imitative verbal tasks are simple presentations designed to quickly determine mathematical majority. Meyer (2004) indicated that "the clinician should decide the number of times a stimulus will be presented prior to requesting the client to respond" (p. 303). To determine whether the majority of imitative verbal tasks were correct, it is recommended that the SLP stimulates using either three *or* five stimulus words. This makes it easy to quickly determine the mathematical majority for either correct or incorrect verbal imitative responses. If the majority of the responses are correct, the client works at the planned level of therapy for the session; if the majority of imitative verbal responses are incorrect, the SLP may choose to begin the client's work at an easier, ideally, more successful level for the first portion of the session, then return to the planned levels of work as the session progresses, if supported by successful client responses to the easier, or prior, levels of work. Figure 7–2 illustrates a typical progression for the establishment phase of the body of therapy.

The following are suggested guidelines regarding the establishment phase of the body of therapy.

1. Maintain a "minutes matter" attitude, and try to establish the beginning levels for the session for each client as quickly as possible, using three or five stimulus items per client.

2. The objective is to determine the best beginning level of work for the session so there is never any correction of client responses or teaching in the establishment phase.

3. Make a note of how much the client seems to regress between sessions as indicated by how often the client is placed at an easier or prior level of work at the beginning of a session. This information is helpful for decisions regarding homework between sessions, and is possibly helpful for administrative decisions regarding the need to either increase the frequency or duration of therapy over time.

Clinician	Client
Establishment Phase of the Body (Example for Heterogeneous Group)	
Everyone, let's see how well you are holding on to your sounds.	
Jacob, you're working on /s/. Tell me "Soup"	Jacob: Thoup.
Sip	Jacob: Sip.
Safe	Jacob: Safe.
You gave me <u>th</u> instead of a /s/ in the word *soup*, Jacob, but overall, you did well. You got two out of three right. Let's keep you on words for initial /s/ for today.	Jacob: Okay.
Reginal, you're working on vocabulary for transportation. Tell me, "I ride in a car."* (*Note: This stimulus sentence suggests that Reginal does not yet have a good grasp of the vocabulary for transportation, so only one imitative verbal task will be presented. If Reginal were more advanced in the skill, the clinician might ask him to name one, two, or three things that we ride in to establish his starting level for the session.)	Reginal: I ride in a car.
Very good, Reginal. You will continue learning the vocabulary for transportation today.	Reginal: Okay.
Megan, you're working on /k/ in the initial positions of words. Tell me "Keep"	Megan: Keep.
Kiss	Megan: Kiss.
Kit	Megan: Kit.
Wonderful, Megan. You made a good /k/ in all three of your words. We'll continue working on /k/ in initial positions of words today.	Megan: Okay.

Figure 7–2. Establishment phase of the body of therapy.

4. Remember that *establishment* is the place to *begin* therapy. The SLP may move across levels as logically desired, but there will need to be a separate data collection line for each level addressed. For example, the SLP may determine that the initial positions of words is the correct or established level for beginning work on /s/ for the session. However, 15 minutes into the session, the SLP may realize that the client is achieving approximately 98% correct production of /s/ in initial positions of words and, based on prior client productions, and pre-established criteria for advancing to another level, decides to advance the client's level of work to /s/ in final positions of words. The SLP needs to keep one data line for /s/ in initial positions of words and a separate data line for /s/ in final positions of words for this session. Data are transferred onto a data reporting sheet in similar fashion: one data entry for results of /s/ in initial positions of words and a separate data entry for results of /s/ in final positions of words.

Once the clinician has established the beginning places or levels for each client for the session, the SLP moves to the second phase of the body of therapy: eliciting and recording.

Eliciting and Recording Phase of the Body

The second phase in the body of the session is *eliciting and recording*. **Eliciting** is defined as bringing forth or drawing out (Nicolosi, Harryman, & Kresheck, 2004). Bringing forth or drawing out responses from clients is a major task during therapy. During the eliciting segments of therapy, the SLP models or demonstrates skills desired for the client's production. For example, if the SLP wants to hear the client correctly produce /s/, the SLP may elicit /s/ by modeling the sound, showing the client a written example of the *s* sound, using flash cards representing the /s/, or by offering other prompts designed to the help the client successfully produce /s/. **Recording** is writing down a tally of correct and incorrect client responses. Recording often is used synonymously with data collection, although in a stricter sense **data collection** comprises all actions of the SLP for gathering information that indicates the client's levels of performances across various tasks in therapy. Data collection may include recording the client's productions of responses, making informal mental notes of performances, observing the client in various settings, and so forth. However, the written accounts of the client's performances, the recordings of performances, are the more objective accounts.

The SLP needs to perform the following four tasks for each client (whether group or individual therapy) in order to implement the requirements of the eliciting and recording phase of the body of therapy.

1. Model and elicit the target of the objective at the established beginning level of therapy.

2. Record each response as it occurs using a consistent data recording notation system.

3. Reinforce (verbally or nonverbally) client's responses on a predetermined schedule of reinforcement (typically using a continuous schedule of reinforcement for beginning level teaching of skills and an intermittent schedule of reinforcement for intermediate and final stages of teaching skills. (See Chapter 6 at Positive Reinforcers.)

4. Provide corrective feedback regarding the nature or quality of the client's response. (Continue activities at items 1 through 4 until an error response occurs, or until a pre-established number of correct responses is produced.)

Eliciting and recording is often easily accomplished by manually making tick marks or other notations of correct or incorrect responses on a sheet of paper, prepared before therapy begins, or on more formalized data collection forms. Regardless of whether informal or formal data collection sheets are used, the SLP will need to select a notation system that is both easy to use and systematic. Meyer (2004) noted that, "When a clear-cut response is required, a choice of the following notations would be appropriate: 1 (correct) or (0) incorrect, + (correct), or − minus (incorrect), and Y(es) (correct) or N(o) (incorrect)" (p. 173). However, simple tick marks, using a | (correct) and X (incorrect) in a grouping of five tallies, works well, also. For example, ||||| for five correct responses is easily determined on quick visual inspection. Similarly, it is easy to see that ||||X represents four correct and one incorrect response in this grouping. Using this system of collecting data, 25 client responses for producing /s/ in the initial positions of words might look like this: ||||| ||||X |X||| X|||X |||||, for a total of 21 correct of 25 responses, with an accompanying percentage of 84% correct production for this example.

Meyer (2004) discussed two methods of keeping data for SLP clients: horizontal notations and vertical notations. ***Horizontal notations*** require a left-to-right progression in taking data across the page (e.g., ||||| ||||X |X|||), whereas ***vertical notations*** require a top-to-bottom orientation and method of data collection. In horizontal notations, the SLP begins taking data toward the left margin of the data collection sheet and moves to the right across the page as notations for either correct or incorrect client responses are made. Meyer (2004) discussed the difficulty in using a horizontal notation system because of the inability of the horizontal method to allow defined analysis of client's responses on second and third attempts. Meyer, instead, suggested that the beginning SLP adopt the practice of using a vertical notation system, whereby second and third client attempts to produce the objective may be more accurately noted and analyzed. Meyer's (2004) concepts regarding analysis of second and third client attempts at correct production are understandable; however, for purposes of this discussion, each client response during the eliciting and recording phase is treated as a single response for data collection purposes. For example, if a client produces an error, then self-corrects to a correct production, the client is recorded as having produced one incorrect, followed by one correct, response; there are essentially no second or third attempts toward correct productions when collecting data in this fashion. However, second, third, fourth, and beyond attempts at correct production do exist during the teaching phases of therapy. This concept is explained more fully in the teaching phases of the body of therapy. Because second and third attempts at correct production are not recorded in the eliciting and recording phase of therapy, SLPs are encouraged to try a horizontal method of data collection for this phase of therapy. As other types of therapy that necessitate analysis of second and third responses are learned, the SLP is encouraged to use data collection methods appropriate for those therapies, for example, Meyer's (2004) recommendation for vertical data collection. However, because of the nature of the eliciting and recording and its relationship to the teaching phase of therapy, once a client produces an error response, all data collection stops, and the teaching phase of therapy begins; there are just no opportunities for the client to produce second and third responses in this phase of therapy. As mentioned earlier, even when a client produces an error, then immediately self-corrects, he or she is given credit for one incorrect response and one correct response. However, even though the client self-corrected, he or she enters the teaching phase of the body of therapy because of the error response.

Students often are asked to collect samples of **data collection forms**, forms used to (a) notate the individual and specific responses of clients during therapy, or (b) report the overall totals for correct performances on objectives at the end of the session. Professionals often interchangeably use the term *data collection form* to refer to the form used in *data collection* and in *data reporting*. However, technically, *data collection* and **data reporting**, an indication of the *total* percentages of productions for the session, are two different activities and may be indicated on two different forms. For example, the SLP might take notes of correct and incorrect client responses on one sheet (a data collection sheet), then transfer the final percentage number onto another sheet (a data reporting sheet). However, this separation of forms is not always necessary because often one form contains a section for indicating both the ongoing tallies of data collections during the session and the final overall percentages of productions for data reporting at the end of the session. For ease of discussion, the term *data collection form* is used to indicate both *data collection* and *data reporting* activities, unless otherwise specified.

Data collection forms may be informal and basic with a simple base-10, or other consistent numerical base to help students easily calculate percentages of correct productions per client, per objective, per session. **Base-10 forms** are recording forms for notating client responses in multiples of 10. There are 10, 20, 30, 40, 50, and so forth spaces for making tick marks to indicate correct or incorrect client productions. Other data collection forms are commercially available, more oriented toward a theme (apples on a tree, feathers on a bird, etc.), and are associated with various programs or commercial publications. Students often are confused by the range of data collection forms available and are uncertain about how to actually use these forms in therapy, particularly in group therapy when data is being kept for several clients within a session. For ease in managing data collection with a high degree of consistency, SLPs are encouraged to do the following.

1. Use paper of any type for collecting data within the session. Some SLPs have been observed using a sheet of paper for collecting data that was so informal that the paper had been thrown in the trash can, but was retrieved from the trash and used for data collection for a therapy session. Of course, data collection forms that are this informal typically end up in the trash, anyway,

once the data has been calculated and transferred onto a more formal data reporting form that is kept in the client's working folder.

2. Use a consistent format of collecting data (e.g., +/−; 1/0; ✓/✗; ⊞; etc.) *for the first response only.* (Stop data collection and begin "teaching" once the client makes an error.)

3. Write each client's name along the left margin of the data collection paper in vertical fashion (e.g., one name is at the top of the page on the left margin, the second name is 8 to 10 spaces down the page on the left margin, and the third name is another 8 to 10 spaces down the page on the left margin. The 8 to 10 spaces between names allow space for listing the phoneme(s) or other objectives each client is working on under his or her name without crowding the space. To the right of each phoneme or other objective, the SLP will note pertinent information about how the data was collected, for example, imitated words, modeled sentences, approximated syllables, and so forth. Data will be recorded beside each phoneme or other objective for each client, using a left–right orientation along a horizontal line. (See Figure 7–3 for an example of a simple data collection form developed by an SLP for an articulation session.)

Ree

/k/ (I, W)   ⊞ IIIIX IXIII XIIIX ⊞

/l/ (F, W)   ⊞ IIIIX IXIII ⊞ IIIIX IXIII

/t/ (I, Syl)   ⊞ IIIIX IXIII XIIIX ⊞

Ambi

/s/ (Sen)   ⊞ IIIIX IXIII ⊞ IIIIX

/z/ (M, W)   ⊞ IIIIX IXIII XIIIX ⊞

/r/ (Place)   ⊞ IIIIX IXIII ⊞ IIIIX IXIII

Janice

/k/ (Sen)   ⊞ IIIIX IXIII XIIIX ⊞

/g/ (F, W)   ⊞ IIIIX ⊞ IIIIX IXIII

Legend: I = Initial position; M = Medial position; F = Final position; Syl = Syllables;
          W = Words; Sen = Sentences; Place = Placement

Figure 7–3. An example of a simple data collection format, using a horizontal data line. The SLP uses a sheet of paper to develop a "recording sheet" before each session. Once the session ends, the percentages are tallied, entered onto a more formal record or data reporting form, and the raw data is discarded. (*Note:* When writing data on a simple informal sheet such as this, always enter a date on the sheet in case it has to be stored for a day or so before the data are transferred onto a formal data reporting form in the official files.) Legend: *I* = Initial position; *M* = Medial position; *F* = Final position; *Syl* = Syllables; *W* = Words; *Sen* = Sentences; *Place* = Placement

4. Block responses in easy-to-read groups of 5 or 10 responses per grouping (5 responses per group appear to be easier to read quickly). Indicating groupings of responses makes it easy for the SLP to quickly determine when the client has been given ample opportunities to respond to the stimulus. For example, using the groupings of 5 responses, the SLP may quickly determine that each client was given 25, 30, 35, 40, or even 50 opportunities to respond to a stimulus during the therapy session. *(Although not as many responses are required for various types of therapy, when using traditional and other therapies based on traditional stimulation, the SLP should always aim for a minimum of 25 to 30 responses per phoneme addressed, per client if the client is working on no more than 3 to 4 phonemes. If fewer phonemes are being addressed, a minimum of 35 or 40 responses per sound should be obtained, depending on the number of clients in the session and the levels at which clients are working.)* Once the session ends, the SLP quickly tallies the percentage of correct production for each phoneme. This percentage number is then entered in the data reporting section of the data collection form, or if a separate form, the percentage for the session is entered on the *data reporting form* and dated. Just as SLPs are encouraged to indicate responses in groupings of 5 for ease in determining the number of response opportunities during data collection, SLPs are also encouraged to make data recording easier by predetermining the percentages of correct production for 25, 30, 35, 40, and 50 response opportunities and list these in a handy chart. This way, the SLP simply refers to the percentage chart to quickly access the correct percentages of productions while clients are transitioning in and out of the therapy setting. (Tip: *Always date the data collection sheet so that data results can be entered in the data reporting form section of the sheet or on a more formal data reporting form at a later time if the transition time is not sufficient for entering percentages for clients immediately following the therapy session.)*

During the eliciting and recording phase of the body of therapy, the primary tasks are to stimulate the client at appropriate levels and record the client's responses. This exchange continues under the concept of the "client's turn" until the client makes an error or produces a predetermined number of successful responses. Typically, 5 to 10 correct responses equals a client's turn. However, because of the interactive nature of therapy, an individual client's turn is not reserved for that client only, particularly when client responses are in error. During all phases of therapy, but particularly following an error response when the teaching phase begins, other clients are engaged in each client's turn in order to (a) enhance the interactive nature of the therapeutic process, and (b) keep all clients involved in the communicative aspects of the therapeutic process, regardless of whose "turn" it is by ensuring that all clients serve as models or evaluators for others as appropriate. In this way, SLPs learn to monitor client participation in therapy and encourage all clients to *contribute to therapy every 15 to 20 seconds.* This frequency of client participation ensures that the session is interactive and is, in fact, interactive group therapy, and not individual therapy in a group as discussed by Meyer (2004).

Once the client responds with an error, the SLP records the error response and immediately dispenses with further data collection for this client for this "turn" because the session now progresses to the *teaching phase* of the body for this client. Again, this is why there are no second or third trials per response attempt to record when collecting data.

Teaching Phase of the Body

The **teaching phase of the body** is the segment of therapy in which the *concepts* associated with the target are taught. The **concepts** associated with the speech-language targets are the actual constructs being taught in therapy and include any specific required underlying mental or physical actions or processes needed to change communication behavior. The physical or mental processes needed to change communication behavior might include *changing physical movements of the articulators, manipulating tension of the vocal folds to achieve a different desired pitch, determining similarities among three stimulus items*, and so forth. The SLP uses descriptions, demonstrations, learning modalities, or other teaching tools such as modeling, peer-modeling, placement, drills, and so forth to help the client achieve success with the underlying concepts or constructs associated with the target skills in therapy. The SLP needs to perform the following nine tasks for each client (whether group or individual therapy) in order to implement the requirements of the *teaching phase of the body of therapy.*

1. Verbally reinforce the client's *effort (effort only)* exhibited when the preceding error was made. For example, "I saw your tongue working hard to make the /t/ sound at the beginning of that word."

2. Provide corrective verbal feedback regarding the error response. For example, "But, you made the /k/ sound instead of the /t/ sound."

3. Demonstrate or model the target at lower or lowest *tolerance level* to teach or reteach the target. **Tolerance level** is that level of work at which the client experiences success. For example, the lowest tolerance level for the production of /t/ might be the isolation or placement level for a particular client. In this instance, the SLP demonstrates, models, teaches, or reteaches /t/ at the level of placement as follows: "The /t/ is made with the tongue tip up, slightly against the alveolar ridge right behind the front top teeth. Watch while I make the sound: /t/."

4. Use others in the session to add peer-modeling and the interactive effect to the teaching or re-teaching event. For example, "Sandra, show Kay how you get the tongue tip up behind the front top teeth." "Great, Sandra, your tongue was in the perfect place up behind your front top teeth." "Leslie, show Kay how to get the tongue up behind the front top teeth." "Wonderful Leslie, your tongue was exactly right."

5. Elicit the target from the client whose turn it is, the client receiving the direct "teaching" for the target based on peers' examples, if possible. (If the peers are unable to produce the target structure, the SLP models or shows the client the correct structure.)

6. Use *successive approximations* or *shaping techniques* (see Chapter 6) to bridge between the desirable target and the undesirable production and to rebuild the production to the desired target level.

7. Once successive approximations are complete and the client is back at target level, provide one slowly presented final opportunity for the client to accomplish his or her objective for this teaching phase. For example, "Slowly tell me 'time.'"

8. Give corrective feedback for the effort with the last slowly produce target. For example, "Wonderful /t/, Jason; your tongue was in up behind the front top teeth exactly right. Good work."

9. Return to eliciting and recording for the next client.

   (Note: Constantly monitor time during the teaching phase of the body of therapy and make concerted efforts to "bring the other clients into the session" under the concept of interactive group therapy by using them as peer models or evaluators. Do not allow more than approximately 15 to 20 seconds to pass without involving other clients interactively as models, evaluators, or as other supports for the client whose targets are being addressed at the moment.)

The teaching phase of the body of therapy is the underlying, bottom line level of work for the SLP. It is the place where the SLP best demonstrates his or her knowledge of the exact aspects of communication production that need to be addressed or "corrected" if the client is to achieve communication success on a consistent basis. *Clients are never asked to "try it one more time" as a part of "teaching" the underlying concepts needed for correcting communication behavior because trying it one more time does not add enough to the client's processing to impact the needed behavioral changes.* Asking the client to try it again does serve as a signal to the client that the first production was not correct, and it serves as a reminder that something needs to be done differently on second or third trials. However, asking the client to change communication behavior by having him or her try the production a second or third time without intervening (or "teaching") the underlying concepts that *help the client learn what to do to change communication behavior between trials* does not offer enough information for the client to make those changes independently. The processes of *teaching*, on the other hand, help the client learn what to do to independently change communication behavior. *Skills in teaching the concepts associated with changing communication behavior is what separates SLPs from other professions* who also have input into the client's communication behavior (classroom teachers, other related services professionals working with the client, parents, spouses, etc.). (See Chapter 10 Guided Practice in Articulation Therapy for an example of both the eliciting and recording and the teaching phases of therapy.)

Closing of the Session

The *closing of the session* constitutes the activities at the end of the session designed to review and reiterate objectives, and end the session. **Approximately 2 to 3 minutes are**

committed for the closing of the session. The SLP needs to perform the following four tasks for each client (whether group or individual therapy) in order to execute the requirements of the *closing of the session.*

1. Review the session's activities.

2. Summarize each client's progress for the session.

3. Give assignments and instructions or demonstrations of homework, if any.

4. Give rewards (if desired, or dictated by behavior management strategies) and dismiss the session.

(See Chapter 10 Guided Practice in Articulation Therapy for an example of the closing phase of the body of therapy.)

Summary

Just as it is important for SLPs to implement excellent clinical skills during each therapy session, it is equally important that the correct management and therapy component structures of the session are properly addressed. Scheduling the client for the appropriate amount of time in therapy, within an appropriate intervention setting, individual or group, is crucial for client successes in therapy. Regardless of the time and setting for therapy, it is important that the SLP understands and uses the constructs for the three divisions of therapy: the introduction, the body, and the closing.

Learning Tool

1. List at least three indicators that suggest the amount of time a client should be seen in therapy each week.

   _____

   _____

   _____

2. Briefly discuss your concepts related to group versus individual therapy.

   _____

   _____

   _____

3. List advantages of both heterogeneous and homogeneous groupings for therapy.

_____

_____

_____

4. List each component of the major divisions of a speech-language therapy session and briefly tell what should transpire within each section of those major components.

_____

_____

_____

References

Backus, O., & Beasley, J. (1951). *Speech therapy with children.* Cambridge, MA: Riverside Press.

Eisenson, J., & Ogilvie, M. (1977). *Speech correction in the schools* (4th ed.). New York, NY: Macmillan.

Hegde, M. N. (2008). *Hegde's pocketguide to treatment in speech-language pathology* (3rd ed.). Clifton Park, NY: Delmar.

Hegde, M. N., & Davis, D. (2005). *Clinical methods and practicum in speech-language pathol-ogy* (4th ed.). New York, NY: Thomson Delmar Learning.

Meyer, S. M. (2004). *Survival guide for the beginning speech-language clinician* (2nd ed.). Austin, TX: Pro-Ed.

Nicolosi, L., Harryman, E., & Kresheck, J. (2004). *Terminology of communication disorders: Speech-language-hearing* (5th ed.). Baltimore, MD: Lippincott Williams & Wilkins.

8

Peripheral Speech-Language Therapy Management Issues

Introduction

Often, the beginning speech-language pathology professional is overwhelmed with the daily management requirements of the profession: clients must be assessed; treatment decisions must be made; therapy must be scheduled; paperwork must be completed; materials must be selected, cleaned, and stored; and phone calls must be made—and all of this is often required *before* the clinician begins seeing the client for therapy. The SLP is often supported by administrative, clerical, or other professional personnel in the management of many peripheral tasks that must be accomplished for therapy to be successful. However, occasionally, the SLP him- or herself must manage these responsibilities without benefit of others. This chapter provides suggestions and strategies for managing the tasks that are not in and of themselves therapy, but are tasks that, without proper management, make therapy significantly less effective.

Transition from Diagnostic Assessment into Therapy

Clients may receive diagnosis of their speech-language disorder from a number of sources, including SLPs from private agencies, hospitals, or schools not affiliated with the SLP designated as the service provider for therapy. In these cases, the SLP responsible for therapy should accomplish several tasks before beginning therapy with the new client. Following is a list of rudimentary steps that should be accomplished for client management prior to therapy. (*Note:* Numerous other steps may also be necessary, depending on office procedures and support staff.)

1. Obtain written permission from the client, a guardian, or a caretaker to secure the files on the client per the ***Health Insurance Portability and Accountability Act of 1996 (HIPAA)***, national standards designed to protect individuals' medical records and other personal health information and to give patients more control over their health information.

2. Forward the appropriate written permission(s) to the prior service provider(s) along with a request for copies of the files on the client. Be prepared to pay for photocopying associated with obtaining those files.

3. Establish a current file for the client that is maintained in a secured location, with access to the files stipulated according to HIPAA laws.

4. Once prior files are received, log in the date the files were received and review them for pertinent information related to the following:
   - date of diagnostic assessment
   - findings of the assessment
   - recommendations
   - personnel completing the assessment

5. Determine whether the information received is sufficient for planning an adequate intervention program or whether additional diagnostic information is required.

6. Schedule and conduct any additional diagnostic measures necessary to obtain information needed for adequately preparing an intervention plan.

In cases in which the client is one that the SLP service provider was also the diagnostician for the client's speech-language diagnostic assessment, the SLP will have complied with all HIPAA requirements during initial assessment, leaving the SLP now able to proceed with decisions regarding the nature of therapy for the client.

Treatment Plans, Schedules, Progress Notes, and Dismissals

The SLP providing therapy, acting alone, often determines the goals and objectives of therapy for the client. However, occasionally, the SLP is part of a team that determines the goals and objectives for the client. In either case, the SLP should be prepared to serve as the expert in communication disorders so that as others suggest or question suggestions, the SLP will be able to provide the perspectives of the communication disorders profession on the client's behalf.

Treatment Plans

Goals and objectives are written in a number of formats and styles. Each employer typically has an established prototype for the way treatment plans are to be written to satisfy the requirements of third-party payers (insurance companies and governmental programs such as Medicaid and Medicare). School-based SLPs will find that SLP services are provided under the auspices of an Individualized Educational Plan (IEP). Each school system also has an established format for the way goals and objectives must be written to comply with requirements of the school system's interpretation and implementation of the laws affecting services to children under the system's IEP. SLPs are encouraged to inquire about the prototypes for established treatment plans per employment setting; writing the plans inappropriately may result in poorly communicated professional directions for the client and nonpayments for services.

Schedules

Schedules for speech-language therapy are determined based on the client's needs for intervention as discussed in Chapter 7 (*Time Frames for Therapy*) for frequency and duration of services. However, for ease in management, most therapy sessions are prescribed from a choice of time blocks, including 30-minute, 45-minute, and 60-minute sessions. Variability on those time blocks is possible, of course, as clients' needs dictate. Additionally, the SLP must determine the frequency of therapy for each client, whether once, twice, or three or more times weekly. The severity of the client's disorder, often classified as either mild, moderate, severe, or profound, is a primary determinant of the frequency of therapy for individual clients.

Progress Notes

Similarly, *progress notes* are written in a number of formats and styles. Each employer, whether private practice, hospitals, clinics, or public schools, typically has an established prototype for the way progress notes must be written to satisfy the requirements of federal laws and for acceptance by third-party payers. SLPs are encouraged to inquire about those prototypes for established progress notes per employment setting to avoid poorly communicated client progress and current status information.

Dismissals

Dismissal criteria, the standard used to determine if a client should be dismissed from therapy, varies from client to client and is dependent on several parameters:

1. the client's success in accomplishing all established goals on the treatment plan, including maintenance of the goals and objectives outside of therapy for a specified period of time

2. the client's plateau in progress at a place professionally judged to be the point of "maximal progress" at the time for the client

3. the client's or caregiver's expressed desire to discontinue therapy at the time

4. any other circumstance that precludes the client from continued benefit from speech-language services, for example, medical or related difficulties.

Start-Ups

SLPs rarely find themselves in a position of having to "start up," or establish from the beginning, a therapy program. Most often, the program and its caseload are inherited from a prior professional, and the SLP simply begins services as pre-established, making necessary changes as needed over time. In those instances when the SLP must start up a program, several considerations impact the decisions that must be made. Some of the considerations for the start-up of a program follow:

1. Compliance with applicable federal, state, and local laws and regulations

2. Fiscal responsibilities for personnel, physical plant, operations, and maintenance costs

3. Health and safety concerns for employees, clients, and visitors to the site

4. Employee relations and employee qualifications

5. Internal management systems for daily operations

6. Advertisement and public relations needs

In less requiring situations, for example, if devising a new speech-language program within an existing administrative order within a school, the SLP may only be responsible for ordering materials, assessing, placing, serving, and maintaining the caseload of clients. However, the American Speech-Language-Hearing Association (ASHA) developed a number of publications devoted to helping the SLP with establishing and maintaining successful speech-language programs. Professionals responsible for start-ups that are more requiring are encouraged to refer to these sources (ASHA, 2003; Golper & Brown, 2004).

Health and Safety Issues

The issues of infection control and practices in the speech-language pathology profession are not new. Flowers and Sooy (1987) were among the first to express concern with disease transmission by SLPs and introduced the profession to information regarding AIDS and the role of SLPs and audiologists in evaluating and treating patients with AIDS. McMillan and Willette (1988) further addressed infectious disease for SLPs and developed guidelines for avoiding such diseases. Additionally, initiatives by ASHA's Committee on Quality Assurance (1989, 1990, 1991) addressed the issues of infection control procedures for SLPs in accordance with the Centers for Disease Control (CDC) procedures (Smith, Brandell, Poynor, & Tatchell, 1993). Grube and Nunley (1995) noted that ASHA's guidelines included the following:

(a) during diagnostic procedures, hands should be washed before and after glove use; (b) glove use is recommended for any examination involving intraoral contact, using new gloves for each person; (c) glove use during treatment is not recommended unless intraoral contact is anticipated; (d) hand washing before and after each treatment session is recommended; (e) care should be taken to prevent the contamination by saliva of records and other items that do not lend themselves to disinfections; and (f) all surfaces and items, including equipment, toys, and materials, should be cleaned or disinfected following each evaluation or treatment session. (p. 15)

Grube and Nunley (1995) noted that no professional mandate or requirement for infection control for SLPs exists and that ASHA's Committee on Quality Assurance recommendations represented a "good faith" effort on the part of the profession "to do no harm" (p. 20). However, Smith, Brandell, Poynor, and Tatchell (1993) reported inconsistent compliance with ASHA recommendations on infection control. Surprisingly, however, 87% of SLPs trained on the job in infection control, and 62% of those not trained, took infectious control precautions in the evaluation and treatment of clients with communicable diseases (Grube & Nunley, 1995). Even though SLPs cite time constraints as a major issue in adhering to recommendations regarding infection control, Logan (2008) offered another incentive for SLPs to take precautions to avoid infectious diseases. Logan found that "adults die 300 times more often than children from diseases that are vaccine preventable" (p. 318). SLPs are urged to adhere to ASHA's Committee on Quality Assurance and work toward controlling infectious diseases in all aspects of professional practice.

Creating the Therapeutic Environment

Therapeutic environment is defined as the physical and psychological climate designed for the client's maximal involvement in the intervention process. This environment includes arranging the *physical setting* so that the client's best performances are promoted. Features of the therapeutic setting integral to the physical and psychological support of the client are:

- seating arrangements (addressed in Chapter 6)
- room size
- size and shape of furniture in the room
- colors of walls
- types and amounts of materials displayed on walls or otherwise visible in the therapy setting
- temperature of the room
- appropriate ventilation

- lighting in the room (overhead and direct vs. diffuse and indirect lighting)
- sounds inherent in the room (neighboring noises, fans or other ventilation system noises, lighting noises, etc.)
- odors/fragrances in the room

Considerations and manipulations of these features in settings for each client and each therapy session help create a supportive learning environment for the client and the clinician as well. Although creating a suitable therapeutic climate may appear superfluous, for some clients it is essential. For example, clients with TBI, autism, or aphasia may not tolerate certain sounds or direct lighting. Consideration of the psychological needs of these clients in the therapy setting is important. For others, decorating halls and other spaces with items that appeal to young children who come into the clinic may increase their feelings of comfort and familiarity with the therapy setting, and providing a waiting room furnished with comfortable chairs, current reading material, and adequate light for reading is viewed as not only thoughtful and caring, but as professional as well.

Client Files and Documentation

Often practicing SLPs are unsure how to structure client files for daily caseload management. Several options for arranging or structuring client files, from relatively simple hard-copy files, to more advanced computer-based file management systems, are available to the SLP. Regardless of the system selected, client files should be easily maintained and capable of adequately reflecting caseload management activities for the client. Typically, reflecting the caseload activities and needs of the client is accomplished through *documentation*, notations regarding activities associated with daily intervention and management of the client that often serve as an official record of professional–client interactions.

Client Files

Client file systems vary, but most often are selected based on work setting issues that dictate the kinds and amounts of information that should be maintained for each client. For example, an SLP working in schools may be required to maintain a file for each child on *due process*, documentation that the child's parents, or guardians, were informed, and gave their informed consent for the child to be assessed, labeled, and placed in speech-language therapy services as prescribed by law (Hallahan & Kauffman, 2000). Due process dictates that not only certain actions and activities are necessary to ensure proper treatment under the law, but also dictates time constraints that must be met for compliance. Because of seriousness of the legal issues that accompany due process paperwork for each child served in speech-language therapy in schools, officials often keep due process files under lock and key, with limited numbers of persons approved for access to the files. In these situations, SLPs often find it advantageous also to maintain "working files" for each child. Working files contain rudimentary information about daily attendance, progress toward goals, contacts with parents/guardians, and so forth, and are maintained in the SLP's physical work location, under lock and key, for quick and easy access by the SLP. Some information contained in the working files (contact with parents/guardians, and information on yearly progress toward goals, for example), is periodically transferred to the official due process files for review by appropriate committees. SLPs working under HIPAA laws may find it helpful, as well, to maintain working files, or daily charts related to client services and progress, in addition to the HIPAA charts maintained by office managers in hospitals, clinics, and skilled nursing facilities, depending on requirements or policies and procedures of the employing agent.

Documentation

A paraphrased concept among service providers working with special needs populations is that *"Documented equals done. Not documented equals not done!"* This is a simplistic, yet powerful, reminder of the importance of documentation. For the SLP, a cursory view of a client's working file, or daily chart, should indicate readily the following information:

1. service date for therapy

2. attendance: absences, and ideally, reasons for absences noted

3. goals/objectives addressed during each session attended

4. notation regarding client performances during the session (percentage correct productions; number of times objective attempted, with number of successes noted; clinician's subjective judgments regarding the proficiency, etc.)

5. brief note regarding recommendations for the next session (continuation; moves toward dismissal, etc.)

6. conversations with caregivers or other authorized service providers regarding the client, his or her progress, or lack thereof

7. any other information pertinent to tracking contact, communications, or other occurrences related to the client

Documentation records range from simplistic to elaborate, depending on work setting requirements. However, regardless of the nature of the documentation record, SLPs are encouraged to systematically document information related to client management. (See Figure 8–1 for an example of a simple documentation form.)

Materials Management

The concept of *"minutes matter"* in therapy was briefly mentioned toward the end of Chapter 2, and again in Chapter 6 under the concept of pace for therapeutic momentum. The discussions indicated that it is important to note how much time is spent getting out,

	Service File Documentation	
Client: _____	DOB: _____	File # _____
Date	**Activity**	**Service Provider**

Figure 8–1. Service file documentation form.

setting up, and putting away materials for therapy. In this section on Materials Management, it is important to note not only the time frame for handling materials in therapy, but also the type of materials chosen for therapy and the presentation of those materials.

Basic Therapy Kit

The *basic therapy kit* is a compilation of materials and items useful to the SLP in a wide range of therapeutic interactions with clients. For example, just as a physician might typically use a stethoscope when examining a wide range of patients, regardless of eventual diagnosis, so does the SLP use basic materials and items when interacting with a wide range of clients, regardless of disorder. Although specific assessment and treatment materials and equipment will be used by the SLP for particular activities of assessment and intervention, some materials serve as "staples" for the SLP who must quickly arrange interaction with clients, or in situations when the SLP travels from place to place in an itinerant position providing services and must collect and transport essential items rather than cart everything available. Figure 8–2 provides a materials list of basic items important to the SLP in providing services to clients for either informal cursory screenings or rudimentary exploratory initial therapy sessions.

Use of Games in Therapy

Speech-language pathologists were placed in schools after the 1975 implementation of P.L. 94-142 more so than in prior years. Along with the broad-based placement of SLPs in the educational setting, partly prompted by psycholinguistic models of speech and language development, came the professional practice of infusing the use of games into the therapeutic process. Weisberg, Zosh, Hirsh-Pasek, and Golinkoff (2013) reported four characteristics of play that tend to link play and language skills:

1. Many forms of play enlist symbolic thinking.

2. The social interaction inherent in many types of play may also feed language development.

3. The amount of language input available in play contributes to language development.

4. When children are in control of an interaction [such as play or a game], they are engaged. (pp. 43–44)

Webster's (1996) defined *game* as a way of diverting oneself through amusement. In a second definition, *Webster's* further defined a game as a competitive activity governed by specific rules. Results of an unpublished national survey of 1,000 experienced SLPs indicated that 68% of more than 700 respondents reported the use of games in therapy with children (Dwight, 2004). Based on these findings, it is likely that SLPs will continue using games in therapy. However, SLPs are encouraged to consider the following concepts when selecting and using games in therapy.

1. Be sure the game is designed to address the goal/objective being addressed in therapy.

2. Help clients remain focused on the communication event being addressed in therapy rather on concepts of the game itself.

3. Choose games that either have no specific rules or have rules that may be manipulated by the clinician to best address the communicative goal/objective of the client.

MATERIALS LIST
BASIC SPEECH-LANGUAGE THERAPY KIT FOR SLPs

Following is a list of materials that the SLP should collect and maintain.

1. **Large tote bag** (large enough to hold all items below with enough space left for maneuvering items in and out of bag easily)

2. **Mirror** (large enough for you to see both your face and the face of your client at the same time; nonbreakable mirror recommended if working with young clients)

3. **Tongue depressors** (sterile, and carefully maintained in a separate zip lock bag)

4. **Pen light**

5. **Tissues**

6. **Alcohol** (for cleaning materials)

7. **Hand sanitizing gel** (for personal use)

8. **Sterile gloves** (nonlatex; nonpowdered)

9. **Writing pad/paper** (blank)

10. **Water-based markers of various colors**

11. **Small hardcover picture book of common items** (animals, colors, transportation, foods, clothing, etc.)

12. **Interesting items for adolescents** (music DVDs, sports cards, celebrity photos, fashion photos, model autos, etc.)

13. **Interesting items for adults, particularly older adults** (era memorabilia, coins, photos of collectibles, but no guns, knives, or other items such as hammers or garden tools that could be used as a weapon, even if they are collectible)

14. **Small, interesting toys** (nothing small enough to fit into the inside of a roll of bathroom tissue; nothing pointed, sharp, or fragile; no latex items; no balloons, or other nonsafe items, or items manufactured for a child below age 3 years)
    - Trucks/cars
    - Figures of popular characters
    - stuffed animals
    - blocks or other stacking toys
    - form boards

15. **re-inforcers/rewards** (stickers and washable ink stamps work well; avoid very small items that might be swallowed)

16. **Any other objects likely to help elicit speech from a client** (remember that clients vary in ages and ability levels)

Figure 8–2. Materials list for basic speech-language therapy kit.

4. When working with groups using a game, make the game communicatively functional, time-efficient, and noncompetitive. Make three changes to traditional games to accomplish this.

   a. Eliminate secondary references for actions to be taken in the game. For example, do not have the client throw the die, and based on the throw, move spaces and *do what's indicated at that space*. Remove this secondary reference and have the client throw the die and perform his or her speech-language task or objective based on the number obtained on the initial die action. This saves time and allows more communicative productions or practices.

   b. Use one game board, one die or spinner, and only one game piece for advancing through the game. Each person throws the die or turns the spinner and everyone takes advantage of the throw or spin for producing his or her communication objective. This eliminates the idea of competition and allows clients to focus on goals of speech, not goals of the game.

   c. Further remove the competition by allowing all clients to perform during everyone's turn (see *Interactive Group Therapy* in Chapter 7. For example, if client *A* throws the die and gets a 5, have client *A* move the game piece five spaces and perform his communication task five times (saying the /k/ sound five times), but also allow everyone else in the group to listen, model, and evaluate interactively as client *A* performs his communication task. Everyone in the group performs his or her communication task five times also, immediately following *A*'s performance, one after the other. When all clients in the group have produced their speech tasks or objectives based on the number obtained on *A*'s die throwing, this constitutes the end of client *A*'s turn. Then, client *B* rolls the die and the cycle begins again, with *B* moving the game piece and performing her communication task for the number of times indicated by the die, followed immediately by every other client in the group who also performs his or her communication task the number of times indicated by *B*'s roll. This ends client *B*'s turn, and the third client in the group now rolls the die, moves the game piece, and performs his or her communication task, with others following suit. Once all clients in the group have rolled the die once, this completes a cycle, or round. The cycle then begins again, as in the previous manner, and so forth.

These three simple changes probably more than triple the number of opportunities the game offers for clients to practice their communication event, and it removes the competition because all clients perform the same number of tasks for each turn. When the game ends, everyone has worked diligently on communication skills, not on winning. The reward at the end is the same for all. Because the competition is removed, clients focus more on communication, and the clinician is able to stimulate interaction using models, examples, and feedback from other clients as each one works on his or her communication task.

5. Learn to adapt games in any ways possible to (a) increase the numbers of opportunities for clients to respond, (b) eliminate the element of competition, and (c) decrease wasted time.

Sanitizing Materials

Discussions earlier in this chapter addressed Health and Safety Issues and information related to the recommendations of ASHA's Committee on Quality Assurance that "all surfaces and items, including equipment, toys, and materials, should be cleaned or disinfected following each evaluation or treatment session" (Grube & Nunley, 1995, p. 15). This is quite a requiring recommendation, particularly when sessions for treatment often are separated by less than 5 minutes. However, one solution may be for SLPs to consider purchases of items that are easily and quickly wiped with a sanitizing cloth or, perhaps, items conducive to a quick sanitizing spray, then a quick wipe down. Another concept to consider is, perhaps, that fewer materials in therapy are better for some clients. With adequate use of some of the therapeutic-specific skills discussed in Chapter 6 (preparation, pace, animation, volume manipulations, etc.), perhaps the clinician may "become the therapy material" him or herself, thereby eliminating the need for large amounts of materials that require sanitizing. Another thought is that several of the items most popular in therapy might be purchased in duplicate and rotated for use throughout the day. This way, one item might be in use while its duplicate is being sanitized, particularly for sanitizing processes that require more than a few minutes.

Work Setting Issues

SLPs are often trained with the thought in mind that he or she may be the only SLP in a designated work setting. For example, in schools there may be 25 teachers, but only one SLP. Similarly, in a hospital setting, there may be numerous physicians, nurses, and other therapy professionals such as an occupational therapist, or a physical therapist, but only one SLP. To that end, the SLP must become proficient and efficient as a stand-alone professional capable of representing the views and perspectives of the communication disorders profession. However, the SLP must also function as a member of a team, regardless of work setting.

The SLP will function as part of a professional team responsible for assessments, services, and basic management of clients needing global services that include speech-language therapy. But, the SLP will serve as part of a larger team, a team that is comprised of the full spectrum of employees in the workplace. Receptionists, physical therapists, physicians, nurses, teachers, principals, housekeepers, occupational therapists, bus drivers, administrators, assistants, and so forth, comprise the full slate of team members of which the SLP will be a part. Typically, to the degree that a team member works well within the milieu of the team, the daily work tasks of the individual team member are more palatable; SLPs are no exception to this rule. Beginning SLPs often are told at the end of a clinical management course, "Remember, as a member of the workplace team, you must do your part to ensure the quality of services clients receive; often your part equals more than 50%."

Communication for Professional Collaboratives

SLPs will need to become proficient in writing a number of communications on behalf of clients seen in therapy. These include diagnostic reports, treatment plans, lesson plans, Individualized Education Plans (IEPs), Individual Family Service Plans (IFSPs), referral reports, requests for information from various sources as guided by HIPAA, progress reports, and discharge summaries. Most facilities or employers have established formats and prototypes for each of these written communications. However, Shipley and McAfee (2009) presented information on the development of written reports and offered examples of several different reports and requests for information from additional sources. Additionally, Hegde and Davis (2005) listed several suggestions related to enhancing written reports. They noted that, "although content is the most important element of your report, clear, concise presentation, neatness, and accurate use of vocabulary, grammar, spelling, and punctuation also are important" (p. 155). SLPs are encouraged to obtain prototypes of various reports from appropriate agencies (employers), to write the applicable report, proof the work, then ask someone from the agency to proofread it also. Make the necessary corrections before sending it out or before filing it.

Summary

The peripheral concerns of speech-language therapy addressed in this chapter impact the quality of therapy in several ways: preparedness for therapy, health and safety issues, quality and care of materials, and the quality of the relationships in the workplace. SLPs interested in providing good speech-language therapy to clients should ensure that the peripheral matters associated with therapy are properly managed.

Learning Tool

1. Discuss and list ideas related to sanitation of materials for therapy.

_____

_____

_____

2. Develop at least two new ways to use a game that (1) increase response opportunities for the client using the game, and (2) remove competition from the game. List below and share with peers.

_____

_____

_____

3. List ways that the environment within a therapy setting might be improved.

_____

_____

_____

References

American Speech-Language Hearing Association Committee on Quality Assurance. (1989). AIDS/HIV: Implications for speech-language pathologists and audiologists. *Asha, 31*(6), 33–38.

American Speech-Language Hearing Association Committee on Quality Assurance. (1990). AIDS/HIV: Implications for speech-language pathologists and audiologists. *Asha, 3*(11), 46–48.

American Speech-Language Hearing Association Committee on Quality Assurance. (1991). Chronic communicable diseases and risk management in the schools. *Language, Speech, and Hearing in the Schools, 22*, 345–352.

American Speech-Language Hearing Association. (2003). Knowledge and skills in business practices needed by speech-language pathologists in health care settings. *ASHA Supplement, 23*, 87–92.

Dwight, D. M. (2004, November). *SLPs' use of games in the therapeutic process.* Poster session presented at the American Speech-Language Hearing Association Annual Convention, Philadelphia, PA.

Flowers, W. M., & Sooy, C. D. (1987). AIDS: An introduction for speech-language pathologists and audiologists. *Asha, 29*(10), 25–30.

Golper, L. A. C., & Brown, J. E. (2004). *Business matters: A guide for speech-language pathologists.* Rockville, MD: American Speech-Language-Hearing Association.

Grube, M. M., & Nunley, R. L. (1995). Current infection control practices in speech-language pathology. *American Journal of Speech-Language Pathology, 4*, 14–23.

Hallahan, D. P., & Kauffman, J. M. (2000). *Exceptional learner: Introduction to special education* (8th ed.). Boston, MA: Allyn & Bacon.

Hegde, M. N., & Davis, D. (2005). *Clinical methods and practicum in speech-language pathology* (2nd ed.). New York, NY: Thomson Delmar Learning.

Logan, J. (2008). Adult vaccination: A commentary. *American Journal of Health Education, 39*(5), 318–320.

McMillan, M. O., & Willette, S. J. (1988). Aseptic technique: A procedure for preventing disease transmission in the practice environment. *Asha, 30*(10), 35–37.

Shipley, K. G., & McAfee, J. G. (2009). *Assessment in speech-language pathology: A resource manual* (4th ed.). New York, NY: Cengage.

Smith, K., Brandell, M. E., Poyner, R. E., & Tatchell, R. H. (1993). Infection control procedures in universities. *Asha, 35*(6), 59–62.

Webster's II New Riverside dictionary (Revised ed.). (1996). Boston, MA: Houghton Mifflin.

Weisberg, D. S., Zosh, J. M., Hirsh-Pasek, K., & Golinkoff, R. M. (2013). Talking it up: Play, language development, and the role of adult support. *American Journal of Play, 6*(1), 39–54.

PART

Introduction

Dreyfus and Dreyfus (1986) presented a model for learning that discussed five stages of perception that students go through in learning. These five stages include (1) novice, (2) advanced beginner, (3) competent, (4) proficient, and (5) expert levels of learning and perception in acquiring new skills. Dreyfus and Dreyfus indicated that the novice learner has little or no perception regarding the learning task, is analytical in decision making, and essentially does what he or she is told to do in the learning event. For example, one clinician remarked how, as a novice in her first clinical session, she was told to take the client, a 4-year-old boy, into the therapy room and play "Go Fish" for 30 minutes. The clinician reported having done what she was told to do, but years later she felt that she had no clue of what she was doing in therapy in that first session, nor did she understand why she was doing it. This is understandable. According to Dreyfus and Dreyfus (1986), it takes consistent and often guided mental processing for a learner to actually learn new information and to make the learning meaningful.

The information presented in Part II of this text has application for all levels of the Dreyfus and Dreyfus Model, except, perhaps, the expert level. The information presented in Part II is intended to help the student and professional acquire skills for moving into expert status in the profession; however, the nature of the text is such that the acquisition of expertise, itself, is not the focus of the text. It is believed, however, that even the expert who intuitively exemplifies the knowledge and skills of any one aspect of the profession may benefit from information in this text related to areas in which expertise has not yet been attained.

How to Use Part II of the Text

The specific examples or scenarios presented in the therapeutic progressions in Part II of this book were selected to highlight various aspects for professional development; each presents a possible therapeutic progression that helps the student and professional transition from novice to proficiency in understanding the skills necessary to promote client advances in communicative competence. Readers are encouraged to work through aspects of the guided practice in Part II in order to (a) develop an understanding of the concepts addressed in the specific therapy presented; (b) develop an understanding of the progression of therapy; (c) become comfortable with the flow of the therapy per area addressed; and (d) move toward competence, proficiency, and eventually expertise in conducting speech-language therapy. As mentioned earlier, much more study in any specific area is needed to acquire the knowledge and skills for expertise in any given area of therapy than is offered in this text. However, the practice opportunities offer a good start toward the clinician's eventual goals.

To maximize learning in each chapter of Part II, the clinician is encouraged to work through each chapter, one at a time, in the following manner.

1. Be prepared to read each chapter *several times* (reading through five to six times is customary) in order to begin developing a comfort level with, and an understanding of, the material being presented.

2. Read *aloud* to support the "think-out-loud" concept of learning promoted in Chapter 6 of this text as you work through each chapter. Reading aloud may seem silly, but numerous beginning SLPs reported it to be helpful in the early stages of practicing procedures associated with learning to do therapy. Practice reading the scripts aloud either (a) in front of a mirror, (b) using a large doll (one clinical instructor routinely passes out large Raggedy-Ann dolls in class when students are learning to do therapy so that they get the feeling of actually learning the script in relation to a client.), or (c) in front of a peer or other supporter, once the comfort level reaches the level of being ready for live *pseudo-interaction*. **Pseudo-interaction** is defined as interaction in which the clinician talks to another person who poses as a "client" for the SLP's learning purposes. However, the client's only contribution to the interaction is to model as a client so that the SLP's practice and learning of specific skills is enhanced. It is common to hear SLP's working with a live model or a doll say something along the lines of, "Oh, wait a minute. I should have said . . . hold on; let me go back to . . . ." The value of that kind of interaction is the belief that the SLP is thinking, processing, learning as she or he works through that type interaction without responsibility for what the client does or says at that point.

3. Focus on thoughts or concepts related to the 14 therapeutic-specific skills groups listed at the beginning of each chapter in Part II of the text. There are 28 different therapeutic-specific skills, grouped into 14 units for ease of discussion. A total of 21 of the 28 skills are addressed on the accompanying DVD for this text. As you read aloud the script provided for each chapter in Part II, think through your skills in demonstrating each of the 14 therapeutic-specific skills groups and try to determine whether your skills and thoughts are approaching effective levels of therapeutic intervention. As you proceed through repeated readings of the scripts in Part II, work toward achieving acceptable performances on two or three different therapeutic-specific skills during each reading. You will not always fully achieve the desired skills

level at first attempt, so do not despair if 5 to 6 minutes into the session, you realize you were not thinking about your skills in one of the selected areas of focus. After several readings of the procedures, when your comfort levels have increased, *you may choose to audio or video record yourself to get a clearer picture of your facial expressions, your general nonverbal communication patterns, and your verbal skills as you proceed through reading the scripts and learning the therapeutic-specific skills needed for success in therapy.* Remember, read aloud as you work and try to infuse the following therapeutic skills into your readings over time.

- Motivation
- ☺ **Communicating Expectations**
- ☺ **Enthusiasm, Animation**, and **Volume** in the Therapeutic Process
- ☺ **Seating Arrangements, Proximity**, and **Touch** in the Therapeutic Process
- ☺ **Preparation, Pacing**, and **Fluency** for Therapeutic Momentum
- ☺ Antecedents: **Alerting Stimuli, Cueing, Modeling**, and **Prompting**
- ☺ Direct Teaching: **Learning Modalities**, Describing/Demonstrating, **Questioning**, and **Wait-Time**
- ☺ Stimulus Presentation: **Shaping (Successive Approximations)**
- ☺ Positive Reinforcers: **Verbal Praise, Tokens**, and **Primary Reinforcers**
- ☺ **Corrective Feedback** in the Therapeutic Process
- ☺ **Data Collection** in the Therapeutic Process
- Probing in the Therapeutic Process
- Behavioral Management in the Therapeutic Process
- Troubleshooting in the Therapeutic Process

4. Remember the Dreyfus and Dreyfus (1986) model of learning and the five stages of perception for the learner (novice, advanced beginner, competent, proficient, and expert). Remain focused on increasing skills from one perceptual stage to the next over time. Practicing the scripted information does help the SLP learn the necessary therapeutic sequences for advancing toward proficiency, and the practice does transfer to new learning situations over time.

5. *Showtime!*

Reference

Dreyfus, H. L., & Dreyfus, S. E. (1986). *Mind over machine.* New York, NY: The Free Press.

9

Guided Practice in Language-Based Therapy

Selected General Concepts for Language-Based Therapy

Language therapy in its purest form may include a plethora of goals, objectives, and activities. Any therapy that addresses client needs for improving aspects of language, from very fine, specific, and minute concepts related to identified needs across semantics, syntax, morphology, phonology, or pragmatics (and any combinations thereof), technically qualifies as language therapy. However, for purposes of this discussion, clarity is being offered to introduce another concept that is somewhat distinguishable from language therapy, in its purest sense. Language-based therapy is a therapy design whereby the SLP establishes naturalistic conversational interaction that serves as the stimulus for all goals and objectives in therapy. Language-based therapy requires the SLP to use a conversational sentence as the basic stimulus, with therapy progressions based on, at a minimum,

(a) a teaching situation that is structured to provide a corrective "emotional" experience, such as a client receiving something in exchange for using language (or attempting to use some aspect of language), and

(b) a teaching experience that is structured to involve conversational speech so that the client perceives the give and take of conversational interaction in forms other than questions–answers. (Backus & Beasley, 1951)

Numerous researchers contributed concepts related to language therapy with dozens of invaluable techniques and countless ideas for therapy stemming from their efforts (Bates, 1976; Bloom & Lahey, 1978; Brown, 1973; Chomsky, 1957; Piaget, 1926; Skinner, 1957). However, for purposes of this discussion, the following are selected concepts that appear to be integral to language-based therapy.

1. Clients may require language therapy for *receptive language disorders, expressive language disorders,* or *both receptive and expressive language disorders.* Whenever receptive and expressive language disorders are present as part of the client's language difficulties, typically it is best to focus on receptive language skills first: give the client an *understanding* (reception) of concepts, vocabulary, and so forth, before asking the client to *use* (express) the vocabulary or talk about the concept. This will, of course, vary with some clients because of the nature of the disorder. Also, when broad-based disorders, such as articulation and language disorders, or language and fluency disorders, are present for an individual client, it may be advantageous to begin addressing both disorders simultaneously, depending, of course, on client skills and tolerance levels.

2. Language therapy may be conducted as *indirect language therapy* or as *direct language therapy.* **Indirect language therapy** is designed for very young children and other clients who operate essentially as nonverbal, even if the client uses a few one-word utterances occasionally. Hegde (2008) and Paul (2011) described indirect language therapy as a more naturalistic, less structured, play-oriented therapy based on the assumption that variables observed in normally developing children are effective clinical treatment strategies for children who are reluctant talkers. Hegde (2008) added, however, that more research is needed to support the use of indirect language therapy techniques. Although the research base for determining the effectiveness of SLP's use of indirect language stimulation techniques with the developing child may not be as prevalent as desired, the naturally occurring indirect communicative interactions typically observed between a young child and an adult are well documented (Becker, 1994; Bryant, 1999; Gleason, 2005) and form the basis of indirect language stimulation techniques for the SLP. Naturally occurring indirect communication interactions between a young child and an adult involve the adult's use of the following communicative techniques: *descriptions, self-talk, parallel-talk, expansions, extensions,* and *recasts.* Descriptions, self-talk, parallel-talk and, as the client begins using a few more words, expansions, extensions, and recasts are ideal techniques for beginning interactions with young clients who have not yet become proficient enough with communicative interactions to verbally impact their environment (Polloway, Patton, & Serna, 2001).

Descriptions are very elementary communicative interactions in which the adult labels or describes what he or she believes the child is *seeing.* This is a systematic attempt to connect the child with the environment by bringing to focus elements in the environment that may momentarily command the child's attention or focus. For example, the child may briefly look at or focus on a toy car placed on the floor. Once the clinician notes that the child is looking at the car, the clinician says, "You see the car," and perhaps, repeats the sentence for emphasis, *"You see the car."* As the child's gaze focuses on another item within the environment (whether contrived as when the SLP places the item in the child's environment or whether occurring more naturally as when the child focuses on an item of clothing worn by the SLP), the SLP again expresses a sentence to connect the child's focus to a labeled item in the environment. For example, when someone closes a door in the next office, and the child looks toward the sound, the clinician says, "You heard the door close." Hegde (2008) described *self-talk* as an indirect language technique in which the SLP describes what he or she is doing as the child looks on. For example, the SLP stacks blocks while at the same time says, "I'm stacking blocks." Hegde further discussed indirect language therapy and noted that *parallel-talk* requires the SLP to describe or comment on what the *child* is doing. For example, when the child picks up a car and touches a tire, the SLP says, "You're picking up the car; you're touching the tire." Description, self-talk, and parallel-talk are useful when the child is not using words. Later, however, when even one word is used by the child, the SLP may use expansions, extensions, and recasts.

Expansions are additions to the child's one- to two-word utterances to approach more *grammatical correctness*. For example, the child says, "Doggie." The SLP then says, "Doggie big," or "Doggie is barking," depending on objectives and language skills of the child. For example, often in language therapy, the objective is to expand a child's mean length utterance (MLU) to a level of 1 unit beyond the child's customary utterance. In this case, if a child produces an MLU of 1 in most expressions, the SLP may choose to stimulate the child with an MLU of 2 units. In other cases, the SLP may choose to expand all utterances to grammatically more correct utterances with minimal regard for the MLU expressions of the client. *Extensions*, sometimes referred to as *expansion-plus* are expansions of the child's utterance, plus the expression of an additional unit of information. For example, when the child says "Doggie," the SLP says, "Doggie is barking. The doggie is big." During use of *recasts*, Fey, Long, and Finestack (2003) indicated that the SLP changes the child's utterance into a different *type* of utterance. For example, if the child says, "Doggie big," the SLP says, "Wow, the doggie is big," or "Is the doggie big?" Both Hegde (2008) and Fey et al. (2003) suggested that SLPs using indirect therapy (a) arrange play situations and materials that are relevant for the desired target response, (b) allow the child to lead the interaction based on his or her desired play interests, and (c) refrain from requiring the child to imitate modeled responses. Indirect therapy techniques are seen as nonintrusive, interactive, and therapeutic when used correctly for appropriate clients.

Although typically reserved for use with clients who are very young, nonverbal, or very near nonverbal (MLU sporadically may equal 1.0), indirect therapy has been used successfully with older verbal clients who presented with behavioral or other difficulties that negatively impacted interactions during speech therapy sessions. Note the following scenario:

> A fourth-grade child who was intellectually advanced, but who also had a diagnosis that manifested in oppositional defiance behaviors was seen in school-based therapy for difficulty with the central vowel /ɝ/. During routine group therapy sequences for the introduction of therapy, clients were always asked what they were working on in therapy. For each therapy session, twice weekly, when asked what he was working on in therapy, this client routinely responded with the word, "Nothing." Rather

than set up a mental battle, or disciple challenge for the client, the SLP immediately incorporated indirect therapy techniques for this very verbal, very bright, and very oppositional client, by responding, "You're working on /ɝ/. /ɝ/ is made by . . . [with the SLP describing the many aspects of placement in order to properly make /ɝ/], and it sounds like this: /ɝ/, in words such as *her, girl, were, shirt, hurt. /ɝ/.*" The SLP conducted therapy in this indirect manner for this client twice weekly for an entire school year with the client never having practiced the /ɝ/during therapy. During the body of therapy, when it was this client's "turn" to pointedly practice his phoneme, the SLP provided the same indirect techniques, using preselected exemplar words for therapy for that week. The only change in the SLP's behavior was a change in the list of different exemplar words over time so that the client was able to hear a large repertoire of words containing the /ɝ/ phonemes. This repertoire included first, one-syllable words containing /ɝ/, then two-syllable exemplars, and so forth. Eventually, the SLP also added a list of exemplars that included the unstressed /ɚ/ such as *painter, butter, runner,* and so forth. Toward the end of the school year, the exemplar list included combined uses of both /ɝ/ and /ɚ/ in sentences for words such as *worker, flirter,* and *shirker.* As would be expected in any progression of traditional articulation therapy, the uses of both the /ɝ/ and the /ɚ/ were modeled and exemplified by the SLP for the client in placement, isolation, syllable, word, phrase, and sentence levels in the typical progression, the same as if the client were actually producing the responses himself. Occasionally, the SLP incorporated aspects of the interactive nature of therapy into indirect therapy by asking other members of the group to correctly model /ɝ/ without ever insisting that the target client (the oppositional client) repeat the words or sentences. Of course, there was no data to collect on the oppositional client's productions, but notes were kept regarding the SLP's indirect technique presentations so that plans for successive sessions could be appropriately made from week-to-week for therapy.

At the end of the school year, during a parent conference (with the oppositional client present), the SLP reviewed the goals and objectives for the client, reported the format of therapy, and added that the client had not made any productions of the phoneme during therapy, but that he attended well and listened well during therapy. The client then interjected that he could make those sounds, and proceeded to do so—with 100% accuracy—using approximately 15 of the words that had been used as exemplar words in therapy over the school year. Of course, the SLP was delighted and immediately established new goals and objectives for the client, with the full intent of continuing to use indirect therapy techniques, if needed.

Indirect language techniques are typically used in individual language therapy sessions. However, as shown in the scenario (above), it is possible to successfully use indirect therapy in group settings, with proper understanding of the uses of the techniques, and with proper planning.

Direct language therapy is for clients who routinely use verbal expression as the primary mode of communication, but with significant delays or disorders in language skills. Direct stimulation across all areas of language, such as the areas discussed in this chapter, is appropriate for this type of client in either individual or group settings. In direct language therapy, "the clinician selects specific language targets, designs a treatment environment and implements the treatment; uses specific stimuli such as modeling, prompting, and manual guidance; uses explicit reinforcement contingencies; expects the child to imitate or produce specific targets upon stimulation; moves through a planned sequence of treatment stages" (Hegde, 2001, p. 331). Additionally, Fey et al. (2003) presented principles of grammar facilitation for children with specific language impairments. Among the principles presented by Fey et al. (2003) was the concept of manipulating the child's social, physical, and language-learning environment in order to provide opportunities for the child to use the targeted forms/concepts of the language session. These "manipulated environments" are often referred to as "contrived" (planned and devised) language-learning settings. More information related to the therapy will be presented later in this chapter under *"planning for the session."*

3. Clients in language therapy may be of developmental age (birth through early adolescence) or of adult ages (adolescence through old age).

4. Selection of materials for teaching language concepts depends on the objectives addressed; however, the age of the client, regardless of the nature or severity of the language disorder, should also be addressed. To the degree possible, always select age-appropriate materials for clients.

5. *Use sentences as the basic level of stimulation for your client when possible.* For example, in articulation therapies, the sound, the word, or even bi-syllables, may be the basic unit of stimulation, but in direct language-based therapy, the stimulation is generally given in sentences when possible. For example, the SLP stimulates the client, by using the sentence, a command, or a directive such as, "Tell me, 'The ball is blue,'" or "Tell me, 'She is running,'" or "Ask me, 'May I get one?'" However, for clients working on certain objectives (increasing MLU, for example), giving a complete sentence may not be possible because the client may only be capable of one- or two-word utterances at a time. For example, it may only be possible to stimulate with, "Tell me, 'See car,'" rather than, "Tell me, 'I see the car,'" for the client who has an MLU of 1.0, and is being stimulated at an MLU level of 2.0 as an appropriate goal.

6. When trying to increase a client's MLU in therapy, stimulate the client at one morpheme higher than the client typically produces during spontaneous speech. For example, if the client says, "Doggie bye-bye," the stimulation from the SLP is generally one unit more, such as, "Dog go bye-bye."

7. Goals for clients in language therapy often center on the following skills.

☑ **Semantics:** Concepts, vocabulary, relationships, events, and so forth related to an object, idea, person, or place (Bloom & Lahey, 1978). For example, *ice-cream cake, Mardi Gras, elephant* are all concepts that have associated with them vocabulary, events, and so forth that a client may address, depending on individual needs, of course. For this reason, selecting a "theme" through which to introduce, discuss, and teach concepts, vocabulary, relationships, and so forth often works well. For example, the theme "Birthday Party" may work well for teaching the concept and vocabulary associated with *ice-cream cake*.

☑ **Syntax:** Rules governing the order of words in a sentence (Bloom & Lahey, 1978). Syntax addresses grammar and parts of speech, subject–verb agreement, and understanding and use of sentence types (declarative, interrogative, etc.), and question forms.

☑ **Morphology:** Understanding and use of the smallest meaning units in language (Bloom & Lahey, 1978). Brown (1973) discussed 14 grammatical morphemes. However, because of the relationship between some morphological expressions and the phonemes used for those expressions, of particular importance for receptive and expressive morphological skills in therapy are the following five grammatical morphemes.

  - *Plurals* (regular forms are expressed by use of /s/, or /z/ at ends of words). For example, *books* where the s is pronounced as /s/ and *boys* where the s is pronounced as /z/.

  - *Possessives* (regular forms are expressed by use of /s/, or /z/ at ends of words). For example, *Beth's house* where the s is pronounced as /s/ and *John's house* where the s is pronounced as /z/.

  - *Third-person singular* (regular forms are expressed by use of /s/ or /z/ at ends of words). For example, *walks* where the s is pronounced as /s/ and *begs* where the s is pronounced as /z/.

  - *Past tense* (regular forms are spelled using ed at the ends of words and expressed as /t/ or /d/). For example, *looked* where the ed is pronounced as /t/ and *hugged* where the ed is pronounced as /d/.

  - *Present progressive* (expressed by use of /ŋ/). For example *running* where the ing is expressed primarily as /ŋ/.

☑ **Phonology:** Study of the sound system associated with language (Bloom & Lahey, 1978). Of particular importance are the sounds that are used as morphemes, as just discussed (/s/, /z/, /t/, /d/, and /ŋ/), although all sounds hold importance in communication.

☑ **Pragmatics:** The appropriate use of language in context (Bloom & Lahey, 1978). Pragmatics addresses intent to communicate, attention and focus, topic skills such as topic maintenance and topic change, and turn-taking skills.

Of course, for each area described there are other concepts and many more examples that might be offered. However, drawing from the information given in these selected general concepts, it is hoped that the reader understands the text well enough to process the information and examples throughout the remainder of this section on language therapy.

Selected Language Objectives

Semantics

Following are examples of semantics objectives for language therapy.

1. Client will correctly identify/point to 8 of 10 fruits when named by the clinician.
2. Client will correctly label/name five body parts when presented by the clinician.

Syntax

Following are examples of syntax objectives for language therapy.

1. Client will correctly identify four of five complete sentences spoken by the clinician.
2. Client will correctly use four-word sentences to express desires.

Morphology

Following are examples of morphology objectives for language therapy.

1. Client will correctly identify/point to 8 of 10 pictured regular plural nouns.
2. Client will correctly use the morphological inflections /s/ or /z/ to name four of five pictured plural nouns.

Phonology

Following are examples of phonology objectives for language therapy.

1. Client will correctly identify final consonant deletions (open syllables) in 8 of 10 occurrences in spoken words.
2. Client will eliminate final consonant deletion in 8 of 10 spoken words.

Pragmatics

Following are examples of pragmatic objectives for language therapy.

1. Client will correctly identify appropriate topics for four of five presented scenarios using pictured prompts.
2. Client will correctly exhibit appropriate turn-taking behaviors during four of five conversational exchanges.

Selecting Appropriate Materials for Therapy Based on Identified Objectives

One of the 28 therapeutic-specific skills identified for the SLP is *preparation,* whereby the SLP appropriately plans the session and selects materials that best support the identified objectives of all clients in the session. This type preparation is sometimes not customary for the SLP, so care must be taken to ensure that appropriate materials support the SLP's desired stimulus sentences for each client.

In planning and preparing for language-based therapy, it is common to present stimulation based on a *theme* or a *global topic* that allows the clinician to weave in numerous concepts around a central theme. This theme is often referred to as a **thematic unit**, a topic selected as the foundation for discussion and presentation in language-based therapy. For example, *transportation, body parts,* and *summer vacations* are all global topics from which a theme may be developed, thereby, allowing the introduction of numerous concepts related to the topic or theme. Materials and stimulus techniques may center on the theme as the SLP addresses specific language goals for the client. It is common for the goals of *direct language therapy* to center on improvements in semantic, syntactic, morphological, phonological, or pragmatic language skills, but in *language-based therapy* it is also possible to focus as well on fluency, voice, or resonance difficulty, once planning and material selections for the session are understood.

Preparation and Therapy Progression for the Language-Based Therapy Session

Ultimately, the goal of therapy should be to improve communication skills, not simply increase skills in isolated aspects of language. Each clinical supervisor or instructor likely has a preferred way of teaching SLP students to plan for respective aspects of therapy. However, the purpose of this discussion is to perhaps add clarity to the specifics of planning to help with implementation of language-based therapy, particularly as related to language-based therapy for heterogeneous groups of clients.

The key to planning language-based therapy for heterogeneous groups is to first plan for addressing the client who is working on a semantic unit (vocabulary, concepts, etc.), then, add-on considerations for the remaining clients in the session. For example, in a session that includes (a) a client working on the concept of "red," (b) a client working on increasing MLU to 3.0 (the client is currently speaking at an MLU of 2.0), and (c) a client working on the /k/ phoneme, the SLP should plan first for how to offer the stimulus sentence or command for the client working on the color *red.* Three things need to be considered in designing the therapy session to address, first the needs of the child working on the semantic concept, and then the needs of the remaining clients:

1. Consider the materials needed to support teaching the concept of *red* (or any other semantic concept to be addressed). The SLP selects materials that

offer multiple opportunities for client exposure to the concept of red. *This exposure should have a very low reliance on questioning the client. Instead, SLPs are encouraged to make deposits in the client's semantic learning by expanding client experiences rather than using questions to teach the client.* The materials selected may be centered around a theme where red is a dominant color (holidays, fruits, ball clubs, etc.), or the materials may be an accumulation of various (seemingly random) materials that are all, or are mostly, red in color; for example, *red* car, *red* ball, *red* box, *red* telephone, *red* cookie cutter, and so forth. It is recommended that approximately 15 items related to the semantic concept are accumulated for a 30-minute therapy session involving a group of three clients. This allows each client to participate in a minimum of five different "turns" using a different item of material for each client's "turn." If items are exhausted prior to the end of the session, the SLP simply re-cycles items for the remainder of the session. The term "re-cycles" is used because once a client selects an item from a container, and the SLP works with the item with each client in the session, the item is deposited in a separate container so that the next client does not run the risk of selecting the same item that a prior client selected. Materials are managed in this way simply as a matter of interest for the session in that it's more interesting if, on every client's "turn," a different item is selected.

2. Once the materials needed for the session are accumulated for the client working on a semantic concept, consider the needs of the remainder of the clients to be sure that appropriate sentence stimulations will work in conjunction with the materials selected for the client with semantic needs. For example, it is customary for the client working on semantics to be given a stimulus sentence such as, "Ask me, 'May I get one?'" as a way of giving the client the language to command the environment in order to get what he or she wants. The actual focus of therapy for the concept of *red* begins *after* the semantics client has selected something from the container, whereas the focus of therapy for the MLU client and for the phoneme client (the /k/ client in this example) begins *before* they select something from the container. As the SLP considers a number of stimulus sentences and determines that several sentences will work for the semantics client, the next consideration is for determining the stimulus sentence (part sentence) that is needed for the MLU client, and the stimulus sentence that is needed for the /k/ client.

3. Focus on the interactive nature of language-based therapy progression. Typically, it is very easy to manage the needs of remaining clients once the appropriate materials are selected for the client working on semantics. For example, for the client working on *red*, with an accumulation of 15 red items, all placed in a bag, box, or some other container, it becomes easy for the SLP to stimulate the semantics client using the stimulus sentence, "Ask me, '<u>C</u>an I get one?'" (Of course, "*Can* I get one?" is not grammatically correct, but *"Can I"* is

being stimulated instead of *"May I"* in order to offer more opportunities for the client who is working on the /k/ phoneme to hear multiple correct productions of /k/. Once the semantics client correctly imitates the question and correctly says, "Can I get one?" the SLP answers the question by saying, "You certainly *c*an get one," emphasizing both normal conversational interaction, and emphasizing the /k/ for the benefit of the client working on /k/. The SLP then encourages the client to reach into the container and get one. [*Important:* The correctness of the semantics client's imitation of the stimulus sentence is not as important because the work of intervening for semantics does not begin until *after* the client chooses something from the container.] Of course, because of prior planning, regardless to what is picked from the container, the color of it will be red, to which the SLP says, "Wow! Look at that; you got a *red car*" (or whatever chosen). The SLP instructs the semantics client by saying, "Tell me, 'I have a *red car,*'" and the client repeats. The SLP then expands by quickly talking about the color red, other things in the room that might be red, or where *red* might be seen in the community, and so forth. *(without asking a question about the color red!).* The SLP then offers verbal praise for the semantics client's work on *red* and looks to immediately pull the other clients into the semantics client's "turn." [*In language-based therapy, every client works on every other client's turn.*] To get the other clients involved in communication learning on the semantics client's "turn," the SLP then says to the client working on MLU, "Tell me, 'I see car,' or 'See red car,'" (whichever serves the greater good for all clients) and proceeds to *reinforce communication attempts* according to the response of the MLU client. *(However, the SLP <u>does not correct the MLU client's productions until his or her respective "turn."</u> This is to support increased involvement in therapy and reduce the feeling that every time something is said in therapy, there will be an evaluative comment from the SLP.).* For the third client who is working on the /k/ phoneme, the SLP says, "Tell me, 'I see car,' or 'I see the red car'"—again, whichever serves the greater good for all clients. The SLP reinforces communication attempts according to the response of the /k/ client, and the SLP may let the client know that something was a little amiss about the /k/ production, if applicable, but the SLP *<u>does not target correction for this client until it's his or her turn</u>* for targeting his or her objective. The SLP goes back to the client whose "turn" it is (in this case, the semantics client who is working on *red*), finishes up that client's "turn" by offering the client more opportunities to process *red* through expansions using conversation ("Look at the red on that door," or, "Point to something red for me."), remote experiences ("I saw a red clown on my way to work"), and so forth. Corrective feedback and verbal praise are offered to this target client (the semantics client, in this case) as appropriate, and the SLP prepares to go to the next client for his or her "turn." The SLP begins the next client's "turn" by offering the client an opportunity to choose something from the container by modeling a sentence (or part sentence) stimulus for the next client, in this case, the client working on MLU.

An appropriate sentence (part sentence) stimulus for the MLU client in this case would be, "Ask me, 'Can I pick?'" [***Important:*** *The SLP allows the client to get something from the container <u>only after having worked on his or her objective</u> because the work of the client addressing MLU begins in the communicative act of using language to control the environment to actually get something he or she wants. The client's production does not have to be exactly correct, but the client must try to use language <u>before</u> getting something from the container. This is part of the emotional experience referenced by Backus and Beasley (1951). This requirement of working on the objective before getting something from the container is different than for the client working on semantics.*]. Once the MLU client responds, the SLP provides whatever therapeutic measures deemed appropriate (corrective feedback, verbal praise, shaping, etc.), remembering to also allow the client working on /k/ and the client working on semantics for *red* to work during the MLU client's "turn" as well. After allowing other clients to also work during the MLU client's "turn," the SLP goes back to the MLU client, allows him or her several opportunities for focused work on MLU by modeling several units with an MLU of 3 for the client to imitate. The SLP ends the MLU client's "turn" with verbal praise as appropriate. The SLP then moves to the client working on /k/.

An appropriate sentence (part sentence) stimulus for the client working on /k/ in this case would be, "Ask me, '<u>C</u>an I get one?'" [***Important:*** *The SLP allows the client to get something from the container <u>only after having worked on his or her /k/ objective</u> because the work of the client addressing a phoneme begins in the communicative act of practicing and using the phoneme to control the environment to actually get something he or she wants. The client's production of the phoneme does not have to be exactly correct, but the client must try to use the phoneme <u>before</u> getting something from the container. This is different from the client working on semantics.*] Once the /k/ client responds with efforts to correctly use the /k/, the SLP provides whatever therapeutic measures deemed appropriate (corrective feedback, verbal praise, shaping, etc.) for quickly teaching the phoneme. After a brief period of working on the phoneme, the SLP says to the /k/ client, "Good working on that /k/. Reach in and get something from the bag" (or something similar). Remember, the work for the phoneme client begins *before* reaching into the bag, if needed. The SLP also remembers to allow the client working on semantics for *red*, and the client working on MLU to have a time to work on his or her objectives during the /k/ client's "turn." After allowing the other clients to also work during the /k/ client's "turn," the SLP goes back to the /k/ client, allows him or her several opportunities for focused work on the /k/ using word lists with /k/, or cards with /k/, and so forth. The SLP always ends a client's turn with corrective feedback and verbal praise, as appropriate.

Working in this interactive way, with each client working during each other client's "turn," the SLP accomplishes the objectives of all client's therapy, working to make sure that each client speaks in some manner (as a peer model, as a peer evaluator, or simply as an integral part of the group) at a minimum of every 20 seconds, or so—more often if possible.

The above information at item (3) constitutes one round of therapy. Of course, several aspects of therapy (peer modeling, peer tutoring, shaping, etc.) were not written into the above sequences, but hopefully these sequences make clearer the nature of planning and implementation of language-based therapy for heterogeneous groups.

Here's How to Do Language-Based Therapy

Note to Reader: The information in the following script is designed to help you learn the progression of language-based therapy as related to specific language objectives. Of course, if different objectives were selected, the script would, accordingly, be different as well.

Listed in Figure 9–1 are the 14 therapeutic-specific skills groups and appropriate boxes for you to check off each time you read through the therapy sequence. Check off each skill as you practice it. Once you comfortably feel you have demonstrated a skill well enough for clinical use of the skill, note the date in a remaining box. Continue to read through the therapy progression until you have indicated a "comfort-level" date for all 14 skills groups. Do not become discouraged if it takes several readings for you to feel you have adequately demonstrated the 14 skills groups with appropriate comfort levels.

(DVD Vignette 12 demonstrates a complete mini-language-based session to help you understand the kinds of therapeutic skills intended for use in a basic language-based therapy session. However, not every therapeutic-specific skill is demonstrated in Vignette 12 of the DVD. Although the script in this chapter and the session in Vignette 12 are purposely different [you should go through your own learning processes and develop your own style based on as many different samples of therapy as possible], please view DVD Vignette 12 as often as needed, in addition to reading the script in this chapter, to help with increasing your skills.)

Advance Organizer (Three Questions to Note)

Focus on the 14 therapeutic-specific skills groups as you read the given script of language-based therapy written for a group of three kindergarten-age children. For each of the 14 therapeutic-specific skills groups listed in Figure 9–1, ask these advance organizer questions.

- ❏ How will I implement this therapeutic-specific skill?
- ❏ How will I sound when I implement this therapeutic-specific skill?
- ❏ As I practice the therapeutic-specific skills, what can I do to improve my clinical skills?

Spaces are provided for multiple practices of the 28 therapeutic-specific skills (14 skills groups) below associated with language-based therapy. Check off or date a block each practice time for the skill or skills groups. You may need several practice sessions to become comfortable with language-based therapy. Once you comfortably feel you have demonstrated a skill or skills groups well enough for use in actual therapy, note the date in a remaining box. (Note: *Skill to be practiced in actual therapy, not in the script.)

☐ ☐ ☐ ☐ ☐ ☐ ☐ ☐ ☐ ☐ Motivation

☐ ☐ ☐ ☐ ☐ ☐ ☐ ☐ ☐ ☐ Communicating Expectations

☐ ☐ ☐ ☐ ☐ ☐ ☐ ☐ ☐ ☐ Enthusiasm, Animation, Volume

☐ ☐ ☐ ☐ ☐ ☐ ☐ ☐ ☐ ☐ Seating, Proximity, Touch

☐ ☐ ☐ ☐ ☐ ☐ ☐ ☐ ☐ ☐ Preparation, Pace, Fluency

☐ ☐ ☐ ☐ ☐ ☐ ☐ ☐ ☐ ☐ Alerting, Cueing, Modeling, Prompting

☐ ☐ ☐ ☐ ☐ ☐ ☐ ☐ ☐ ☐ Modalities, Describing/Demonstrating, Questioning, Wait-Time

☐ ☐ ☐ ☐ ☐ ☐ ☐ ☐ ☐ ☐ Shaping (Successive Approximations)

☐ ☐ ☐ ☐ ☐ ☐ ☐ ☐ ☐ ☐ Praise, Tokens, Primary Reinforcers

☐ ☐ ☐ ☐ ☐ ☐ ☐ ☐ ☐ ☐ Corrective Feedback

☐ ☐ ☐ ☐ ☐ ☐ ☐ ☐ ☐ ☐ Data Collection

☐ ☐ ☐ ☐ ☐ ☐ ☐ ☐ ☐ ☐ Probing*

☐ ☐ ☐ ☐ ☐ ☐ ☐ ☐ ☐ ☐ Behavioral Management*

☐ ☐ ☐ ☐ ☐ ☐ ☐ ☐ ☐ ☐ Troubleshooting*

Figure 9–1. Practice chart for sample language-based therapy.

Here's How to Do Language-Based Therapy
15-Minute Scripted Session for Language-Based Therapy
(Group Therapy Session)

INTRODUCTION

Clinician	Clients
Greeting and Rapport	
Hi, Marlon. Great sneakers today.	Marlon: Hi.
Hi, Sam, what a nice smile today.	Sam: Thank you.
Hi, Crystal. Good to see you today.	Crystal: Hi.
Review of Previous Session	
Marlon, tell me what you've been working on in here.	Marlon: Words for cars and things. (Semantics)
Right, you've been working on words for transportation. Sam, tell me what you've been working on.	Sam: My /s/ sound. (Phoneme)
Excellent! You're working on /s/ in words. Crystal, how about you; what have you been working on?	Crystal: My words. (MLU)
Great, Crystal. Yes. You've been working on using more words to make longer sentences. *(Crystal is increasing MLU to 3.0.)* Way to go, guys. Everyone remembered today.	
Collection of or Mentioning of Homework	
Marlon, you didn't have homework today, but Sam, you did. Did you bring your homework for today?	

Clinician	Clients
	Sam: No, I forgot.
Okay, but try to remember to bring it the next time, deal?	
	Sam: Deal
Crystal, did you bring your homework?	
	Crystal: Yes.
Good remembering, Crystal *(takes homework and puts it aside).* Very good.	

BODY

Clinician	Clients
Establishment Phase	
Alright, everyone let's see where we should begin for today. Marlon, you're working on transportation. Name these items. *(Shows toy bus.)*	
	Marlon: "Bus."
(Shows toy car.)	
	Marlon: "Car."
(Shows toy truck.)	
	Marlon: "Truck."
Very nice work, Marlon. All three of those were right. Let's try to get 8 out of 10 of your transportation words correct for today. *(Place stimulus items in the therapy bag, or place aside if not interested in using stimulus items as part of this session.)*	
Sam, you're working on/s/. Tell me these one-syllable words: <u>s</u>it.	
	Sam: "<u>S</u>it."
<u>S</u>ale.	
	Sam: "<u>S</u>ale."

continues

continued

Clinician	Clients
<u>S</u>oup.	Sam: "<u>S</u>oup."
Wonderful, Sam. Those were all easy for you. Let's try for 4 out of 5 correct /s/ words today.	Sam: "Okay."
Crystal, you're working on making your sentences longer. Tell me, "I see truck."	Crystal: "See truck."
Almost (*no correcting or teaching in establishment phase of therapy*). Tell me, "I see bus."	Crystal: "I see bus."
Wonderful. "I see pie."	Crystal: "I see pie."
Good trying, Crystal. You had trouble with one of those, but let's stay on making our sentences 3 units long, and let's see if we can make 7 out of 10 of your sentences at least three words long today.	
Let's get started!	
Eliciting and Recording	
(Most often, there is no daily recording for language-based therapy because the clinician needs to keep conversational interactions going. Occasionally, it may be possible to loosely record client responses during language-based therapy, but often the session moves so quickly that accurate recording is not possible. For this reason, more formal data collection is done once every 7 to 10 days, as desired, within a few minutes of time set aside at the end of a session specifically for data collection for each client. The daily task for the clinician	

Clinician	Clients
in the body of therapy for language is to teach the concepts, which entails defining; describing; characterizing for function, size, shape; comparing; contrasting; relating to familiar current or remote experiences; modeling; eliciting; etc. These tasks are accomplished by making as many deposits into the clients' experience base as possible.)	
Everyone, take a look at this! (*Shows items to all, pointing to various parts as describing, defining, characterizing, etc.*) This is a **bus**. It's a **bus**. The **bus** is yellow; the **bus** has wheels, and the **bus** has a long top. The **bus** takes children to school each morning, and the **bus** brings children home each afternoon. This is a **bus**." Now. Let me hear everyone. Tell me, "I see bus."	
	All Clients: "I see bus."
Good talking. "I see bus." Now, everyone, watch me. I'm putting the bus into my bag. There are lots of other things in my bag also. Everyone will have a turn taking things out of the bag, but first, you must use your words to get something out of the bag. Marlon, let's begin with you. Ask me, "May I see one?"	
	Marlon: "May I see one?"
Excellent, Marlon. You used all four words, and you got the /s/ in *see* exactly right. Sam, did you hear that good /s/ sound? And, Crystal, did you hear all those words Marlon used? (*These two questions are used rhetorically for emphasis on attending/focus, peer evaluation, and interactive nature of*	

continues

continued

Clinician	Clients
language—with no real waiting for a response, but with clinician surveying Sam and Crystal and using nonverbal cues such as smiling, head nodding, etc. to keep Sam and Crystal focused and interested while Marlon selects from the bag.)	
	(Marlon reaches into bag.)
Wow, Marlon! Look at what you got, you got the bus. We just talked about the bus a few minutes ago. *(Immediately takes item retrieved from the bag, not only for Marlon's turn, but for all clients' turns)* Marlon. Tell me, "I hear the bus go vroom, vroom."	
	Marlon: "I hear the bus go vroom, vroom."
Excellent work, Marlon. You used lots of words: "I hear the bus go vroom, vroom." Crystal, tell me, "I hear bus."	
	Crystal: "Hear bus."
Good trying, Crystal. You told me two words: *"hear bus."* We'll try for all three *(three fingers held up)* words in a few minutes when you have your turn. Sam, tell me, "I <u>s</u>ee the bus."	
	Sam: "I <u>t</u>ee the bus."
Good trying, Sam, you got all the words, but you had a little trouble with the /s/ in <u>s</u>ee. We'll work on that in just a few minutes. Marlon, back to you to end your turn. Tell me, "The bus has lots of wheels."	
	Marlon: "The bus has lots of wheels."
Nice job, Marlon. The bus has lots of wheels. Show me two of them. *(Holds bus up for Marlon to touch wheels.)*	
	Marlon: *(Touches two wheels.)*

Clinician	Clients
Good touching, Marlon. Way to go! Now, everyone, let's think for a moment. Where are some places we can go on a bus other than just school? Hum, let's think, think, think (*Points to head to support thinking.*) Where do you remember going on a bus that was a fun place to go see animals? (*Rhetorical question; don't wait for an answer. Question posed to support expansion and remote experiences.*) Who has been to the zoo on a bus to see zoo animals? Wow! Who, who, who?	
	Clients: All or some jump in with "Me," or "I have," or hand raises, etc.
Marlon, tell me, "I ride the bus to the zoo."	
	Marlon: "I ride the bus to the zoo."
Wonderful, Marlon! And, I'll bet at the zoo, you saw all sorts of fun animals like monkeys, and bears, and . . . (*Helps 1–2 clients remember a zoo animal and tell it to the group*) . . . what's another fun animal at the zoo, Sam?	
	Sam: "A tiger."
Yeah, a tiger can be fun to look at, but we try not to get too close to tigers. Everyone, tell me, "I ride the bus to the zoo."	
	Clients: "I ride the bus to the zoo."
Good talking, everyone; good work, Marlon. Crystal, tell me, "I ride bus."	
	Crystal: "I ride bus."
Wonderful, Crystal; you got all the words: "I ride bus." Did everyone hear all of Crystal's words? (*Surveys the group, showing a thumb's-up for Crystal.*) Yeah, that was a thumb's-up, Crystal; you used all your words, "I ride bus." Easy for you.	

continues

continued

Clinician	Clients
Good talking, everyone. (*Places bus in a side container positioned on the floor away from clients.*) Sam, it's your turn to get something from the bag. Ask me, "May I <u>s</u>ee one?"	
	Sam: "May I <u>t</u>ee one?"
I saw you trying, Sam, but instead of saying /s/, you gave me a /t/. /s/ is made by putting the tongue tip up behind the front top teeth and letting the air go out in a long skinny stream like a snake sound. It sounds like this: /s/. Crystal, show Sam your /s/.	
	Crystal: /s/.
Good work, Crystal, easy for you. Marlon show Sam your /s/.	
	Marlon: /s/.
Great job, Marlon, easy for you. Sam, remember, /s/ is made by putting the tongue tip up behind the front top teeth, and letting the air go out in a long skinny stream like a snake sound. It sounds like this: /s/. Let me hear your /s/.	
	Sam: /s/.
Excellent /s/, Sam. Your /s/ is exactly right; it's long and skinny. Now, let's take your /s/ and put it back into your word in two parts: (*This begins successive approximations, or shaping*) /s/-----ee. (*Use hand motions to show a visual of "putting sound back in the word in* **two parts.***" Hand motions will proceed from the client's left to right, the order of words as they appear in the written form of English. The SLP will use hand motions to accompany the verbal presentations of both the SLP and the client during the teaching*	

Clinician	Clients
phases of successive approximations or shaping, always presenting and eliciting the approximations from the client's left to right, not the SLP's left to right.)	
	Sam: /s/------ee
Great job, Sam. Let's put the sounds a little closer together: /s/---ee *(Remember, as the verbal presentations get closer [more approximated], so do the visual hand motions that accompany the verbal presentations.)*	
	Sam: /s/---ee
Great! Now, let's blend your sounds altogether in one long word, nice and slow: <u>s</u>ee. *(The hand motion when verbally blending the sounds into one continuous word is now one continuous motion for the client to see, going from left-to-right, of course.)*	
	Sam: <u>s</u>ee
Good work, Sam; your tongue was in the right place. Way to go! Marlon, let me hear your "see."	
	Marlon: "See."
Excellent! Crystal, let me hear, "See."	
	Crystal: "See."
Perfect, Crystal. Alright, Sam. Let me hear one last word, nice and slow, "Song."	
	Sam: "Song."
Perfect, Sam on that "Song." You did a lot of good work. Sam, reach into the bag to <u>s</u>ee one. *(Surveys the group, asking them to show a thumb's-up for Sam as he reaches into the bag.)* Yeah, that was a thumb's-up, Sam; you said your sound exactly right; your tongue was in the right place for that /s/.	
	(Sam reaches into the bag.)

continues

continued

Clinician	Clients
Wow! Look at what you got. You got a motor-cycle, yeah! (*Takes motorcycle for all to see.*) Tell me, Sam, "I see the motorcycle"—and watch for the /s/ sound in two places, listen: <u>s</u>ee, and motor<u>c</u>ycle. (*Pronounces both slowly so that Sam can clearly hear the /s/ sounds*). Tell me, "I see the motorcycle." Everyone, listen for Sam's /s/ words.	
	Sam: "I <u>s</u>ee the motor<u>c</u>ycle."
Wow! Sam, you got both /s/ sounds exactly right. Was that a thumb's-up, guys?	
	Marlon and Crystal: "Yes" (*both show thumb's-up*)
Yeah, it was a thumb's-up, Sam; your /s/ was perfect. Marlon, tell me the motorcycle goes very fast.	
	Marlon: "The motorcycle goes very fast."
Easy for you, Marlon. Crystal, tell me, "I see motorcycle."	
	Crystal: "See motorcycle."
Good trying, Crystal. "See motorcycle." That's still a lot of words for you. We'll make your words longer in just a moment when it's your turn. Sam, let me hear a few /s/ words to end your turn. Tell me, "<u>S</u>oup."	
	Sam: "<u>S</u>oup."
Great, "<u>S</u>ome."	
	Sam: "<u>S</u>ome."
"<u>S</u>ail."	
	Sam: "<u>S</u>ail."
Easy for you, Sam. Very nice work. Crystal, it's your turn. Ask me, "See one please."	
	Crystal: "See one."
You're really trying, Crystal, but instead of giving me three words, you gave me two words. I need to hear three words, like this: "See – one – please" (*holding up one finger for each word as it is slowly spoken*).	

Clinician	Clients
Marlon, tell Crystal, "See one please."	Marlon: "See one please."
Good talking, Marlon. Sam, tell Crystal, "See one please."	
	Sam: "<u>T</u>ee one please."
You had a little trouble with the /s/, Sam, but you got all three words, "See one please." Crystal, watch me, "See one please." You try, one word at a time. (*This begins successive approximations or shaping.*) Tell me, "See" (*holding up one finger for each word as it is slowly spoken*).	
	Crystal: "See."
Perfect. "One."	
	Crystal: "One."
Good. "Please."	
	Crystal: "Please."
Wonderful, Crystal. Now, let's put two words together, "See – one" (*holding up one finger for each word as it is slowly spoken*).	
	Crystal: "See one."
Very nice, now let's put it all together, "See – one – please" (*holding up one finger for each word as it is slowly spoken*).	
	Crystal: "See one please."
Excellent, Crystal. You got all three words: "See one please." Way to go! Marlon, let me hear, "I'd like to see one."	
	Marlon: "I'd like to see one."
Great, Marlon, and Sam, tell me, "See one please."	
	Sam: "See one please."
Way to go, Sam. You got the /s/ that time. Awesome everyone. Crystal, reach in the bag to see something. (*Surveys group, commenting on how well Crystal did with her words as Crystal reaches in the bag.*)	
	(*Crystal reaches in the bag.*)

continues

continued

Clinician	Clients
Wow! Look at what you got. You got an airplane. (*Takes airplane for all to see.*) Tell me slowly, "I – see – plane."	
	Crystal: "I – see – plane."
Wonderful. Marlon, tell me three places you can to go to on a plane. Everyone, let's think. Where are places we can go on the plane? Marlon, tell me three places we can go on a plane.	
	Marlon: I can go to my Granddaddy's house. And I can go to see my friend, and . . . " (*pauses to think*)
That's two good places, Marlon. Good thinking. Think of another place we can go on an airplane. (*Waits 5 seconds, surveying everyone in the group.*) Alright, let's think, Marlon can go see his granddad on a plane, and he can go see his friend on a plane. Sam, where is someplace you can go on a plane.	
	Sam: "I can go to the beach on a plane."
Oh, fun, fun, fun. "I can go to the beach on a plane," yeah! Marlon, let me hear that, "I can go to the beach on a plane."	
	Marlon: "I can go to the beach on a plane."
Wonderful, Marlon. Sam, tell me, "The airplane is safe."	
	Sam: "The airplane is safe."
Good /s/ sound, Sam. Very nice work. Crystal, tell me these things to end your turn: "Go to beach."	
	Crystal: "Go to beach."
Easy for you, Crystal. "Go to beach." Good talking. Tell me, "Plane is safe."	
	Crystal: "Plane is safe."
Excellent, Crystal. Tell me, "I like plane."	
	Crystal: "I like plane."

Clinician	Clients
Awesome, Crystal! Did everyone hear all of Crystal's words? Way to go, Crystal. Was that a thumbs-up or a thumb's-down, guys? *(Showing a thumb's-up to give others a clue.)*	
	(Marlon and Sam both showing a thumb's-up for Crystal's work.)
Way to go, Crystal! *(Gives a high five to Crystal)*	
	Crystal: *(High five)*
Marlon, it's your turn, again. Ask me, "May I see one?"	
	Marlon: "May I see one?"
You certainly, may; reach right in. *(Surveys other clients, saying: "Did you hear that good /s/ in see, and did you hear all those words?" as Marlon reaches into the bag.)*	
	(Marlon reaches into the bag.)
Wow, Marlon, look at what you got! It's a train. *(Takes train from Marlon, holding it up for all to see.)* Tell Sam something fun about this train.	
	Marlon: *(Looks at Sam, but says nothing.)*
Everyone, let's put on our thinking caps, and think of something fun to say about the train. *(Surveys all clients, and touches head to emphasize thinking.)* *(Waits about 5 seconds, continuing to survey everyone.)* I can think of something fun about the train; listen for me: "I saw a fun train at Disney World! Wow! How about that?! Marlon, What do you know about a fun train at Disney World?"	
	Marlon: "Oh, you ride the train to get to different places."
You certainly do. Tell that to Sam: "I ride the train to get to different places."	

continues

continued

Clinician	Clients
	Marlon: (*Turns to Sam.*) I ride the train to get to different places."
	Sam: I know, I <u>t</u>aw a train like that when my mom took us to the park.
Good remembering, Sam. You <u>saw</u> a train like that (*emphasizes correct production of /s/ without mentioning Sam's error*), and Marlon, good talking to Sam. Crystal, tell Marlon, "I ride train."	
	Crystal: "I ride train."
Way to go, Crystal. You got all the words: "I ride train." Everyone, listen for Crystal's words and let's see how well she does. Crystal, tell us again, "I ride train."	
	Crystal: "I ride train."
Yeah! Is that a thumb's-up, or a thumb's-down for Crystal's words?	
	Marlon and Sam: (*Both hold thumb's-up for Crystal.*)
Yeah, that's a thumb's-up, Crystal. (*Holds thumb up.*) Very good talking, Crystal; you got all the words: "I ride train." Marlon, it's still your turn. You told Sam something fun about the train, but guess what? I have three trains in this room for everyone to find. Ahhh! Now, everyone let's look around the room. Look, look, look, look (*holding hands to eyes, emphasizing the looking or visual scanning function*). Everyone, let's get up quietly from our seats and use our eyes to find three trains. When you find a train, pick it up and bring it to your seat so that we can talk about it.	

Clinician	Clients
	All Clients: (*Mill around the room until all three have found a train and returned to his or her seat with it.*)
Wonderful! Now, we each have a train. Now, listen. These are the kinds of things we can talk about for our trains. We can talk about the color, or the size of our trains. We can talk about some of the numbers we see on our trains, or we can talk about some place we would like to visit on a train, and on, and on. Marlon, let's begin with you because it's still your turn. Tell us something about your train.	
	Marlon: "I saw one like this on TV. It had smoke coming out of the top, though."
The one on T.V. had smoke coming out of the top?	
	Marlon: "Yeah, it was a puffy train."
Good thinking, Marlon. Yeah, sometimes trains do have smoke; they sort'a huff and puff along. Now who knows what sound a train makes when smoke is coming out of the top and the train is huffing and puffing along? (*Moves arm in an up-and-down position suggesting the "choo-choo" sound.*)	
	All Clients: "Choo-choo!!" (*Arms all move in an up-and-down position suggesting the "choo-choo" sound*).
Yeah! Choo-choo! (*Continues arm in an up-and-down position suggesting the "choo-choo" sound*). Alright! Everyone tell me, "The train says 'choo-choo!'"	
	All Clients: "The train says 'choo-choo.'"
Very nice, Everyone. Sam, let's begin your turn. Tell me, "I see the train," and watch for your /s/ sound.	
	Sam: "I see the train."

continues

continued

Clinician	Clients
Wonderful! Great /s/, Sam. Everyone, was that a thumb's-up for Sam on his /s/?	
	Marlon and Crystal: (*Both show thumb's-up.*)
Yeah! That was a thumb's-up, Sam. The /s/ sound was exactly right. Good talking. Crystal, tell me, "I see train", and let's try for all the words, Crystal, nice and slow. Watch me: "I – see – train" (*holding up one finger for each word as it is spoken*).	
	Crystal: "I see train."
Way to go, Crystal. Great talking. Everyone, was that a thumb's-up for Crystal?	
	Marlon and Sam: (*Both show thumb's-up.*)
It surely was a thumb's-up, Crystal (*holding a thumb up for Crystal*). Great job, Crystal! Sam, tell us one thing about your train before we go.	
	Sam: "It's got <u>t</u>ome numbers on it, just like her train."
Yeah, your train has numbers on it, just like Crystal's train, and really, just like Marlon's train also. Good thinking, and good talking, but I want you to work on your /s/ sound for a moment now that it's your turn. I saw you trying for your /s/, but instead of giving me an /s/, you gave me a /t/. /s/ is made by putting the tongue tip up behind the front top teeth and letting the air go out in a long skinny stream like a snake sound. It sounds like this: /s/. Crystal, show Sam your /s/.	
	Crystal: /s/.
Good work, Crystal, easy for you. Marlon show Sam your /s/.	
	Marlon: /s/.

Clinician	Clients
Great job, Marlon, easy for you. Sam, remember, /s/ is made by putting the tongue tip up behind the front top teeth, and letting the air go out in a long skinny stream like a snake sound. It sounds like this: /s/. Let me hear your /s/, Sam.	
	Sam:/s/.
Excellent /s/, Sam; it's long and skinny, and it sounds exactly right. Now, let's take your /s/ and put it back into your word in two parts: (*This begins successive approximations.*) /s/-----ome. (*Use hand motions to show a visual of "putting sound back in the word in* **two parts.**" *Hand motions will proceed from the client's left to right, the order of words as they appear in the written form of English.*)	
	Sam: /s/-----ome.
Great job, Sam. Let's put the sounds a little closer together: /s/---ome. (*Remember, as the verbal presentations get closer [more approximated], so do the visual hand motions that accompany the verbal presentations.*)	
	Sam: /s/---ome.
Great! Now, let's blend your sounds altogether in one long word, nice and slow: <u>s</u>ome. (*The hand motion when verbally blending the sounds into one continuous word is now one continuous motion for the client to see, going from client's left-to-right, of course.*)	
	Sam: <u>s</u>ome.
Good work, Sam; your tongue was in the right place. Way to go! Marlon, let me hear your "some."	
	Marlon: "some."
Excellent! Crystal, let me hear, "some."	
	Crystal: "Some."

continues

continued

Clinician	Clients
Fabulous, Crystal, good /s/ sound. Alright, Sam. Let me hear one last word, nice and slow, "Sack."	
	Sam: "Sack."
Perfect, Sam on that "sack." You did a lot of good work for you /s/ sound related to your train. (*Surveys the group, asking them to a show thumb's-up for Sam for his /s/ sound.*) Yeah, that was a thumb's-up, Sam; you said your sound exactly right; your tongue was in the right place for that /s/.	
	Marlon and Crystal: (*Both show a thumb's-up.*)
Alright, everyone. We won't have time to finish with the trains today. Crystal, you didn't have a turn to talk about your train, but maybe we can revisit the trains again on another day. You guys have done really good work today.	

CLOSING

Review of Objectives	
Marlon, you worked on transportation today. You talked about *bus, motorcycle, airplane,* and *train.* We didn't talk a lot about each one, but you started working on these very nicely.	
Sam, you worked on the /s/ sound in words like *see, safe,* and *some.*	
Crystal, you worked on making your sentences with three words and you told us "I see bus," and "I see plane." Good work for everyone.	

Clinician	Clients
Summarize Client's Performances	
Everyone, I'll take data the next time you come to therapy, but Marlon, it looks like every one of your transportation words were correct today. Sam, it looks like your work on /s/ was near 80% correct today, and Crystal, you worked hard today; I think you got a lot better toward the end of the session, but overall, it looks like you got your three words the best when you had some help. Way to go everyone!	
Homework	
No homework for anyone today, but Sam, please remember to bring back your homework from last time.	
Rewards	
Stickers for everyone today! Crystal, here's a sticker.	
	Crystal: Thank you.
Sam, here's your sticker.	
	Sam: (*Holds out hand, smiles*)
Marlon, here's a sticker for you.	
	Marlon: Thanks.
Everyone, enjoy the rest of the day, and I'll see you on Wednesday. Bye-bye.	

Summary

Language therapy in its basic foundation takes many forms because of the many constellations of language disorders. *Language-based therapy* as presented in this chapter lends itself to interactive group work, especially when heterogeneous grouping is employed. Knowledge of the basic concepts of language-based therapy supports good speech and language therapy services.

Learning Tool

List each component of the major divisions of a speech-language therapy session and briefly tell what should transpire within each section of those major components for language-based therapy.

_____

_____

_____

_____

_____

_____

References

Backus, O., & Beasley, J. (1951). *Speech therapy with children.* Cambridge, MA: Riverside Press.

Bates, E. (1976). *Language and context: Studies in the acquisition of pragmatics.* New York, NY: Academic Press.

Becker, J. (1994). Pragmatic socialization: Parental input to preschoolers. *Discourse Processes, 17,* 131–148.

Bloom, L., & Lahey, M. (1978). *Language development and language disorders.* New York, NY: John Wiley & Sons.

Brown, R. (1973). *A first language: The early stages.* Cambridge, MA: Harvard University Press.

Bryant, J. B. (1999). Perspectives on pragmatic socialization. In A. Greenhill (Ed.), *Proceedings of the 23rd Annual Boston University Conference on Language Development* (Vol. 1, pp. 132–137). Boston, MA: Boston University Press.

Chomsky, N. (1957). *Syntactic structures.* The Hague, the Netherlands: Mouton.

Fey, M., Long, S., & Finestack, L. (2003). Ten principles of grammar facilitation for children with specific language impairments. *American Journal of Speech-Language Pathology, 12,* 3–15.

Gleason, J. B. (2005). *The development of language* (6th ed.). New York, NY: Pearson Allyn & Bacon.

Hegde, M. N. (2001). *Hegde's pocketguide to treatment in speech-language pathology* (2nd ed.). San Diego, CA: Singular Thompson Learning.

Hegde, M. N. (2008). *Hegde's pocketguide to treatment in speech-language pathology* (3rd ed.). Clifton Park, NY: Delmar.

Paul, R. (2011). *Language disorders from infancy through adolescence* (4th ed.). St Louis, MO: Mosby Elsevier.

Piaget, J. (1926). *The language and thought of the child.* New York, NY: Harcourt Brace Jovanovich.

Polloway, E. A., Patton, J. R., & Serna, L. (2001). *Strategies for teaching learners with special needs* (7th ed.). Columbus, OH: Merrill Prentice Hall.

Skinner, B. F. (1957). *Verbal behavior.* Englewood Cliffs, NJ: Prentice-Hall.

10

Guided Practice in Articulation Therapy

Selected General Concepts for Articulation Therapy

Clients experiencing difficulty with clearly producing the sounds of language often qualify for articulation therapy. Levels of articulation difficulty range from mild to severe or profound disorders. Clients experiencing severe and profound articulation disorders often benefit from intervention using specific articulation programs or techniques. However, skills highlighted in this chapter address generalized articulation therapy.

1. Several articulation therapies are founded in the traditional articulation approach to therapy as presented by Van Riper as early as 1939. Although revisited, changed, and embellished over the years (Van Riper, 1939, 1978; Van Riper & Emerick, 1984; Van Riper & Erickson, 1969, 1996), traditional articulation remediation is often considered to be fundamental for articulation therapy (Peña-Brooks & Hegde, 2000). Although traditional articulation therapy involves several stages of work to be performed in specific ways (Van Riper & Erickson, 1996), the premise of traditional articulation therapy most applicable to this discussion is the following progression of therapy.

   a. Begin with *ear training* or *auditory discrimination* as needed with a high level of correct productions established as criteria for advancement.

   b. Teach the phoneme in *isolation* with a high level of correct productions established as criteria for advancement.

   c. Teach the *phoneme in syllabic contexts* to include consonant–vowel (CV), vowel–consonant (VC), vowel–consonant–vowel (VCV), and consonant–vowel–consonant (CVC) configurations with a high level of correct productions established as criteria for advancement.

d. Teach the *phoneme in initial, final,* and *medial* positions of the *sound in words* with a high level of correct productions established as criteria for advancement.

e. Teach the phoneme in *words in phrases* (all positions of words) with a high level of correct productions established as criteria for advancement.

f. Teach the phoneme in *words in sentences* (all positions of words) with a high level of correct productions established as criteria for advancement.

g. Teach the phoneme in *words in conversation* (all positions of words) with a high level of correct productions established as criteria for advancement.

h. Teach the phoneme in *words in generalized communication contexts* (all positions of words) with a high level of correct productions established as criteria for completion or dismissal.

2. Make sure that traditional articulation therapy is the better choice of intervention approaches for the client, especially if multiple articulation errors are present in the client's repertoire. For example, if the client exhibits numerous articulation errors with accompanying poor conversational intelligibility, another approach other than traditional articulation therapy may be a better choice for the client. Clinical work in the areas of distinctive features and phonological processes influenced development of intervention techniques aimed at addressing more than one error sound at a time (Creaghead, Newman, & Secord, 1989) and supported the use of an articulation intervention approach other than traditional articulation therapy for many clients. The SLP may, therefore, wish to consider the use of the following types of therapy approaches for clients for whom traditional articulation therapy is inappropriate.

    a. Multiphonemic Articulation Therapy (McCabe & Bradley, 1975)

    b. Distinctive Features Therapy (Blache, 1978)

    c. Phonological Processes Therapy (Hodson & Paden, 1983; Ingram, 1986)

    d. Sensory-Motor Approach to Therapy (McDonald & August, 1970)

    e. Other approaches aimed at intervention for the client with severely or profoundly impaired articulation or phonology.

3. Establish high percentages for correct productions of sounds during traditional articulation therapy and require clients to meet these criteria for *two consecutive therapy sessions* before advancing to the next level of work:

    • 100% correct production of sounds in isolation

    • 100% correct production of sounds in all syllabic contexts (CV, VC, VCV, CVC)

    • 90% correct production of sounds in all positions in words (initial, medial, final)

    • 80% correct production of sounds in all positions in words in sentences

- 80% correct production of sounds in all positions in words in conversational speech, and

- 80% correct production of sounds in all positions in words in generalized communication contexts.

Often SLPs are reluctant to establish criteria at high levels, particularly when working with children in schools because of parents' concern that too high a standard is required for children in therapy, specifically when 100% correct productions are the required criteria. However, often those thinking along these lines fail to consider that clients are being treated in therapy, and as such, standards and levels of activities customary to typical populations often are not high enough to positively impact performances for those needing therapy. An important point to remember is that if a client fails to work at very high criteria at the foundational levels for learning a phoneme (isolation and syllabic context levels), often progress beyond the word level is hampered. For example, if a client is unable to correctly produce ba- in CV syllables, it is unlikely that the client will be able to correctly produce words that begin with the ba- combination (*bake, bait, baby,* etc.). Omitting even one or two correct productions at the syllabic level leads to difficulty in producing words represented by the syllabic combination, and this difficulty leads to slowed progress at the word level of production and beyond.

4. Work on articulation skills within the context of groups as often as possible to benefit from the interactive nature of communication (Backus & Beasley, 1951).

5. Use clients within the group as models, as communicating partners, or as evaluators of productions for each other.

6. Collect data for each client, each session, and avoid what is termed "***data mixing,***" collecting data on more than one task, task level, or task objective within the same data batch. For example, do not collect data on /t/ in the initial position of words and /t/ in the final position of words in the same set of data so that how well a client is progressing in a specific aspect of therapy is more accurately determined. There are times, however, when the objective of data collection is to determine client skills in varying syllabic or word contexts, in which case, of course, the productions of sounds in initial and final positions of syllables, and in initial, medial, and final positions of words in the same data set is expected; other than those times, do not combine data for "mixed" productions.

7. Decide on a format for data collection and be consistent in the application of that format, particularly in the determination of how to handle self-corrections. For example, some SLPs count self-corrections as correct, whereas others count them as incorrect. Still another option, and perhaps a more accurate account of actual performance, is the practice of counting self-corrections as first, incorrect, then as correct, which is essentially what happens in a self-correction.

Regardless of the format chosen, consistency in accounting for client productions is important for decision making and client management in the therapeutic process.

8. Although most beginning level therapy depicts a clinician–model and client–imitation format for stimulus–response, as clients achieve higher levels of proficiency, especially at the word level and beyond, it is common to stimulate the client using flash cards, toy models, or other therapeutic materials that add interest and variety to stimulations without detracting from the number of client response possibilities. Be careful to ensure that the materials introduced in therapy do not detract from the client's focus on correctly producing sounds and that the stimulus item does not require so much management and manipulation as to decrease the number of responses the client is able to produce in therapy.

Numerous other concepts and guidelines apply for articulation therapy. However, based on the information given in these selected general concepts, it is hoped that the reader understands the text well enough to process the information and examples throughout the remainder of this section on articulation therapy.

Selected Articulation Objectives

Following are examples of objectives for articulation therapy:

1. Client will correctly produce /l/ in initial positions of words 9 out of 10 opportunities.

2. Client will correctly produce /s/ in final positions of words in sentences 8 out of 10 opportunities.

3. Client will correctly produce /k/ in CVC syllables 100% of opportunities.

Here's How to Do Articulation Therapy

Note to Reader: The information in the script below is designed to help you learn the progression of articulation therapy as related to specific articulation objectives. Of course, if different objectives were selected, the script would, accordingly, be different as well.

Listed in Figure 10–1 are the 14 therapeutic-specific skills groups and appropriate boxes for you to check off each time you read through the therapy sequence. Check off each skill as you practice it. Once you comfortably feel you have demonstrated a skill well enough for clinical use of the skill, note the date in a remaining box. Continue to read through the therapy progression until you have indicated a "comfort-level" date for all 14 skills groups. Do not become discouraged if it takes several readings for you to feel that you have adequately demonstrated the 14 skills groups with appropriate comfort levels.

Spaces are provided for multiple practices of the 28 therapeutic-specific skills (14 skills groups) below associated with articulation therapy. Check off or date a block each practice time for the skill or skills group. You may need several practice sessions to become comfortable with articulation therapy. Once you comfortably feel you have demonstrated a skill or skills group well enough for use in an actual therapy session, note the date in a remaining box. (Note: *Skill to be practiced in actual therapy, not in the script.)

☐ ☐ ☐ ☐ ☐ ☐ ☐ ☐ ☐   **Motivation**

☐ ☐ ☐ ☐ ☐ ☐ ☐ ☐ ☐   **Communicating Expectations**

☐ ☐ ☐ ☐ ☐ ☐ ☐ ☐ ☐   **Enthusiasm, Animation, Volume**

☐ ☐ ☐ ☐ ☐ ☐ ☐ ☐ ☐   **Seating, Proximity, Touch**

☐ ☐ ☐ ☐ ☐ ☐ ☐ ☐ ☐   **Preparation, Pace, Fluency**

☐ ☐ ☐ ☐ ☐ ☐ ☐ ☐ ☐   **Alerting, Cueing, Modeling, Prompting**

☐ ☐ ☐ ☐ ☐ ☐ ☐ ☐ ☐   **Modalities, Describing/Demonstrating, Questioning, Wait-Time**

☐ ☐ ☐ ☐ ☐ ☐ ☐ ☐ ☐   **Shaping (Successive Approximations)**

☐ ☐ ☐ ☐ ☐ ☐ ☐ ☐ ☐   **Praise, Tokens, Primary Reinforcers**

☐ ☐ ☐ ☐ ☐ ☐ ☐ ☐ ☐   **Corrective Feedback**

☐ ☐ ☐ ☐ ☐ ☐ ☐ ☐ ☐   **Data Collection**

☐ ☐ ☐ ☐ ☐ ☐ ☐ ☐ ☐   **Probing***

☐ ☐ ☐ ☐ ☐ ☐ ☐ ☐ ☐   **Behavioral Management***

☐ ☐ ☐ ☐ ☐ ☐ ☐ ☐ ☐   **Troubleshooting***

Figure 10–1. Practice chart for sample articulation therapy.

(DVD Vignette 11 demonstrates a complete mini-articulation and language session to help you understand the kinds of therapeutic skills intended for use in a basic articulation therapy session. However, not every therapeutic-specific skill is demonstrated in Vignette 11 of the DVD. Although the script in this chapter and the session in Vignette 11 are purposely different [you should go through your own learning processes and develop your own style based on as many different samples of therapy as possible], please view Vignette 11 as often as needed, in addition to reading the script in this chapter, to help with increasing your skills.)

Advance Organizer (Three Questions to Note)

Focus on the 14 therapeutic-specific skills groups as you read the given script of articulation therapy written for a group of three elementary school-age children. For each of the 14 therapeutic-specific skills groups listed in Figure 10–1, ask these advance organizer questions:

- ❑ How will I implement this therapeutic-specific skill?
- ❑ How will I sound when I implement this therapeutic-specific skill?
- ❑ As I practice the therapeutic-specific skill, what can I do to improve my clinical skills?

Here's How to Do Articulation Therapy 15-Minute Scripted Session for Articulation Therapy (Group Therapy Session)	
INTRODUCTION	
Clinician	Clients
Greeting and Rapport Hi, Anthony. Great to see you today. Jacob, How are you? Great hair cut. Hi, Joe. Good to see you today.	Anthony: Hi. Jacob: Thank you. Joe: Hi.

Clinician	Clients
Review of Previous Session Anthony, do you remember what you've been working on in here?	Anthony: /k/ and I can't remember.
Good remembering for the /k/, Anthony, and your other sound is the /t/. You're working on /k/ in sentences, and /t/ is still at syllables. Good remembering for the /k/ sound, Anthony. Jacob, what have you been working on?	Jacob: /f/ and /l/.
Excellent! You're working on /f/ in the beginning of words, and /l/ in sentences. Good remembering, Jacob. Joe, how about you; what have you been working on?	Joe: /s/ and /l/.
Good remembering, Joe. You're working on the /s/ in the beginning of words and the /l/ in sentences. In fact, Jacob and you are both working on /l/ in sentences. Way to go guys. Good remembering your sounds. **Collection of or Mentioning of Homework** No one had homework for today, so let's get started.	
BODY	
Establishment Phase Everyone let's see where we should begin for today. Anthony, you're working on /k/ in sentences and /t/ in syllables. Let's start with /k/. Tell me "I see the car.	Anthony: I see the <u>c</u>ar.

continues

continued

Clinician	Clients
"The cup is full."	
	Anthony: The <u>c</u>up is full.
"Keep the change."	
	Anthony: /t/-<u>k</u>eep the change.
Very nice effort Anthony. You changed the /t/ to /k/ on your own, and the other two sentences were exactly right. Let's try to get 9 out of 10 of your /k/ sounds in sentences correct today. Now, let's check for the /t/ is syllables: Tell me, "ta."	
	Anthony: <u>T</u>a.
"Te."	
	Anthony: <u>T</u>e.
"To."	
	Anthony: <u>T</u>o.
Great, Anthony; you got the /t/ right in all beginning parts of syllables, so we'll start there today. Let's see if we can get 90% correct for /t/ today. Jacob, you're working on /f/ in the beginning of words. Tell me, "fun."	
	Jacob: <u>F</u>un.
"Foot."	
	Jacob: <u>F</u>oot.
"Face."	
	Jacob: <u>F</u>ace.
Good work on /f/, Jacob; we'll start on /f/ in the initial positions of words, and let's try for 90% on /f/ today. Now, let's check on the /l/ in sentences: Tell me, "The light is on."	
	Jacob: The <u>w</u>ight is on.
Almost (**no correcting or teaching in establishment phase of therapy**). Tell me, "Look at the teacher."	
	Jacob: <u>W</u>ook at the teacher.

Clinician	Clients
I saw you trying, but watch my mouth closely this time; "The puppy is lost."	
	Jacob: The puppy is l̲ost.
Good /l/ that time, Jacob, but you had a little trouble with /l/ in the other sentences; you only got one of three correct, so let's drop back to the word level at the beginning of the session, and if you do well at that level within the first few minutes of therapy, we'll move you up to sentences before the session is over. Let's try for 9 of 10 correct words using /l/ in initial positions of words for a few rounds before taking a look at your /l/ in sentences today. Joe, you're working on /s/ in words. Tell me, "sun."	
	Joe: S̲un.
"Soup."	Joe: S̲oup.
"See."	Joe: S̲ee.
Good work on /s/ Joe. You got all /s/ sounds right at the beginning of words, so let's start there today; we'll try to get 9 of 10 of your /s/ sounds correct in the beginning of words. Now, let's take a look at /l/ in sentences. Tell me, "Look at the toy."	
	Joe: L̲ook at the toy.
"The light is green."	Joe: The l̲ight is green.
"This is the last one."	Joe: This is the l̲ast one.
Good work, Joe. You got the /l/ right in all sentences, so we'll start there for you today. Let's try to get 8 of 10 /l/ sounds correct in your sentences for today.	
	Joe: Okay.

continues

continued

Clinician	Clients
Eliciting and Recording	

Let's get started! (All responses will be recorded, with a separate data collection line/set for each child, each phoneme, per level of work. For example, if collecting data in a horizontal format, there will be two lines of data for Anthony, one data line for the /k/ in sentences, and one data line for /t/ in syllables. There might be three data lines for Jacob: one for the /f/ in words, one for the /l/ in words, and if the data indicates high percentages of correct production of /l/ in words, a third data line, a line for /l/ in sentences will be added as the session progresses. The task in this section of the body of therapy for articulation is to [1] teach the phonemes, using placement, modeling, cueing, prompts, etc. as necessary to ensure correct production of the sound; [2] record all productions—both correct and error productions; and [3] obtain as many responses as possible within the session, preferably a minimum 25–30 responses per phoneme addressed per child, per session—more, of course, is better.) Anthony, let's start with your /k/ in sentences. Tell me, "The trash can is full."

Anthony: The trash <u>c</u>an is full.

Great, the /k/ in can was exactly right. Let's speed it up a little. Tell me, "She came to town."

Anthony: She <u>c</u>ame to town.

"The ice is cold."

Anthony: The ice is <u>c</u>old.

Clinician	Clients
"I want to keep the puppy."	
	Anthony: I want to <u>k</u>eep the puppy.
"They went camping yesterday."	
	Anthony: They went <u>c</u>amping yesterday.
Wow, Anthony, you got all five correct. Good job. Everyone, thumb's up for Anthony's /k/, yeah! Jacob, let's try your /f/ in words. Tell me, "Food."	
	Jacob: <u>F</u>ood.
"Fill."	
	Jacob: <u>F</u>ill.
"Fold."	
	Jacob: <u>F</u>old.
"Fast."	
	Jacob: <u>P</u>ast.
(Immediately stop recording and proceed to the Teaching Phase of the Body of Therapy. To help with data collection, note that at this point, Jacob has 3 correct and 1 incorrect responses for this round.) You're working hard on the /f/, Jacob, but on that one, I heard a /p/ instead of an /f/. I need you to continue the sound by placing your top teeth lightly on your bottom lip to let the airstream flow between the top lip and the bottom teeth, like this: /f/ (*SLP demonstrates then solicits models from other clients*). Watch Joe. Joe, show Jacob your /f/.	
	Joe: /f/.
Great job, Joe. Jacob, watch how Anthony makes the /f/. He's going to let his top teeth touch his bottom lip, then, he'll let the airstream out to make /f/.	

continues

continued

Clinician	Clients
Watch, Jacob. Anthony, show Jacob how to make /f/.	
	Anthony: /f/.
Good job, Anthony, good /f/. Jacob, you try; place your top teeth gently on your bottom lip, and let the airstream pass between them in a long stream: /f/.	
	Jacob: /f/.
Very good work, Jacob. Now, let's put that /f/ sound back into your word, but we'll break it up into two parts *(successive approximations) (Using hand motions to help demonstrate "two-parts")*. Tell me, "F --- ast."	
	Jacob: F̲ --- ast.
Good job, /f/ was exactly right. Now, let's make the sounds a little closer in the word: "f - ast."	
	Jacob: F̲ - ast.
Excellent, Jacob. Now let's blend the sounds into one slow word: "Fast."	
	Jacob: F̲ast.
Wonderful! You got the /f/ exactly right. Joe, tell me, "Fast." *(This pulls Joe into therapy and keeps him from being idle too long.)*	
	Joe: Fast.
Perfect. Anthony, tell me, "Fast." *(This pulls Anthony into therapy and keeps him from being idle too long.)*	
	Anthony: Fast.
Good job, Anthony. Jacob, tell me one last word, nice and slow, "Fade."	
	Jacob: F̲ade.
Excellent work, Jacob. Joe, your turn, tell me, "Sail."	
	Joe: S̲ail.

Clinician	Clients
"Some."	
	Joe: Some.
"Safe."	
	Joe: Safe.
"Sit."	
	Joe: Sit.
"Sew."	
	Joe: Sew.
Great job, Joe, you got all five right. High five to Anthony and Jacob on that!	
	Joe: Gives Anthony and Jacob a "high five."
(Note: This is the beginning of round two. You have a choice of continuing a second round of the phoneme that was addressed for each child in round one, or you may proceed to each child's second phoneme. Also, in each round, each child is most often elicited and recorded for five responses or until an error occurs. Five responses per child is used simply to keep other children from having to wait too long before a turn, especially when others are not needed for helping to model an error sound. However, as therapy progresses over weeks and months, and the pace increases, it is possible to elicit up to 10 short responses from each client, if desired, without others having to wait too long.) Anthony, it's your turn again; you're doing well with /k/ in sentences. Let's work on /t/ in syllables. Tell me, "/te/."	
	Anthony: /te/.
Good; "/ti/."	
	Anthony: /ti/.

continues

continued

Clinician	Clients
"/to/."	Anthony: /to/.
"/tu/."	Anthony: /tu/.
"/tæ/."	Anthony: /kæ/.
(Immediately stop recording and proceed to the Teaching Phase of the Body of Therapy. To help with data collection, note that at this point, Anthony has 4 correct and 1 incorrect responses for this round.) Oh, you got most of those /t/ sounds, Anthony, and I saw you working hard. But, on the last one, you said /k/ instead of /t/. You made a /k/ in the back of the mouth, the same as for your words in sentences, but for these sounds, you should be making a /t/ in the front of the mouth, with the tongue tip up behind the front top teeth, like this: /t/ (*demonstrates*). Watch Jacob. Jacob, show Anthony the /t/ sound.	
	Jacob: /t/.
Good job, Jacob. Now, Anthony, watch how Joe's tongue goes up behind his front top teeth when he makes the /t/. Joe, show Anthony the /t/.	
	Joe: /t/.
Excellent, Joe. Now, Anthony, you try; put the tip of your tongue up behind your front top teeth and make the sound like this: /t/.	
	Anthony: /t/.
Great /t/ sound, Anthony; your tongue was in exactly the right place. Show Jacob the /t/.	

Clinician	Clients
	Anthony: (Turns to Jacob) /t/.
Great! Show Joe the /t/.	Anthony: (Turns to Joe) /t/.
Wonderful, Anthony. Now, let's take your /t/ and put it back into the syllable, in two parts: "t --- æ." (*hand motions to help*).	
	Anthony: t̲ --- æ.
Great job, good /t/ sound. Let's put the sounds a little closer together: t -- æ.	
	Anthony: t̲ -- æ.
Good work, Anthony. Now, let's blend your syllable, very slowly: /tæ/.	
	Anthony: /t̲æ/.
Nice job, Anthony /tæ/. Everyone, listen. Give Anthony a thumbs-up if the sound is correct. Anthony, tell Jacob /tæ/.	
	Anthony: /t̲æ/. Jacob: (Thumbs-up)
Great job, Anthony. Good listening, Jacob. Anthony, tell Joe /tæ/.	
	Anthony: /t̲æ/. Joe: (Thumbs-up)
Great job, Anthony. Good listening, Joe. Anthony, tell me one last syllable, nice and slow: /ta/.	
	Anthony: /t̲a/.
Very nice work, Anthony. Jacob, let's try your /f/ in words again. Tell me, "Feed."	
	Jacob: F̲eed.
"Full."	Jacob: F̲ull.
"Found."	Jacob: F̲ound.
"Feet."	Jacob: F̲eet.

continues

continued

Clinician	Clients
"Fist."	Jacob: <u>F</u>ist.
Perfect, Jacob. You got all five of the <u>f</u> sounds right! Way to go! High five for me! *(Holds up open hand for high five from Jacob!)* Joe, your turn. Tell me, "Said."	
	Joe: Said.
"Soon."	Joe: Soon.
"Save."	Joe: Save.
"Sick."	Joe: Sick.
"Set."	Joe: Set.
Great job, Joe, you got all five right again. High five to Anthony on that!	
	Joe: *(Turns and gives Anthony a high five.)*
(Note: This is the beginning of round three.) Anthony, let's go back to your /k/ in sentences. Tell me, "The candy box is empty."	
	Anthony: The <u>c</u>andy box is empty.
Great, the /k/ in candy was exactly right. Let's speed it up a little. Tell me, "She caught the ball."	
	Anthony: She <u>c</u>aught the ball.
"Kiss mommie goodnight."	Anthony: <u>K</u>iss mommie goodnight.
"He cares for us."	Anthony: He <u>t</u>ares for us.
(Immediately stop recording and proceed to the Teaching Phase of the Body of Therapy. To help with data collection, note that at this point,	

Clinician	Clients
Anthony has 3 correct and 1 incorrect responses for this round.) Anthony, you are really working hard on the /k/ in sentences, but I heard a /t/ instead in the word *cares*. Pull your tongue back and hump it up back there (*touches Anthony's face near the ear*) to make a good /k/ sound. Listen: /k/. Jacob, make /k/ for Anthony.	
	Jacob: /k/.
Excellent, Jacob. Anthony, listen for Joe. Joe, make /k/ for Anthony.	
	Joe: /k/.
Good work, Joe. Anthony, you try; pull your tongue back into a hump toward the back and let the air flow over the hump: /k/. Tell me /k/.	
	Anthony: /k/.
Very nice work, Anthony; the /k/ is exactly right. Now, let's put your /k/ back into your word very slowly, into two parts: "C --- ares." (*Hand motions to help demonstrate.*)	
	Anthony: C --- ares.
Wonderful. Now, closer together: "C--ares."	
	Anthony: C--ares.
Excellent. Now, let's blend your word very slowly, "Cares."	
	Anthony: Cares.
Good work, Anthony. Jacob, let me hear *cares*. (*This pulls Jacob into therapy and keeps him from being idle too long.*)	
	Jacob: Cares.
Good work, Jacob. Joe, let me hear *cares*. (*This pulls Joe into therapy and keeps him from being idle too long.*)	
	Joe: Cares.

continues

continued

Clinician	Clients
Excellent, Joe. Now, Anthony, let's put your word back into your sentence very slowly; watch me: "He cares for us."	
	Anthony: He <u>c</u>ares for us.
Wonderful, Anthony! He cares for us. Joe, let me hear: "He cares for us."	
	Joe: He <u>c</u>ares for us.
Great job Joe. Jacob: "He cares for us."	
	Jacob: He <u>c</u>ares for us.
Good work, Jacob. Very nice work, guys. Anthony, one last sentence, slowly. Watch me for your /k/. "I see the cup."	
	Anthony: I see the <u>c</u>up.
Very good work, Anthony; you tongue was in the right place for a perfect /k/ sound. Jacob, let's continue your /f/ in words. Tell me, "First."	
	Jacob: First.
"Four."	
	Jacob: Four.
"Fit."	
	Jacob: Fit.
"Fed."	
	Jacob: <u>P</u>ed.
(Immediately stop recording and proceed to the Teaching Phase of the Body of Therapy. To help with data collection, note that at this point, Jacob has 3 correct and 1 incorrect responses for this round.) You're working hard on the /f/, Jacob, but on the last one, I heard a /p/ again, instead of an /f/. We make /p/ by stopping the air, but for your /f/ sound, the air keeps going in a long stream. I need you to continue the airstream for the	

Clinician	Clients
/f/ sound by placing your top teeth lightly on your bottom lip to let the airstream flow between the bottom lip and the top teeth, like this: /f/ (*demonstrates then solicits models from other clients*). Watch Joe. Joe, show Jacob how to make /f/.	
	Joe: /f/.
Great job, Joe. Jacob, watch how Anthony makes the /f/. He's going to let his top teeth touch his bottom lip, then, he'll let the airstream out for a long flow to make /f/. Watch, Jacob. Anthony, show Jacob how to make /f/.	
	Anthony: /f/.
Good job, Anthony, good /f/. Jacob you try; place your top teeth gently on your bottom lip, and let the airstream pass between them in a long stream: /f/.	
	Jacob: /f/.
Did everyone hear how well Jacob made the /f/? Was that a thumbs-up or a thumbs-down?	
	Anthony and Joe: (Both show a thumbs-up)
Very good work, Jacob. Now, let's put that /f/ back into your word, but we'll break it up into two parts (**successive approximations**): Tell me, "F --- ed."	
	Jacob: F̲ --- ed.
Good job; /f/ was exactly right. Now, let's make the sounds a little closer in the word: "F -- ed."	
	Jacob: F̲ -- ed.
Excellent, Jacob. Now let's blend the sound into one slow word: Fed.	
	Jacob: F̲ed.

continues

continued

Clinician	Clients
Wonderful! You got the /f/ exactly right. Joe, tell me, "Fed." (*This pulls Joe into therapy and keeps him from being idle too long.*)	
	Joe: F̲ed.
Perfect, Joe. Anthony, tell me, "Fed." (*This pulls Anthony into therapy and keeps him from being idle too long.*)	
	Anthony: F̲ed.
Great job, Anthony. Jacob, tell me one last word, nice and slow, "Fan."	
	Jacob: F̲an.
Excellent work, Jacob. Joe, your turn; tell me, "Sat."	
	Joe: S̲at.
"Same."	Joe: S̲ame.
"Seed."	Joe: S̲eed.
"Set."	Joe: S̲et.
"Sift."	Joe: S̲ift.
Great job, Joe, you got all five right. High five to Anthony and Jacob on that!	
	Joe: Turns and gives Anthony a high five, then gives Jacob a high five.
(Note: **This is the beginning of round four.**) Anthony, it's your turn again; you're doing well with /k/ in sentences; let's work on /t/ in syllables again. Tell me, "/te/." **(Therapy continues in this manner until the end of the time segment for the body of therapy. [Typically, about 24–26 minutes of a 30-minute session is devoted to the body of therapy.] Then, proceed to the closing.)**	

CLOSING	
Clinician	**Clients**
Review of Objectives	
Everyone worked hard today. Anthony, you worked on /k/ in sentences, and /t/ in syllables. Jacob, you worked on /f/ in words, and /l/ in words. Joe, you worked on /s/ in words, and /l/ in sentences. Good work for everyone.	
Summarize Client's Performances	
Anthony, you got 90% correct on /k/ in sentences, and 80% on /t/ in syllables. Great work. We got the percentage we wanted on /k/, but missed it a little on /t/; we'll try harder next time on the /t/, okay?	Anthony: Okay.
Jacob, you got 90% correct on /f/, and 90% on /l/ in words today. Good work, Jacob; we will go to /l/ in sentences next time. Way to go, Jacob.	Jacob: That was good!
That was good work Jacob; you're right about that. And, Joe, you got 100% on /s/. We didn't work on /l/ in words, so we'll start there next time. Great work on /s/ today!	Joe: Thank you.
Homework	
No homework for next time.	
Rewards	
Stickers for everyone today!	

continues

Clinician	Clients
Joe, here's a sticker for you. Jacob, here's your sticker. Anthony, here's a sticker for you. Everyone, enjoy the rest of the day, and I'll see you next Monday. Bye-bye.	

Summary

Traditional articulation therapy is one of several approaches to articulation intervention and is considered to be foundational for articulation intervention. One of the advantages to learning traditional articulation therapy is that several other approaches to articulation therapy either compare or contrast to the traditional model of therapy. SLPs employing the traditional model of articulation therapy experience success with many clients with poor intelligibility, although sometimes not as rapidly as might occur with other approaches to therapy. For this reason, traditional therapy may not be recommended for all articulation clients due to the nature and severity of the disorder. SLPs are encouraged to become proficient with traditional articulation therapy and to venture toward more in-depth approaches to intervention for clients with severe articulation difficulties, particularly when phonological processes intervention or oral motor interventions may be required.

Learning Tool

List each component of the major divisions of a speech-language therapy session and briefly tell what should transpire within each section of those major components for articulation therapy.

_____

_____

_____

_____

_____

_____

References

Backus, O., & Beasley, J. (1951). *Speech therapy with children.* Cambridge, MA: Riverside Press.

Blache, S. (1978). *The acquisition of distinctive features.* Baltimore, MD: University Park Press.

Creaghead, N. A., Newman, P. W., & Secord, W. A. (1989). *Assessment and remediation of articulatory and phonological disorders* (2nd ed.). New York, NY: Macmillan.

Hodson, B., & Paden, E. (1983). *Targeting intelligible speech: A phonological approach to remediation.* San Diego, CA: College-Hill Press.

Ingram, D. (1986). Explanation and phonological remediation. *Child Language Teaching and Therapy, 2,* 1–19.

McCabe, R. B., & Bradley, D. P. (1975). Systemic multiple phonemic approach to articulation therapy. *Acta Symbolica, 6,* 2–18.

McDonald, E. T., & August, L. (1970). Apparent impedence of oral sensory functions and articulatory proficiency. In J. Bosma (Ed.), *Second symposium on oral sensation and perception.* Springfield, IL: Charles C. Thomas.

Peña-Brooks, A., & Hegde, M. N. (2000). *Assessment and treatment of articulation and phonological disorders in children.* Austin, TX: Pro-Ed.

Van Riper, C. (1939). *Speech correction: Principles and methods.* Englewood Cliffs, NJ: Prentice-Hall.

Van Riper, C. (1978). *Speech corrections: Principles and methods* (6th ed.). Englewood Cliffs, NJ: Prentice-Hall.

Van Riper, C., & Emerick, L. (1984). *Speech corrections: An introduction to speech pathology and audiology.* Englewood Cliffs, NJ: Prentice-Hall.

Van Riper, C., & Erickson, R. (1969). A predictive screening test of articulation. *Journal of Speech and Hearing Disorders, 34,* 214–219.

Van Riper, C., & Erickson, R. (1996). *Speech corrections: An introduction to speech pathology and audiology* (9th ed.). Englewood Cliffs, NJ: Prentice-Hall.

11

Guided Practice for Voice Therapy

Selected General Concepts for Voice Therapy

The need for voice therapy may arise from a number of causes ranging from functional misuse of the voice to more invasive surgical procedures. When the need for voice therapy arises, SLPs may choose from specific voice programs or general therapy techniques. The therapy presented in this chapter addresses general techniques for voice intervention.

1. Haynes and Pindzola (2004) devised "An Organizational Schema of Voice Disorders" (p. 276) that presented both *perceptual attributes* and *physical systems* that most directly influence voice production. The *perceptual attributes of voice*, quality, pitch, and loudness, although evaluated often through listener perception, relate to measurable sound wave complexities, frequencies of the sound wave, and the amplitude of the sound wave associated with the speaker's voice. Difficulty in any of the perceptual attributes of voice often results in a need for assessment of voice by the SLP. The physical systems, sometimes referred to as *the systems of speech production* (Seikel, King, & Drumright, 1997), most closely related to voice production are the respiratory, phonatory, and resonatory–articulatory systems (Haynes & Pindzola, 2004). Boone, McFarlane, Von Berg, and Zraick (2013) discussed three causes, or etiologies, of voice disorders: functional, neurological, and organic. Through careful assessment of quality, pitch, and loudness, as related to either the respiratory, phonatory, or resonatory–articulatory systems, in conjunction with the etiology of the voice disorder, either functional, neurological, or organic, it is possible to determine the type of therapy that is likely suitable for the client.

2. "There is no set voice therapy regimen. Rather, voice therapy is highly indi-vidualized, depending on the cause of the problem, its maintaining factors, the motivation of the patient, and the availability of appropriate management

and treatment" (Boone et al., 2013, p. 179). To this end, before prescribing therapy, the SLP is strongly encouraged to determine (a) the voice attribute (quality, pitch, loudness) that is negatively impacted in the client's voice sample, (b) the speech system that appears to be most impacted by the client's voice (respiratory, phonatory, resonatory–articulatory), and (c) the probable etiology of the disorder (functional misuse/abuse of the voice, neurological disorders related to difficulty with the nerves or nervous system, or organic disorders caused by physiological conditions).

3. The SLP may work independently as the professional involved in voice intervention. However, the SLP should be prepared to work with other professionals, (ear, nose, and throat specialists [ENTs], surgeons, psychologists, and others) for assessment and management of some voice clients.

4. It is important that the cause of vocal fold pathology is determined prior to implementation of speech-language therapy for voice disorders. This generally entails assessment by medical professionals such as ENTs in addition to the SLP's clinical assessment.

5. Some clients with resonance disorders may need to be evaluated by a craniofacial specialist to assist with diagnosis and management of resonance disorders.

6. Be prepared to change the course of therapy for the voice client as the physical or nervous system of the client changes over the course of intervention.

Numerous other concepts and guidelines apply for voice therapy. However, based on the information given in these selected general concepts, it is hoped that the reader understands the text well enough to process the information and examples throughout the remainder of this section on voice therapy.

Selected Voice Objectives

Following are examples of objectives for voice therapy:

1. Client will sustain an audible vocal tone using an open vowel sound for 10 consecutive seconds at least 5 times during a 30-minute period.

2. Client will manipulate vocal pitch from lower to higher pitches on command while maintaining a constant moderate-to-low volume 8 of 10 opportunities.

3. Client will decrease vocal tension as exemplified by a reduced pitch using the Yawn-Sigh technique 100% of opportunities.

Here's How to Do Voice Therapy

Note to Reader: The information in the script below is designed to help you learn the progression of voice therapy as related to specific voice objectives. Of course, if different objectives were selected, the script would, accordingly, be different as well.

Listed in Figure 11–1 are the 14 therapeutic-specific skills groups and appropriate boxes for you to check off each time you read through the therapy sequence. Check off

Spaces are provided for multiple practices of the 28 therapeutic-specific skills (14 skills groups) below associated with voice therapy. Check off or date a block each practice time for the skill or skills group. You may need several practice sessions to become comfortable with voice therapy. Once you comfortably feel you have demonstrated a skill or skills group well enough for use in an actual therapy session, note the date in a remaining box. (Note: *Skill to be practiced in actual therapy, not in the script.)

☐ ☐ ☐ ☐ ☐ ☐ ☐ ☐ ☐ ☐ Motivation

☐ ☐ ☐ ☐ ☐ ☐ ☐ ☐ ☐ ☐ Communicating Expectations

☐ ☐ ☐ ☐ ☐ ☐ ☐ ☐ ☐ ☐ Enthusiasm, Animation, Volume

☐ ☐ ☐ ☐ ☐ ☐ ☐ ☐ ☐ ☐ Seating, Proximity, Touch

☐ ☐ ☐ ☐ ☐ ☐ ☐ ☐ ☐ ☐ Preparation, Pace, Fluency

☐ ☐ ☐ ☐ ☐ ☐ ☐ ☐ ☐ ☐ Alerting, Cueing, Modeling, Prompting

☐ ☐ ☐ ☐ ☐ ☐ ☐ ☐ ☐ ☐ Modalities, Describing/Demonstrating, Questioning, Wait-Time

☐ ☐ ☐ ☐ ☐ ☐ ☐ ☐ ☐ ☐ Shaping (Successive Approximations)

☐ ☐ ☐ ☐ ☐ ☐ ☐ ☐ ☐ ☐ Praise, Tokens, Primary Reinforcers

☐ ☐ ☐ ☐ ☐ ☐ ☐ ☐ ☐ ☐ Corrective Feedback

☐ ☐ ☐ ☐ ☐ ☐ ☐ ☐ ☐ ☐ Data Collection

☐ ☐ ☐ ☐ ☐ ☐ ☐ ☐ ☐ ☐ Probing*

☐ ☐ ☐ ☐ ☐ ☐ ☐ ☐ ☐ ☐ Behavioral Management*

☐ ☐ ☐ ☐ ☐ ☐ ☐ ☐ ☐ ☐ Troubleshooting*

Figure 11–1. Practice chart for sample voice therapy.

each skill as you practice it. Once you comfortably feel you have demonstrated a skill well enough for clinical use of the skill, note the date in a remaining box. Continue to read through the therapy progression until you have indicated a "comfort-level" date for all 14 skills groups. Do not become discouraged if it takes several readings for you to feel that you have adequately demonstrated the 14 skills groups with appropriate comfort levels.

Advance Organizer (Three Questions to Note)

Focus on the 14 therapeutic-specific skills groups as you read the given script of voice therapy written for an individual client of young adult age. For each of the 14 therapeutic-specific skills groups listed in Figure 11–1, ask these advance organizer questions:

❑ How will I implement this therapeutic-specific skill?

❑ How will I sound when I implement this therapeutic-specific skill?

❑ As I practice the therapeutic-specific skill, what can I do to improve my clinical skills?

Here's How to Do Voice Therapy **15-Minute Scripted Session for Voice Therapy** **(Individual Therapy Session)**	
INTRODUCTION	
Clinician	Client
Greeting and Rapport Good morning, Lisa. How are you today?	 Hi. (low-tone, weak voice, waving hand also)
Review of Previous Session You've been working on increasing your vocal strength by lengthening the breath stream that you use for speaking and raising your pitch. Remember?	 Yes. (low-tone, weak voice, almost a whisper)

Clinician	Client
Collection of or Mentioning of Homework	
I asked you to bring a cassette recorder so that I could show you how to do your exercises at home. Did you remember to bring it?	
	Um-hmm. (hands the recorder to the SLP)
Good remembering, Lisa. Bringing the recorder was like homework for you, wasn't it? So, you did well in getting your homework done! We, of course have recorders in the clinic, but I wanted to get a feel for the kind of recorder that you have at home to work with, and I wanted to be sure you're comfortable doing the exercises using your own equipment so that it wouldn't be such a big transition for you at home. Does that make sense to you?	
	Um-hmm.

<table>
<tr><td colspan="2" align="center">BODY</td></tr>
</table>

Clinician	Client
Establishment Phase	
Let's get started, Lisa. Let's see if we can achieve 80% correct pitch manipulation and 80% correct maintaining voice in the session today.	
Eliciting and Recording and Teaching Phases (Often eliciting and recording and teaching phases are overlapping in voice therapy for general procedures. When using specific voice programs, these phases may be presented separately.)	

continues

continued

Clinician	Client
The first thing we need to work on is sustaining an audible sound. I'll record you using your recorder while you vocalize for me something you've already done twice today. Do you know what that is?	
	(Shakes head, "No")
It's your *agreement sound*, "Um-hmm."	
	Um-hmm. (smiles)
Let's begin with three, "Um-hmms," one after the other, but try to make each one a little longer than the one before it, like this: "Um-hmm, um-hmmm, um-hmmmm." Now, you try, but let me turn on the recorder first (*presses record*). Okay, ready? You try.	
	Um-hmm, um-hmmm, um-hmmmm.
(*Stops recorder*) Very nice work, Lisa. Your sounds were very well controlled. Let's try the same thing to get your voice ready to work a little harder, except this time, you operate the recorder to get more accustomed to the routine. Let's try it again: Make each one longer than the one before. "Um-hmm, um-hmmm, um-hmmmm." Press record and begin your um-hums. Stop the recorder when finished.	
	(Presses record) Um-hmm, um-hmmm, um-hmmmm. (stops recorder)
Good work, Lisa. Now, let's play it back to see if there's a difference in the way you sound on those two samples. (*Rewinds and re-plays the samples*) Did one sound better than the other to you?	
	Um-hmm.

Clinician	Client
Which one sounded better?	
	Two. (with only /t/ barely audible, holding up two fingers)
Two. Great. I think two was much stronger, also. Good listening, Lisa. Now, let's try something a little different with the "um-hmm" sample. This time, we'll start with "um-hmm," but instead of making the "um-hmms" longer, we will add a one-syllable words such as *may, me, my, more, moot* to the end of the "um-hmm." I have the words written here for you to read so you don't have to remember them. *(Shows Lisa the list of one-syllable words.)* This is what it sounds like: "Um-hmm may, um-hmm me, um-hmm my, um-hmm more, um-hmm moot." Press record, and you try it. Read each word in the list to add to the end of "Um-hmm." Stop the recorder when finished.	
	(Presses record) Um-hmm may, um-hmm me, um-hmm my, um-hmm more, um-hmm moot. (presses stop)
How did that feel to your throat, Lisa?	
	(Thumbs-up; laughs)
It sounded good; it was stronger, clearer, and sounded as if it was easier than last week. Let's try it again, but this time make the last part of "Um-hmm" longer, like this: "Um-hmmmm" before adding the end word, so it will sound like: "Um-hmmmm may, um-hmmmm me, um-hmmmm my, um-hmmmm more, um-hmmmm moot." Press record, then you try, and make sure to project a nice, strong, steady voice while you're working. Stop the recorder when finished.	

continues

continued

Clinician	Client
	(Presses record) Um-hmmmm may, um-hmmmm me, um-hmmmm my, um-hmmmm more, um-hmmmm moot. (presses stop)
Great, Lisa. I heard a lot more clarity and strength in your voice that time; what about you; did it sound good to you?	
	Yes, it was good. (slow rate, but voice stronger and clearer than a few minutes ago)
Good. This time, we'll continue the lengthy "Um-hmm," but we'll add lengthening to the end word also. I'll use a stopwatch to help keep up with the length this time. What I'd like to try is three seconds per unit, so three seconds for "Um-hmm," and three seconds for the end word. Listen to hear how long three seconds is per unit: "Um-hmmmm maaay, um-hmmmm meeee, um-hmmmm myyyy, um-hmmmm moooore, um-hmmmm mooooot." Did you get a feel for the length?	
	Yes.
Great. I want you try in a few seconds, but first, let's practice. I'll start the stopwatch and direct you with hand counting so that you can see when the three seconds are up for the first part and for changing into the second part. Watch my hand movements (*moves hands in counting motion as if directing an orchestra to change from one part of music to another*). Are you able to follow that well enough to know when the three seconds are up?	
	I think so. (voice slightly more audible)
Okay, great. Let me demonstrate again, and after that, you press record and begin.	

Clinician	Client
Be sure to read along so you don't have to remember the end words. Ready? Listen: "Um-hmmmm maaay, um-hmmmm meeee, um-hmmmm myyyy, um-hmmmm moooore, um-hmmmm mooooot." Now you try; press record and watch me; don't forget to stop the recorder when finished. (*directs with hand as Lisa says each unit set*)	
	(Presses record) Um-hmmmm maaay, um-hmmmm meeee, um-hmmmm myyyy, um-hmmmm moooore, um-hmmmm mooooot. (presses stop)
Great work, Lisa. Looks like we stayed on track, and your units sounded good for strength and clarity. This is a little difficult, so let's try it once more before moving on. Listen to me once more: "Um-hmmmm maaay, um-hmmmm meeee, um-hmmmm myyyy, um-hmmmm moooore, um-hmmmm mooooot." Now you try. Press record and watch me. Stop the recorder when finished. (*directs with hand motions*)	
	(Presses record) Um-hmmmm maaay, um-hmmmm meeee, um-hmmmm myyyy, um-hmmmm moooore, um-hmmmm mooooot. (presses stop)
Great work, Lisa! Was that a thumbs-up or a thumbs-down?	
	Thumbs-up. (low volume, but steady voice)
That was a thumbs-up! Way to go! (*holds up thumb for Lisa to see*) This time, Lisa, we'll do the same amount of time and the same format, but we'll change the words. For example, we'll continue to work on the three seconds per unit, but the end words will change.	

continues

continued

Clinician	Client
This time, let's add at the end of "Um-hmmmmm" (*holds three seconds*) these words: *Nate, knee, night, note, new,* so your new units will sound like this: "Um-hmmmm naaaate, um-hmmmm kneeee, um-hmmmm niiiight, um-hmmmm noooote, um-hmmmm neeeew." Here's the list; just read so you don't have to remember the words. Ready?	
	Yes. (voice both stronger and clearer)
Press record and begin. Watch me. Stop the recorder when finished. (*moves hands in counting motion to help keep Lisa on track*)	
	(Presses record) Um-hmmmm naaaate, um-hmmmm kneeee, um-hmmmm niiiight, um-hmmmm noooote, um-hmmmm neeeew. (presses stop)
Excellent, Lisa. Great work. I heard a louder, clearer voice on all units that time! Very nice work.	
	Thanks. (stronger, clearer voice)
Let's try two more things. Let's work on the word list for just a minute, then work on open vowels. We've been working with 10 words today, and I'd like to see how well you do with reading those words, using vocal manipulations. For example, reading the word *may*, I'd like you to say it with a slight wave in pitch (*start, then slight upward inflection, and back to starting*) that sounds a little like you're signing the word like this (*demonstrates on all 10 words, slowly, about 30 seconds to complete all 10*). Now, you try. Take your time, and be sure the change in the middle is upward, if possible. Press record, then begin slowly. Stop the recorder when finished.	

Clinician	Client
	(Presses record) May, me, my, more, moot, Nate, knee, night, note, new. (takes about 30 seconds to complete) (presses stop)
Excellent, Lisa. Very nice work! I heard lots of vocal movement and manipulations in that segment. Let's have you do it once more, but I want you to go a little slower so that you get the feel of how your vocal mechanism is moving when you change the pitch upward. Let's take about 35 seconds to go through all 10 words this time, so you'll really have to slow it down. Start again; press record.	
	(Presses record) May, me, my, more, moot, Nate, knee, night, note, new. (takes about 35 to 50 seconds to complete) (presses stop)
Excellent use of your voice, Lisa. What could you feel happening in your throat as you changed the pitch very slowly?	
	I think my voice box was moving up and down a little. (good voice, with a little fatigue starting to set in due to amount of work in the session)
That's right, Lisa. Your voice box should have been moving slightly up and down as you worked slowly on changing pitch. Good work. Let's try one more thing. I want you to extend a few vowels up to 10 seconds, if possible. Let's use the long vowels that we've been working with today: *a, e, i, o, u*. What I'd like you to do is to take one at a time and simply hold it for 10 seconds while I count for you. For example, *a* will sound like this: aaaaaaaaaaaaaaaaaaaa. Clear?	
	Yes.

continues

Clinician	Client
Alright, start with, *a*, and hold it for 10 seconds, then go to the other four vowels and hold each for 10 seconds. We don't need to record for this part, so just begin when I give you a hand signal. I'll use the stop watch for the 10-second count. Ready?	
	Um-hmm.
Begin.	
	aaaaaaaaaaaaaaaaaaaaaaaaaaaaaaaaaaaaa eeeeeeeeeeeeeeeeeeeeeeeeeeeeeeeeeeeeeeeee iiiiiiiiiiiiiiiiiiiiiiiiiiiiiiiiiiiiiiiiiiiiiiiiiiiiiiii ooooooooooooooooooooooooooooooooooo uuuuuuuuuuuuuuuuuuuuuuuuuuuuuuuuu
Good effort, Lisa. How did that feel?	
	Okay. But, it seemed a little hard on a few of them. (voice good for volume and clarity)
It's good that you noticed that. We'll work on breath control as well next week. **(Session continues in this manner until the time ends, or until the client's voice becomes fatigued as it is becoming in this example. Then, proceed to the closing.)**	

CLOSING

Review of Objectives and Summarize Client's Performances Lisa, you've done well today. You worked on using the *agreement sound (um-hmm)* to transition into one-syllable words, and it looks like you did 90% correct production of those units. Good work. Then, we	

Clinician	Client
worked with one-syllable words for vocal manipulation and open vowels to relax your vocal mechanism. You got 100% of vocal manipulations, but I think you said that some of the vowels were a little difficult to maintain toward the end.	
	Yes.
I didn't take data on those because they were used to help you relax your vocal folds after working so hard today.	
Overall, you did very well today, Lisa. Congratulations on a good session.	
Homework	
Please take the cassette home and listen to the format of the work we've done today and practice the same structures at home for about 8 to 10 minutes each day for the next three days (Friday, Saturday, Sunday). Then on the fourth day, Monday, please record your practices and bring in the tape for me to hear your work. I should be able to hear very nice improvements by Monday, the fourth day. Is all that clear?	
	Yes.
Rewards (No tangible reward given)	
Great. Then, thanks for coming in, and I'll see you next Tuesday. Remember, record your work for me on Monday of next week and bring it in. Thanks, and have a great day.	
	Good-bye.

Summary

SLPs consider the structures and functions of anatomy associated with speech and language for all areas of therapy. However, it is, perhaps, more important to focus on structure and function of the anatomy associated with voice than any other area of speech. It is important for the SLP to consult with medical (ENT) specialists for support in determining the exact nature of voice difficulties before beginning voice therapy. Similarly, a referral to a craniofacial specialist to obtain additional information regarding structures and functioning of the resonance mechanisms is often helpful.

Learning Tool

List each component of the major divisions of a speech-language therapy session and briefly tell what should transpire within each section of those major components for voice therapy.

_____

_____

_____

_____

_____

_____

References

Boone, D. R., McFarlane, S. C., Von Berg, S. L., & Zraick, R. I. (2013). *The voice and voice therapy* (9th ed.). Boston, MA: Allyn & Bacon.

Haynes, W. O., & Pindzola, R. H. (2004). *Diagnosis and evaluation in speech pathology* (6th ed.). Boston, MA: Pearson Allyn & Bacon.

Seikel, J. A., King, D. W., & Drumright, D. G. (1997). *Anatomy and physiology for speech, language, and hearing.* San Diego, CA: Singular Publishing Group.

12

Guided Practice for Resonance Therapy

Selected General Concepts for Resonance Therapy

Resonance difficulties were addressed as subcomponents of voice disorders by the speech-language pathology profession until 2001 when ASHA published a scope of practice statement that acknowledged resonance as a separate area of practice for SLPs (ASHA, 2001). Following are general concepts related to resonance therapy.

1. *Vocal resonance* is the perceptual increases in loudness of the laryngeal tone due to the concentration and reflection of sound waves by the oral, pharyngeal, and nasal cavities during voice production (Boone, McFarlane, Von Berg, & Zraick, 2013).

2. ASHA developed a *Scope of Practice* document (ASHA, 2001) indicating that the practice of speech-language pathology involves providing services to address resonance disorders as an entity separate from disorders of voice. Historically, however, SLPs studied and clinically addressed resonance disorders as an aspect of voice, attributable to difficulty in the resonatory system of speech as represented by Seikel, King, and Drumright (1997). The resonatory system was depicted by Haynes and Pindzola (2004) as well in their "Organizational Schema of Voice Disorders" (p. 276). Prior to ASHA's (2001) separation of voice and resonance disorders, professionals made clinical judgments in conjunction with medical assessments by otolaryngologists, or other medical professionals who worked closely with the vocal mechanism, to determine if a disorder of vocal quality was, in fact, attributable to vocal fold pathology or to difficulties with the velopharyngeal system associated with the resonatory system. Most often, the distinguishing feature of voice disorders associated with resonance

involved nasality or related difficulties as opposed to voice difficulties due to laryngeal or related difficulties (Boone et al., 2013).

3.   It is important that the cause of resonance difficulty is determined prior to implementation of speech-language therapy for resonance disorders. This determination may entail assessment by medical professionals such as ENTs and craniofacial specialists in addition to the SLP's clinical assessment.

4.   Boone et al. (2013) discussed several disorders of resonance including *hypernasality, hyponasality, assimilative nasality*, and *cul-de-sac resonance*. These researchers also discussed two oral pharyngeal resonance disorders: stridency and thin voice quality. Boone et al. defined **hypernasality** as an excessive and undesirable amount of perceived nasal cavity resonance during phonation of normally nonnasal vowels and nonnasal voiced consonants. They described **hyponasality** as reduced nasal resonance for the production of the nasal sounds /m/, /n/, and /ŋ/. **Assimilative nasality** was defined as excessive nasality on sounds adjacent to the three normally nasalized consonants due to extended time that the velopharyngeal port is opened when making the three nasalized sounds; any adjacent sound following the production of the nasal phonemes is perceived as being nasal also because the port remains open long enough for that sound to be emitted nasally rather than orally (Boone et al., 2013). **Cul-de-sac resonance** was defined as a hollow, muffled sounding voice often caused by posterior tongue retraction, or an anterior nasal obstruction (Haynes & Pindzola, 2004; Peterson-Falzone, Hardin-Jones, & Karnell, 2001).

5.   Clinically, the disorders often associated with resonance disorders are cleft palate and craniofacial disorders.

6.   Difficulty in any of the perceptual attributes of resonance often results in a need for assessment of resonance by the SLP. The physical systems, sometimes referred to as *the systems of speech production* (Seikel et al., 1997) most closely related to resonance are the respiratory and the resonatory–articulatory systems described by Haynes and Pindzola (2004).

7.   Boone et al. (2013) discussed three causes, or etiologies, of resonance disorders: functional, neurological, and organic. Through careful assessment of the perceptual quality of oral or nasal resonance, in conjunction with the etiology of the resonance disorder, either functional, neurological, or organic, it is possible to determine the type of resonance therapy that is likely suitable for the client.

8.   Because of the configuration of structural and functional articulations that must work in synchrony for a client to produce acceptable resonance, before prescribing resonance therapy, the SLP is strongly encouraged to determine (a) the type of resonance disorder that is present in the client's speech sample and (b) the probable etiology of the disorder (i.e., functional difficulty related to severe hearing impairment, neurological disorders related to difficulty with the nerves or nervous system, or organic disorders caused by physiological conditions that negatively impact resonance).

9. The SLP may work independently as the professional involved in resonance intervention. However, the SLP should be prepared to work with other professions (craniofacial specialists, ENTs/surgeons, psychologists, and others) for management of some clients with resonance disorders.

10. Intervention services are provided for individuals with resonance or nasal airflow disorders, velopharyngeal incompetence, or articulation disorders caused by velopharyngeal incompetence and related disorders such as cleft lip/palate (ASHA, 2004).

11. Be prepared to change the course of therapy for the client with resonance disorders as the physical or nervous systems of the client change over the course of intervention.

Numerous other concepts and guidelines apply for resonance therapy. However, based on the information given in these selected general concepts, it is hoped that the reader understands the text well enough to process the information and examples throughout the remainder of this section on resonance therapy.

Selected Resonance Objectives

Following are examples of objectives for resonance therapy:

1. (For the client who exhibits *hyponasality*) Client will increase nasal resonance through use of nasal cavity phonemes (/m/, /n/, /ŋ/) in words and phrases with acceptable nasal resonance 8 of 10 opportunities.

2. (For the client who exhibits *hypernasality*) Client will decrease hypernasality by producing oral consonants, vowels, and diphthongs in the oral cavity 90% of opportunities.

3. (For the client who exhibits *functional cul-de-sac resonance*) Client will use tongue-forward positions to increase nasal resonance when reading one- to two-syllable words that include the use of nasal consonants 8 of 10 opportunities.

Here's How to Do Resonance Therapy

Note to Reader: The information in the script below is designed to help you learn the progression of resonance therapy as related to specific resonance objectives. Of course, if different objectives were selected, the script would, accordingly, be different as well.

Listed in Figure 12–1 are the 14 therapeutic-specific skills groups and appropriate boxes for you to check off each time you read through the therapy sequence. Check off each skill as you practice it. Once you comfortably feel you have demonstrated a skill well enough for clinical use of the skill, note the date in a remaining box. Continue to read through the therapy progression until you have indicated a "comfort-level" date for all 14 therapeutic skills groups. Do not become discouraged if it takes several readings for you to feel that you have adequately demonstrated the 14 skills groups with appropriate comfort levels.

Spaces are provided for multiple practices of the 28 therapeutic-specific skills (14 skills groups) below associated with resonance therapy. Check off or date a block each practice time for the skill or skills group. You may need several practice sessions to become comfortable with resonance therapy. Once you comfortably feel you have demonstrated a skill or skills group well enough for use in an actual therapy session, note the date in a remaining box. (Note: *Skill to be practiced in actual therapy, not in the script.)

☐ ☐ ☐ ☐ ☐ ☐ ☐ ☐ ☐ ☐   Motivation

☐ ☐ ☐ ☐ ☐ ☐ ☐ ☐ ☐ ☐   Communicating Expectations

☐ ☐ ☐ ☐ ☐ ☐ ☐ ☐ ☐ ☐   Enthusiasm, Animation, Volume

☐ ☐ ☐ ☐ ☐ ☐ ☐ ☐ ☐ ☐   Seating, Proximity, Touch

☐ ☐ ☐ ☐ ☐ ☐ ☐ ☐ ☐ ☐   Preparation, Pace, Fluency

☐ ☐ ☐ ☐ ☐ ☐ ☐ ☐ ☐ ☐   Alerting, Cueing, Modeling, Prompting

☐ ☐ ☐ ☐ ☐ ☐ ☐ ☐ ☐ ☐   Modalities, Describing/Demonstrating, Questioning, Wait-Time

☐ ☐ ☐ ☐ ☐ ☐ ☐ ☐ ☐ ☐   Shaping (Successive Approximations)

☐ ☐ ☐ ☐ ☐ ☐ ☐ ☐ ☐ ☐   Praise, Tokens, Primary Reinforcers

☐ ☐ ☐ ☐ ☐ ☐ ☐ ☐ ☐ ☐   Corrective Feedback

☐ ☐ ☐ ☐ ☐ ☐ ☐ ☐ ☐ ☐   Data Collection

☐ ☐ ☐ ☐ ☐ ☐ ☐ ☐ ☐ ☐   Probing*

☐ ☐ ☐ ☐ ☐ ☐ ☐ ☐ ☐ ☐   Behavioral Management*

☐ ☐ ☐ ☐ ☐ ☐ ☐ ☐ ☐ ☐   Troubleshooting*

Figure 12–1. Practice chart for sample resonance therapy.

Advance Organizer (Three Questions to Note)

Focus on the 14 therapeutic-specific skills groups as you read the given script of resonance therapy written for an individual client of young adult age. For each of the 14 therapeutic- specific skills groups listed in Figure 12–1, ask these advance organizer questions:

- ❑ How will I implement this therapeutic-specific skill?
- ❑ How will I sound when I implement this therapeutic-specific skill?
- ❑ As I practice the therapeutic-specific skill, what can I do to improve my clinical skills?

Here's How to Do Resonance Therapy
15-Minute Scripted Session for Resonance Therapy (Individual Therapy Session)

INTRODUCTION

Clinician	Client
Greeting and Rapport Good morning, Jared. How are you today?	 I'm fine. (low-tone, hyponasal voice)
Review of Previous Session Do you remember what you've been working on in therapy?	 I'm supposed to be making more sounds through my nose when I speak.
That's right; you've been working on increasing your nasality for /m, n, ŋ/ words and phrases. Good remembering.	
Collection of or Mentioning of Homework How about your homework; did you have time to practice a few minutes each day?	

continues

continued

Clinician	Client
	Well, I practiced, but not each day.
Well, practicing some is better than not practicing at all. How many days do you think you practiced, and how many minutes per day do you think you practiced?	
	Um, about three days, and I think it was about 5 to 6 minutes each day.
Great start for practicing. I'm glad you took the time to work on your speech at home.	

BODY

Establishment Phase	
Today, we're going to use a short-term recorder/playback unit so that you can hear how you sound when you're working on your exercises. Ready?	
	Yes, I'm ready.
Let's see how well you are doing with the /m, n, ŋ/. Try each sound five times for me, like this: "/m, m, m, m, m/, /n, n, n, n, n/, /ŋ, ŋ, ŋ, ŋ, ŋ/."	
	/m, m, m, m, m/, /n, n, n, n, n/, /ŋ, ŋ, g, g, ŋ/.
Very nice effort, Jared. All of your /m/ and /n/ sounds were exactly right, but you had trouble with 2 of the /ŋ/ sounds. Let's see if we can achieve 90% correct production of the nasal sounds /m, n/ and 80% correct production of the /ŋ/ for pushing the sounds through your nose today. Does that sound good?	
	Yes, that's okay.

Clinician	Client
Eliciting and Recording and Teaching Phases	
(Often eliciting and recording and teaching phases are overlapping in resonance therapy for general procedures. When using specific resonance programs, these phases may be presented separately.)	
Great. The first thing we need to work on is sustaining the nasal sounds. Let me hear you hold the /m, n, ŋ/ for 10 seconds each while you focus on how it feels as the sound comes out of your nose. Start with /m/. I'll count off the 10 seconds for you so that you can concentrate on how the /m/ sounds and feels when you make it. Go ahead and begin like this: "/mmmmmmmmmmmmmmmmmm/." *(prepares to silently count showing client the counting process by gentling waving the hand or counting off per finger)*	
	/mmmmmmmmmmmmmmmmmmm/.
Good. Tell me what it felt like as the sound came through the nasal cavity.	
	It felt a little like something was vibrating in my nose.
Good explanation! Actually, that's exactly what it feels like sometimes because the air from your lungs is being channeled through your nose to make the /m/. You may feel slight vibrations in the nasal area as you make /n/ and /ŋ/ as well. Now, try the /n/ for 10 seconds. I'll count the 10 seconds off for you so that you can concentrate on how the /n/ sounds and feels when you make it.	

continues

continued

Clinician	Client
Go ahead and begin like this: "/nnnnnnnnnnnnnnnnnnnnnnnnnnn/." (*prepares to silently count showing client the counting process*)	
	/nnnnnnnnnnnnnnnnnnnnnnnnnnnnn/.
Good effort, Jared! How did the /n/ feel?	
	It felt okay, but I didn't feel as much vibration that time.
Good assessment, Jared. Actually, you may not feel as much vibration because for the /n/ the tip of the tongue touches the alveolar ridge, the bumpy part of the roof of the mouth right behind the front top teeth, and I suspect that touching may reduce the sensation of vibration to some degree. Good work on /n/. Now try the /ŋ/. Same routine: I'll count while you produce the sound and think about it as you make it. Try "/ŋŋŋŋŋŋŋŋŋŋŋŋŋŋŋŋŋŋŋŋŋŋŋ/." (*prepares to count*)	
	/ŋŋŋŋŋŋŋŋŋŋŋŋŋŋŋŋŋŋŋŋŋŋŋŋŋŋ/.
Good. Tell me what it felt like as the /ŋ/ sound came through the nasal cavity.	
	It felt fine, but this time, I felt the back of my tongue sorta touching the top of my mouth back there.
Wow, Jared! You're thinking and focusing well because that's exactly where your tongue is—humped in the back, touching the top of your mouth when you make the /ŋ/ sound. Great work. Keep thinking about how it felt to make those nasal sounds /m, n, ŋ/ as we go into the next steps of therapy. Now, I'd like for you to use each of your nasal phonemes in one-	

Clinician	Client
syllable words, very slowly pronouncing each of the nasal sounds to process how each one feels as you say it. Here's an /m, n, ŋ/ word list for you to read: *man, men, name, main, ring, rang.* I'll record your voice while you slowly read the words, thinking about each sound. Be sure the nasal sounds come out of the nose, like this: (*demonstrates, very slowly pronouncing each word: man, men, name, main, ring, rang*). Ready, begin. (*presses record*)	
	Man, men, name, main, ring, rang. (very slowly pronouncing each)
(*Stops recorder*) Very nice work, Jared. Your sounds were very well controlled and they all sounded as if they came from the nasal cavity. Let's listen to see how you sounded. You tell me how you think it sounds. Try to focus on whether the /m, n, ŋ/ sounds were made through your nose. (*plays back the recorded words while both listen*) How do you think you sounded?	
	I think it was good.
Yes, it sounded like all of the nasals were produced through the nasal cavity. Let's try the same thing, except this time we'll make each nasal sound a little longer so that we have time to really hear them on play back. Try it like this: *man, men, name, main, ring, rang.* (*making each word especially long in order to stretch out the nasal sounds*) Now, you try it and I'll record. (*presses record*)	
	Man, men, name, main, ring, rang. (stretching out each one, especially the nasals)

continues

continued

Clinician	Client
(*Stops recorder*) Good work, Jared. Now, let's play back to see if there's a difference in the way you sound on those two samples—sample number 1 and sample number 2 (*Rewinds and re-plays both samples*) Did one sound better than the other to you?	
	Well, I could hear the /m, n, ŋ/ better on the second one.
I agree, Great! I think the sounds were all coming through the nasal cavity on both samples, but it was much easier to hear them on the second sample. Good listening, Jared. Now, let's try something a little different. This time, we'll start with *man*, but instead of going to the next word *men*, we'll stay with *man* and add the /ɑ/ sound after it, like this: "man a," then repeat it four more times so that it's one long string, like this: "man-a-man- a-man- a-man-a-man-a." Let's start slowly so that you can feel how the articulators are moving as you say the sequence. Listen and feel for the /m, n/ sounds to come out of the nose. Try it. I'll record while you speak. Ready, go. (*presses record*)	
	Man-a-man-a-man-a-man-a-man-a.
How did that feel, Jared?	
	(Thumbs-up; laughs) It felt okay; I think I could hear the sounds coming out of my nose and sometimes I felt the vibrations.
Yes, the sounds were coming out of your nose; it sounded good. Let's try it again, but this time, let's use all six of your words: *man, men, name, main, ring, rang*, adding the /ɑ/ at the end of each word so that it sounds like this for "men":	

Clinician	Client
"men-a-men-a-men-a-men-a-men-a," and so on with each word. Say each part slowly, however, as you go from word to word, like this: "man-a-man-a-man-a- man-a-man-a," "men-a-men-a-men-a- men-a-men-a," and so on, very slowly. Is that clear?	
	Yes.
Good, I'll record, while you speak. Make sure to produce all of the nasal sounds through the nose. Here's the list of the six words so you don't have to remember them; we'll listen when you finish. (*gives client the list; presses record*)	
	Okay. Man-a-man-a-man-a-man-a-man-a, Men-a-men-a-men-a-men-a-men-a, Name-a-name-a-name-a-name-a-name-a, Main-a-main-a-main-a-main-a-main-a, Ring-a-ring-a-ring-a-ring-a-ring-a, Rang-a-rang-a-rang-a-rang-a-rang-a.
Great, Jared. I heard a lot more clarity for those nasals actually coming out of your nose that time! How did it sound and feel to you?	
	It sounded okay, but it was a little hard to remember to make the right sounds come out of my nose sometimes.
I'm sure it gets a little confusing to remember to make the nasals correctly especially when all other sounds should come from the mouth rather than the nose. Hang in there, though; you're doing well. Let's listen to your recording. (*presses rewind and play; both listen*) What do you think?	
	Actually, I think it sounds good!

continues

continued

Clinician	Client
Well, it does sound good. The nasals are coming from the nasal cavity and the other sounds are coming from the mouth, just as they should. Great job, Jared. Way to go! Now, let's try the same sequence again. This time, though, let's speed it up just a little, not so fast that it's hard to remember what sound comes from the nose, but just a little faster to start thinking about how fast sounds actually occur when we speak to others. We're not ready for conversations yet for these sounds, but I do want you to speed it up, just a little, like this. (*demonstrates a slightly faster pace*) "Man-a-man-a-man-a-man-a-man-a, Men-a-men-a-men-a-men-a-men-a, Name-a-name-a-name-a-name-a-name-a," and so forth. I'll record and you try it again using all six of your words. (*presses record*)	
	Okay. Man-a-man-a-man-a-man-a-man-a, Men-a-men-a-men-a-men-a-men-a, Name-a-name-a-name-a-name-a-name-a, Main-a-main-a-main-a-main-a-main-a, Ring-a-ring-a-ring-a-ring-a-ring-a, Rang-a-rang-a-rang-a-rang-a-rang-a.
(*Stops recording*) Good, Jared. What did you think about that sequence?	
	It was good, I think. (slow rate, as if thinking about what he's saying)
It was good. I may have heard one or two nasals that sounded as if they came from your mouth, but overall it was good work. Let's play back this segment so we can listen together. (*plays back the sequence;*	

Clinician	**Client**
both listen) I think it sounded good; most of the nasals were emitted nasally, and that's good, especially since we increased the pace a little; this means that you're really working hard and thinking about what you're doing. Great job!	
	Thanks.
Let's work on the same sequence once more, but this time, we'll change the end a little. Instead of saying each word unit five times, we'll say it only three times, then we'll add the one-syllable word twice at the end, like this: "Man-a-man-a-man-a-man-man," "Men-a-men-a-men-a-men-men," "Name-a-name-a-name-a-name-name," "Main-a-main-a-main-a-main-main," "Ring-a-ring-a-ring-a-ring-ring," "Rang-a-rang-a-rang-a-rang-rang." This will cause the rhythm to change some at the end, and, hopefully, that will help with the transfer into conversations as we get further along in therapy. So, the pattern you'll be doing with every word on the list is: "Man-a-man-a-man-a-man-man." Clear?	
	Yes, I think so.
Use the slower pace this time, to give yourself time to think. I'll record. (*presses record*)	
	Man-a-man-a-man-a-man-man, Men-a-men-a-men-a-men-men, Name-a-name-a-name-a-name-name, Main-a-main-a-main-a-main-main, Ring-a-ring-a-ring-a-ring-ring, Rang-a-rang-a-rang-a-rang-rang.

continues

continued

Clinician	Client
Great work, Jared. Let's listen to the recording to see how well you are doing with the nasals. (*plays back the sequence; both listen*) Great work, Jared! Was that a thumbs-up or thumbs-down on that one?	
	Thumbs-up!
That was a thumbs-up! Way to go! (*holds up thumb for Jared to see*) Excellent, Jared. Very nice work! I heard lots of good nasal sounds in that activity. Excellent use of resonance; very good effort.	
	Thanks.
(**Session continues in this manner until the time ends for the Body of Therapy; then proceed to the closing.**)	

CLOSING

Review of Objectives and Summarize Client's Performances Jared, you've done well today. You worked on using the nasals /m, n, ŋ/ in one-syllable words, then in sequences, and it looks like you achieved 100% correct production on the one-syllable words, and 100% correct production of the sequenced units. Good work. Overall, you did very well today. Congratulations on a good session. If you do as well next week, we will advance your work to the next level.	
	Okay.
Homework Please continue practicing the one-syllable words on your list as we did today at least	

Clinician	Client
4 to 5 minutes per day and we'll work in the same manner next week. Is all that clear?	Yes.
Rewards (No tangible reward given) Great. Then, thanks for coming in, and I'll see you next Monday. Remember: practice at least a few minutes daily, if possible. Thanks, and have a great day. Good-bye.	Good-bye.

Summary

For many years, SLPs addressed resonance as a part of voice disorders. However, as of 2001, the scope of practice for SLPs included resonance as a separate area of practice for the profession. According to ASHA (2004), "individuals of all ages receive intervention and consultation when their ability to communicate effectively is impaired because of a resonance or airflow or related articulation disorder and when there is a reasonable expectation of benefit to the individual in body structure/function and/or activity/participation" (p. 37). SLPs may perform resonance or airflow interventions as members of collaborative, interdisciplinary teams.

Learning Tool

List each component of the major divisions of a speech-language therapy session and briefly tell what should transpire within each section of those major components for resonance therapy.

_____

_____

_____

_____

_____

_____

References

American Speech-Language-Hearing Association. (2001). *Scope of practice in speech-language pathology.* Rockville, MD: Author.

American Speech-Language Hearing Association. (2004). *Preferred practice patterns for the profession of speech-language pathology.* Retrieved from http://www.asha.org/members/desk ref-journal/deskref/default

Boone, D. R., McFarlane, S. C., Von Berg, S. L., & Zraick, R. I. (2013). *The voice and voice therapy* (9th ed.). Boston, MA: Allyn & Bacon.

Haynes, W. O., & Pindzola, R. H. (2004). *Diagnosis and evaluation in speech pathology* (6th ed.). Boston, MA: Pearson Allyn & Bacon.

Peterson-Falzone, S. J., Hardin-Jones, M. A., & Karnell, M. P. (2001). *Cleft palate speech* (3rd ed.). St Louis, MO: Mosby.

Seikel, J. A., King, D. W., & Drumright, D. G. (1997). *Anatomy and physiology for speech, language, and hearing.* San Diego, CA: Singular Publishing Group.

13

Guided Practice for Fluency Therapy

Selected General Concepts for Fluency Therapy

Most people in the public sector readily recognize stuttering as a speech disorder; they know of stuttering and can give examples of what is meant by stuttering. Cluttering, however, another fluency disorder, is less well known. Following are concepts related to both stuttering and cluttering.

1. Fluency disorder is a "term used to describe any interruption in the flow of oral language; not restricted to stuttering" (Nicolosi, Harryman, & Kresheck, 2004, p. 130). In fact, cluttering, rapid utterances with many elisions, transpositions, and omissions of significant speech sounds (Nicolosi et al., 2004), is also considered to be a part of fluency disorders.

2. Although there are numerous systematic programs devoted to fluency intervention (Bloodstein, 1995; Cooper & Cooper, 2003; Ryan, 1974; Schwartz, 1999; Shames & Florance, 1980; Van Riper, 1973), stuttering therapy is highly individualized, just as are many other intervention strategies in the speech-language pathology profession. To this end, before prescribing therapy, the SLP is strongly encouraged to determine (a) the speech systems that appear to be most impacted by the client's fluency disorder (respiratory, phonatory, resonatory–articulatory) and (b) the presenting symptoms (repetitions, hesitations, prolongations, blocks, etc.) that negatively impact the client's fluency skills.

3. The physical systems, sometimes referred to as *the systems of speech production* (Seikel, King, & Drumright, 1997) most closely related to fluency are the respiratory, phonatory, and articulatory systems. From these systems emerge an awareness of some of the underlying physical causes of fluency disorders.

However, many possible causes of stuttering, including neuromuscular, physical difficulty, environmental, and behavioral or faulty learning difficulties were reported (Bloom & Cooperman, 1999).

4. Once the affected presenting systems of speech are determined for the client, in conjunction with a determination of the characterizing features of the dysfluency, the SLP then determines the objectives of therapy, or the *fluency targets* to be addressed. For example, a decision should be made to determine whether the client needs to focus on breathing for speech production, on relaxation of the phonatory mechanism, or on reduction of tension in the articulators. Often a combination of several different objectives is needed for the client with a fluency disorder (Schwartz, 1999).

5. The SLP often works independently as the professional involved in fluency intervention. However, the SLP should be prepared to work with other professionals (psychologists, teachers, parents, and others) for management of some clients with fluency disorders.

6. Be prepared to change the course of therapy for the fluency client as circumstances for the client change over the course of intervention.

Numerous other concepts and guidelines apply for fluency therapy. However, based on the information given in these selected general concepts, it is hoped that the reader understands the text well enough to process the information and examples throughout the remainder of this section on fluency therapy.

Selected Fluency Objectives

Following are examples of objectives for fluency therapy:

1. Client will use "full breath" techniques before beginning vocalizations and at predetermined pauses during reading segments 100% of opportunities.

2. Client will use easy onsets to begin phonation when speaking with 90% accuracy.

3. Client will use light contacts at the ends and beginnings of words to bridge across word boundaries with 80% accuracy.

Here's How to Do Fluency Therapy

Note to Reader: The information in the script below is designed to help you learn the progression of fluency therapy as related to specific fluency objectives for decreasing stuttering. Of course, if different objectives were selected, the script would, accordingly, be different as well.

Listed in Figure 13–1 are the 14 therapeutic-specific skills groups and appropriate boxes for you to check off each time you read through the therapy sequence. Check off

Spaces are provided for multiple practices of the 28 therapeutic-specific skills (14 skills groups) below associated with fluency therapy. Check off or date a block each practice time for the skill or skills group. You may need several practice sessions to become comfortable with fluency therapy. Once you comfortably feel you have demonstrated a skill or skills group well enough for use in an actual therapy session, note the date in a remaining box. (Note: *Skill to be practiced in actual therapy, not in the script.)

☐☐☐☐☐☐☐☐☐☐ Motivation

☐☐☐☐☐☐☐☐☐☐ Communicating Expectations

☐☐☐☐☐☐☐☐☐☐ Enthusiasm, Animation, Volume

☐☐☐☐☐☐☐☐☐☐ Seating, Proximity, Touch

☐☐☐☐☐☐☐☐☐☐ Preparation, Pace, Fluency

☐☐☐☐☐☐☐☐☐☐ Alerting, Cueing, Modeling, Prompting

☐☐☐☐☐☐☐☐☐☐ Modalities, Describing/Demonstrating, Questioning, Wait-Time

☐☐☐☐☐☐☐☐☐☐ Shaping (Successive Approximations)

☐☐☐☐☐☐☐☐☐☐ Praise, Tokens, Primary Reinforcers

☐☐☐☐☐☐☐☐☐☐ Corrective Feedback

☐☐☐☐☐☐☐☐☐☐ Data Collection

☐☐☐☐☐☐☐☐☐☐ Probing*

☐☐☐☐☐☐☐☐☐☐ Behavioral Management*

☐☐☐☐☐☐☐☐☐☐ Troubleshooting*

Figure 13–1. Practice chart for sample fluency therapy.

each skill as you practice it. Once you comfortably feel you have demonstrated a skill well enough for clinical use of the skill, note the date in a remaining box. Continue to read through the therapy progression until you have indicated a "comfort-level" date for all 14 therapeutic-specific skills groups. Do not become discouraged if it takes several readings for you to feel that you have adequately demonstrated the 14 therapeutic-specific skills groups with appropriate comfort levels.

Advance Organizer (Three Questions to Note)

Focus on the 14 therapeutic-specific skills groups as you read the given script of fluency therapy written for an individual client of young adult age. For each of the 14 therapeutic-specific skills groups listed in Figure 13–1, ask these advance organizer questions:

- ❏ How will I implement this therapeutic-specific skill?
- ❏ How will I sound when I implement this therapeutic-specific skill?
- ❏ As I practice the therapeutic-specific skill, what can I do to improve my clinical skills?

Here's How to Do Language-Based Therapy **15-Minute Scripted Session for Fluency Therapy** **(Individual Therapy Session)**	
INTRODUCTION	
Clinician	Client
Greeting and Rapport Good morning, Julius. How are you today? **Review of Previous Session** Tell me what you've been working on in here.	 Hi. Um-ah, I ah, I've been w-working on ah, um ah light contacts. (sentence was spoken with vowel and pitch changes)

Clinician	Client
Right! Good remembering; you've been working on making light contacts at both the ends of words and at the beginnings of words in order to decrease blocks between words and increase fluency. Does that sound right to you?	Yes.
Collection of or Mentioning of Homework Good. For your homework, you were supposed to practice five minutes daily of bridging between two words using your light contacts. How did that work out for you?	Ummm, well, ah, it was Ok-k-kay for the m-most part.
Did you actually get a chance to practice each day?	Yes, I um, I practiced.
Great. Thanks for doing that.	

BODY

Establishment Phase Let's see how well you are doing with your targets for today. Use your light contacts to tell me these phrases, "Upside down cake."	Up-up-upside down cake.
"Water slide."	W-w-water slide.
"Birthday card."	Birthday card.
Good effort, Julius. You did well with one of those phrases, but you had a little problem with the first two.	

continues

continued

Clinician	Client
Let's drop back to a little easier level for today and see if you can achieve 90% correct use of light contacts to bridge for both one- to two-syllable words and in multisyllabic words. If your percentages are strong, we'll return to longer phrases later in the session. We'll start with two-word phrases.	
	Okay.
Eliciting and Recording and Teaching Phases	
(Often eliciting and recording and teaching phases are overlapping in fluency therapy for general procedures. When using specific fluency programs, these phases may be presented separately.)	
I have a list of two-word utterances, such as *base hit*, *ice cream*, *up town*, and so forth for you to read. There are 60 pairs of words on the list, but I want you to read only 20 pairs at a time. We'll compare the sets of 20 pairs to each other to see how you're doing with your light contacts.	
As you read, I'll note whether your light contacts appeared to be present. Also, let's record your work so that we can compare portions of the sets to each other. Ready?	
	Ah, r-ready.
Let's begin. *(gives Julius a copy of the list with the 60 word pairs, presses record, and prepares to take data on a duplicate list for correct or incorrect uses of light contacts)*	
	Base hit, ice cream, uptown, downtown, l-last stop, steak knife, s-side street, ...

Clinician	Client
	(takes approximately 45 to 50 seconds to complete the first 20 word pairs; dysfluencies noted on approximately 10% of the pairs)
(Stops recorder) Very nice effort, Julius. Your ending and beginning sounds were well controlled to create good bridging across words. Tell me how you think you did on that segment.	
	Umm, ah I-I did okay, b-but I had some, some st-stuttered words.
Yes, you did have some dysfluencies on about 10% of the pairs, but that's a good beginning for today. Let's try the same thing to bridge across words. Remember, focus on making the ending sounds of the first words nice and easy, with light contacts for those ending sounds, then go into the first sound of the second word easy, with a light contact also. Let's try one or two examples before your next set of 20. For example, the ending and beginning sounds in the pairs "mat<u>ch</u> <u>p</u>oint" and "sto<u>p</u> <u>s</u>ign" should be pronounced with the lightest articulation touches (tongue to lips, tongue to teeth, etc.) as possible in order to avoid getting "stuck" at the beginning of the second word. Don't forget that you need to also make contacts on the very first word, but I'm not counting that for today. Listen to how "mat<u>ch</u> <u>p</u>oint" and "sto<u>p</u> <u>s</u>ign" sound when you make the light contacts to bridge across the words. *(demonstrates the light contacts on the 2-word pairs)* Clear?	
	Um-hmm. Yes.

continues

continued

Clinician	Client
Good; let me demonstrate once more, then you try. *(demonstrates the light contacts on the same 2-word pairs)* Okay, your turn. Let me hear you practice the same pairs: "mat<u>ch</u> <u>p</u>oint" and "sto<u>p</u> <u>s</u>ign."	
	Mat<u>ch</u> <u>p</u>oint; sto<u>p</u> <u>s</u>ign. (makes light contacts appropriately)
Great job, Julius! The contacts were perfect. Did you have a chance to think about how everything felt as you were doing the light contacts?	
	Ah, well, I-I really ah didn't think about it.
Fair enough because I really didn't ask you to think about it. I wanted you to focus on the light contacts, and you did that very well. Let's try the practice again, but let's use only one pair so that it's a little easier. This time, work on two things as you say the first pair: (1) concentrate on making the light contacts just like you made a few seconds ago, and (2) try to also think of how your articulators feel as you are making the light contacts. Let's use "mat<u>ch</u> <u>p</u>oint" five times so that you have an opportunity to practice the light contacts and think about how the articulators feel without having to add the reading element right now. I'll count for you as you say, "mat<u>ch</u> <u>p</u>oint" five times. Ready?	
	Okay.
Begin. *(counts using fingers to show Julius the number of times)*	
	Mat<u>ch</u> <u>p</u>oint, mat<u>ch</u> <u>p</u>oint, mat<u>ch</u> <u>p</u>oint, mat<u>ch</u> <u>p</u>oint, mat<u>ch</u> <u>p</u>oint.
Good work, Julius. How do you think those sounded?	

Clinician	Client
	(Gives a thumbs-up and smiles)
I agree; those were thumbs-up units, so I'm marking those as correct. They were nice and smooth. How did your articulators feel when you said the pairs?	
	Um, ah they felt good, um, sorta relaxed.
Great! The sample sounded really good. Now, let's get back to the first set of pairs. Let's do them again, remembering to make the light contacts, but also try to think about how the articulators feel as well as you speak. I'll tape record your speech this time, and I'll take data for correct or incorrect productions on my copy of the pairs list as well. Let's erase the first set of 20 word pairs and begin again. Begin when you're ready. *(prepares to press record and to take data on the duplicate copy of the pairs list)*	
	Base hit, ice cream, uptown, downtown, last stop, steak knife, s-side street, ... (takes approximately 45–50 seconds; dysfluencies noted on approximately 10% of the pairs)
Good work, Julius. Before we analyze this section, let's get the second set of word pairs (pairs 21–40) recorded. I'll tape record as you speak, and I'll take data on my copy of the pairs list as well. Remember, the words are new this time, so be careful to remain focused on both the light contacts and how the articulators feel as you speak. Begin when you're ready. *(prepares to press record and to take data on the duplicate copy of the pairs list)*	

continues

continued

Clinician	Client
	Big hug, lost boys, late start, t-trail mix, done deal, ... (takes approximately 45–50 seconds; dysfluencies noted on approximately 5% of the pairs)
Good work, Julius. Now, let's play back to see if there's a difference in the way you sound on those two samples. *(rewinds and replays the samples)* Did one sound better than the other to you?	
	Yes, the second one was b-better.
Great; the second one is much smoother. You got 90% nonstuttered word on the first set of pairs and 95% nonstuttered words on the second set of pairs. Good listening, Julius, and good work on your word list. Now, let's try the third set of pairs (pairs 41–60). I'll record again as you speak, and I'll take data on my copy of the word list as well. Remember at the beginning of the session, I said that we would work on more difficult phrases if you did well at the beginning of the session. Well, you've done well, so we will now go back to phrases that are a little more difficult than the first two sets of words. Again, some of the words are a little different than the ones you've worked on before, so you have to work a little harder on your light contacts; okay?	
	Okay.
Begin when you're ready. *(prepares to press record and to take data on the duplicate copy of the pairs list)*	
	Bubble bath, model-T, western sun, coffee pot, midnight snack. (takes approximately 50–55 seconds; dysfluencies noted on approximately 5% of the pairs)

Clinician	Client
Great work, Julius. Did you notice anything different about those word pairs?	
	Yes, they were a little harder to do.
Yes, they were a little more difficult because all of the first words had two syllables this time and that's something we haven't worked on before. Let's play back to see if there's a difference in the way you sound on the second and third lists. *(rewinds and replays the two samples)* Did one sound better than the other to you?	
	I'm not r-r-really sure. They both sound good to me.
Well, good listening because you read both lists with 95% correct production. Way to go!	
	That's good.
That's very good, Julius; you used light contacts between words for almost all of the pairs; that's wonderful work. Were you able to think about how your articulators felt as you spoke and focused on your light contacts?	
	S-some time I, ah, would think about it, but sometime I didn't. It was a lot t-to, ah, to think about.
I'm sure it is a lot to think about, but you're progressing well. Good session, so far. Let's move on. This time, I'd like for you to read the entire list of 60 word pairs without stopping; it'll take a few minutes to read it all, but don't rush through it. Take time to make the light contacts and to think about how your articulators feel as often as possible as you produce the words.	

continues

continued

Clinician	Client
I'll take notes, but I'm not going to record this segment. *(prepares to take data on the duplicate list, using a different color of ink this time for comparisons as Julius produces the 60 word pairs)* Begin when you're ready.	
	Base hit, ice cream, uptown, downtown, last stop, steak knife, side street, ... Big hug, lost boys, late start, trail mix, done deal, ... Bubble bath, model-T, western sun, coffee pot, midnight snack, ... (takes almost three minutes to complete the list; dysfluencies noted on approximately 10% of the pairs)
Great, Julius. I heard a lot of really good light contacts in those pairs. How did the pairs sound good to you?	
	Ah, thumbs-up for me; I-I thought they, um, they were good.
Excellent analysis. They were good this time. Approximately 90% correct production! Very good work, Julius. Let's expand the work a little. This time, I still want you to make light contacts, but I want you to work for a while within longer words (multisyllabic words), then transition into a second word. The concept of light contacts still applies, but I want you to practice that concept *within words* as well as *across words*. The words will sound like this. *(demonstrates with a four-syllable word followed by a one-syllable word, i.e., motorcycle gang)* Try this combination just a little slower so that you have time to think about the syllables, the light contacts, and how your articulators are feeling.	

Clinician	Client
We'll do these just a little differently because I want you to repeat each one three times like this: "motorcycle gang," "motorcycle gang," "motorcycle gang," Is that clear?	Yes
Great; I want you try in a few seconds, but first, let's practice. You'll be saying more words in running speech, but don't rush; just make sure you take in enough air before beginning. Ready?	Yes
Try three times "motorcycle gang."	Motorcycle gang, motorcycle gang, motorcycle gang.
Good, Julius; that was easy for you! Try these 20 word pairs, but remember, repeat each one three times. I'll tape record while you speak and I'll take data on a duplicate list; then we'll play back part of the recording to see how you sound. Begin when you're ready. *(presses record and prepares to take data on a duplicate list)*	Motorcycle gang, m-motorcycle gang, motorcycle gang; excavation team, excavation team, excavation team, g-graduation day, graduation day, graduation day, ... (takes approximately three minutes; dysfluencies noted on approximately 10% of the pairs)
(Stops recorder) Great work, Julius.	Thanks.
Your phrases sounded good, and your percentages are good: 10% for this segment! Excellent work. Let's listen to a few of the productions so that you get a feel for how good you sound in running speech.	

Clinician	Client
(plays approximately 30 seconds of the recorded sample) What do you think?	I think it w-was good. It sounds like a l-lot of talking to me.
(Chuckles) Well, it is a lot of talking because of the multisyllabic words. I know that sometimes you try to keep your words simple so they will be easier to say, but you're doing well with multisyllabic words. This segment was a little difficult, so let's try it once more before moving on. **(Session continues in this manner until the time ends for the Body of the Session. Then, proceed to the closing of the session.)**	

CLOSING

Clinician	Client
Review of Objectives and Summarize Client's Performances Julius, you've done well today. You worked on using light contacts to transition between one-syllable words, and it looks like you achieved 90% correct production of those units. Good work. Then, we worked on light contacts within multisyllabic words also. You got 90% correct use of light contacts on those as well. Great work! **Homework** Overall, you did very well today, Julius. Congratulations on a good session.	 Thanks.

Clinician	Client
Please take the two-word lists home and practice your light contacts a few minutes each day for the next five days. Is all that clear?	
	Yes, it's um, clear. (uses thumbs-up signal)
Rewards (No tangible rewards)	
Great. Then, thanks for coming in, and I'll see you next Tuesday. Have a great day. Good-bye.	
	You bet. Good-bye.

Summary

Fluency disorders may comprise combinations of difficulties across several speech systems. Most common of the fluency disorders is stuttering, although cluttering also is included among fluency disorders. Several programs addressing fluency disorders are commercially available; however, SLPs are encouraged to consider the individual needs of the client when selecting a fluency intervention program.

Learning Tool

List each component of the major divisions of a speech-language therapy session and briefly tell what should transpire within each section of those major components for fluency therapy.

_____

_____

_____

_____

_____

_____

References

Bloodstein, O. (1995). *A handbook on stuttering.* San Diego, CA: Singular Publishing Group.

Bloom, S. C., & Cooperman, D. K. (1999). *Synergistic stuttering therapy: A holistic approach.* Boston, MA: Butterworth-Heinemann.

Cooper, E. B., & Cooper, C. (2003). *Personalized fluency control therapy for children* (3rd ed.). Austin, TX: Pro-Ed.

Nicolosi, L., Harryman, E., & Kresheck, J. (2004). *Terminology of communication disorders: Speech-language-hearing* (5th ed.). Baltimore, MD: Lippincott Williams & Wilkins.

Ryan, B. P. (1974). *Programmed therapy for stuttering in children and adults.* Springfield, IL: Charles C. Thomas.

Schwartz, H. D. (1999). *A primer for stuttering therapy.* Boston, MA: Allyn & Bacon.

Seikel, J. A., King, D. W., & Drumright, D. G. (1997). *Anatomy and physiology for speech, language, and hearing.* San Diego, CA: Singular Publishing Group.

Shames, G. H., & Florance, C. L. (1980). *Stutter-free speech: A goal for therapy.* Columbus, OH: Merrill.

Van Riper, C. (1973). *The treatment of stuttering.* Englewood Cliffs, NJ: Prentice-Hall.

Appendix

Form 9. Therapeutic-Specific Workshop Form: Positive Reinforcers: Verbal Praise, Tokens, and Primary Reinforcers

Form 10. Therapeutic-Specific Workshop Form: Corrective Feedback in the Therapeutic Process

Form 11. Therapeutic-Specific Workshop Form: Data Collection in the Therapeutic Process

Form 12. Therapeutic-Specific Workshop Form: Probing in the Therapeutic Process

Form 13. Therapeutic-Specific Workshop Form: Behavioral Management in the Therapeutic Process

Form 14. Therapeutic-Specific Workshop Form: Troubleshooting in the Therapeutic Process

Form 1

(No DVD Accompaniment for this Workshop)
Therapeutic-Specific Workshop Form: Motivation

Name: _____ Date Post Organizer Completed: _____

Section A

(Read this section *and* the section on *Motivation* in Chapter 6
of your textbook *before* proceeding to Section B.)

Definition	Rationale	Relevance to SLP Profession
Motivation is providing a stimulus or force that causes the client to act or perform well in therapy.	Clients often need motivation to perform well in therapy because of prior difficulties in communication attempts. *Can you provide an example.*	A client who is motivated to perform well in therapy typically attends more sessions, is prompt, and seeks to benefit from the activities of therapy.

Section B

(Read this section *before* proceeding to Section C.)

Advance Organizer

Topic: Motivation.

Purpose: To increase the SLP's awareness of the importance of motivation to the therapeutic process.

SLP Action: Consider client motivation for participation in therapy and discuss with the client as needed.

Background: Clients may be motivated to perform well in therapy for several different reasons: intrinsic reasons such as the satisfaction of performing well, or extrinsic reasons such as tangible or nontangible rewards.

Links to Prior Learning: Think of times when you were motivated to learn a new skill, and determine the source of your motivation: intrinsic or extrinsic. Be prepared to discuss personal experiences with motivation with the client. *Student give examples*

Objective and Clarification of Skill to be Learned: The objective is for the SLP to consider the impact of motivation on therapy and to determine and use appropriate motivation strategies for clients during therapy.

Rationale: SLPs need to consider and use appropriate motivation strategies because motivation is often directly linked to performance in therapy: clients who are more motivated most often perform better in therapy.

New Vocabulary: Extrinsic motivation—motivated by some outside force (i.e., rewards); Intrinsic motivation—motivated by an internal force (i.e., satisfaction of doing a job well, pride in competence).

Individual SLP Outcomes/Performance Objectives: As a result of experiences in this workshop on Motivation, I will: (Indicate information you would like to learn during this workshop.)

_____

_____

Section C

(Read this section *before* proceeding to Section D.)

Description/Demonstration

Motivation is the stimulus or force that causes the client to act or perform well in therapy. Motivation may be extrinsic—caused by an outside stimulus or force such as rewards that the client receives from the SLP during therapy. Motivation may also be intrinsic—caused by an internal force such as the desire to achieve, or the desire for competence. Researchers agree that intrinsic motivation is stronger for the client's learning. SLPs should try to ultimately establish intrinsic motivators for the client; however, extrinsic motivators may be necessary in the beginning stages of therapy. Note the following examples:

Example 1: (Intrinsic) "Nordo, you are doing a great job of making the /l/ sound. You should be so proud that you're saying that sound correctly in all of your words. Wow! What an accomplishment for you!"

Example 2: (Extrinsic) "Jerome, you remembered all five of your words for today. Here's a gold star for good remembering!"

Section D

(Complete this section *before* proceeding to Section E.)

Think-Out-Loud Questions

☑ **Read questions aloud.**

☑ **Verbalize answers to help with cognitive processing.**

☑ **Write short answers in spaces provided.**

1.   What is the first thing that I must do in order to motivate~~to~~ my client?

have a connection to your previous experience.
show him the relevance of working on it

2.   What is/are the next step(s) that I must take in order to motivate my client?

show progress from session to session.
Find positives even when errors are made.

3.   What vocabulary must I use in order to motivate my client?

Specific feedback!   — Why would "good job" grow old?

4.   What should I say or do in interactions with my client to motivate him/her?
     (To help with authenticity, give your client an imaginary name!)

_____

_____

_____

5.   How will I know that I am appropriately motivating my client?

_____

_____

Section E

(Complete this section *before* proceeding to Section F.)

Prompts for Practice Opportunity

Practice the skills discussed in Sections A–D above. Revisit Sections A–D as needed to increase comfort with this section. *Use SLP peers, friends, parents, other relatives, large dolls positioned in a chair in front of you to pose as the "client(s)," etc., for your practices. If no one is available to serve as your client(s), use yourself as the client(s) by standing or sitting in front of a large mirror as you practice; the effect of "using yourself as client(s)" is the same, and sometimes more powerful, than having another pose as client(s).* Repeat practices until therapeutic features 1–3 *below* are accomplished. (You may require more or less than the practice check boxes provided.) Check one box each time a feature is practiced. Enter date each feature is accomplished to your satisfaction in the date spaces provided. (Dates may/may not be the same for each feature accomplishment.)

1.   ❑ ❑ ❑ ❑   Accuracy in the skill sequence accomplished.   Date: _____

2.   ❑ ❑ ❑ ❑   Personal comfort in the skill sequence accomplished.   Date: _____

3.   ❑ ❑ ❑ ❑   Adequate speed/fluency in the skill sequence accomplished.   Date: _____

Section F

**(Complete this section *before* entering the date for
Date Post Organizer Completed, upper right, page 1.)**

Post Organizer

Review of Related Content: Motivating the client is providing a stimulus or force that causes the client to act or perform well in therapy. A client who is motivated to perform well in therapy typically attends more sessions, is prompt, and seeks to benefit from the activities of therapy. Motivators may be intrinsic or extrinsic. Intrinsic motivation is seen as better for the client, but SLPs may find ways to motivate the client extrinsically until intrinsic motivation is apparent.

What I Accomplished in this Workshop: _____

_____

_____

Importance of My Accomplishment(s) to My Therapy: _____

_____

My Assessment of My Performance of the Skill(s) Presented in this Workshop:

The Easiest Parts for Me: _____

The Most Difficult Parts for Me: _____

Thought Processes/Emotions I Experienced Learning the Skill(s) Presented in this Workshop Compared to What I Ultimately Learned from this Effort (Reflection Exercise):

_____

_____

_____

_____

Date Post Organizer Completed (Enter here and in upper right corner of page 1): _____

Form 2

(DVD Vignette 1)

Therapeutic-Specific Workshop Form: Communicating Expectations

Name: _____ Date Post Organizer Completed: _____

Section A
(Read this section *and* the section on *Communicating Expectations* in Chapter 6 of your textbook *before* proceeding to Section B.)

Definition	Rationale	Relevance to SLP Profession
Informing the client of the anticipated expectations of a relevant aspect of therapy.	Teacher expectations have been shown to impact student performance.	When expectations are communicated, they help guide both client and clinician throughout the activities of the session.

Section B
(Read this section *before* proceeding to Section C.)

Advance Organizer

Topic: Communicating Expectations.

Purpose: To help the SLP learn and set high expectations for accomplishing the goals and objectives of therapy.

SLP Action: Develop and communicate expectations for client behavior and productions in a therapy session.

Background: Do you remember how it helps you to focus and perform better when you know what's expected of you? Well, communicating expectations achieves the same effects for clients.

Links to Prior Learning: At some point, someone has communicated a *positive expectation* to you; you are being asked to do the same thing for your client. student examples

Objective and Clarification of Skill to be Learned: The objective is for the SLP to learn to communicate expectations to clients by (a) *developing a positive expectation for therapy*, and (b) telling the client what this expectation is, particularly in areas of expectations for accomplishing goals and objectives of therapy. It is appropriate to also use encouragement at the same time that expectations are communicated.

Rationale: The reason the SLP needs to learn to communicate expectations to the client is to help the client understand that the SLP is focused on what is being addressed in therapy; this focus typically helps the client and the overall outcomes of therapy as well.

New Vocabulary: Expectation—anticipation for something to happen.

Individual SLP Outcomes/Performance Objectives: As a result of experiences in this workshop on communicating expectations, I will: (Indicate information you would like to learn during this workshop.)

_____

_____

Section C

(Read this section *before* proceeding to Section D.)

Description/Demonstration

Communicating expectations is the act of telling the client what actions, activities, and outcomes are hoped for during the session. The primary purpose for communicating expectations is to set the focus for the session, but communicating expectations often also serves to reiterate the objectives of the session and to motivate the client. As you communicate your expectations, note that it is not always necessary to explicitly use the words "*expect*" or "*expectation*" when addressing the client. Note the following examples:

Example 1: "Jason, you're working on /k/ in initial positions of words. You did well with those words on Tuesday. **I expect** you to do even better today; let's try for 90% correct production of /k/ in the 30 words we'll be working on today."

Example 2: "Mr. Mason, it was a little difficult for you to remember the names of fruits yesterday. However, you seem stronger today, and **I *think you can name*** at least five fruits in three minutes today; let's give it a try."

Section D

(Complete this section *before* proceeding to Section E.)

Think-Out-Loud Questions

☑   Read questions aloud.

☑   Verbalize answers to help with cognitive processing and practice effect.

☑   Write short answers in spaces provided.

1.   What is the first thing that I must do in order to communicate expectations to my client?

     _____

2.   What is/are the next step(s) that I must take in order to communicate expectations to my client?

     _____

3.   What vocabulary must I use in order to communicate expectations to my client?

     _____

4.   What should I say or do in interactions with my client to communicate expectations?
     (To help with authenticity, give your client an imaginary name!)

     _____

     _____

     _____

5.   How will I know that I am appropriately communicating expectations to my client?

     _____

Section E

(Complete this section *before* proceeding to Section F.)

Prompts for Practice Opportunity

Practice the skills discussed in Sections A–D above and demonstrated in Vignette #1. Revisit the DVD demonstrations and Sections A–D as needed to increase comfort with this section. *Use SLP peers, friends, parents, other relatives, large dolls positioned in a chair in front of you to pose as the "client(s)," etc., for your practices. If no one is available to serve as your client(s), use yourself as the client(s) by standing or sitting in front of a large mirror as you practice; the effect of "using yourself as client(s)" is the same, and sometimes more powerful, than having another pose as client(s).* Repeat practices until therapeutic features 1–3 *below* are accomplished. (You may require more or less than the practice check boxes provided.) Check one box each time a feature is practiced. Enter date each feature is accomplished to your satisfaction in the date spaces provided. (Dates may/may not be the same for each feature accomplishment.)

1.   ❑ ❑ ❑ ❑   Accuracy in the skill sequence accomplished.   Date: _____

2.   ❑ ❑ ❑ ❑   Personal comfort in the skill sequence accomplished.   Date: _____

3.   ❑ ❑ ❑ ❑   Adequate speed/fluency in the skill sequence accomplished.   Date: _____

Section F

(Complete this section *before* entering the date for
Date Post Organizer Completed, upper right, page 1.)

Post Organizer

Review of Related Content: Communication of expectations is informing the client of the anticipated expectations of a relevant aspect of therapy. SLPs need to communicate expectations because doing so has been shown to positively impact performance. When expectations are communicated, they help guide both client and clinician throughout the activities of the session.

What I Accomplished in this Workshop: _____

_____

_____

Importance of My Accomplishment(s) to My Therapy: _____

_____

My Assessment of My Performance of the Skill(s) Presented in this Workshop:

   The Easiest Parts for Me: _____

   The Most Difficult Parts for Me: _____

Thought Processes/Emotions I Experienced Learning the Skill(s) Presented in this Workshop Compared to What I Ultimately Learned from this Effort (Reflection Exercise):

_____

_____

_____

_____

Date Post Organizer Completed (Enter here and in upper right corner of page 1): _____

Form 3

(DVD Vignette 2)

Therapeutic-Specific Workshop Form: Enthusiasm, Animation, and Volume in the Therapeutic Process

Name: _____ Date Post Organizer Completed: _____

Section A

(Read this section *and* the section in Chapter 6 of your textbook on *Enthusiasm, Animation, and Volume in the Therapeutic Process before* viewing the vignette on *Enthusiasm, Animation,* and *Volume.*)

Definition	Rationale	Relevance to SLP Profession
Enthusiasm is a strong excitement or feeling for something. Animation is spirit, movement, zest, and vigor.	An enthusiastic communicating partner inspires clients to engage in communication attempts more often.	Enthusiasm has a positive impact on interest, attending, and academic engagement. These skills are all important to speech-language learning.

Section B

(Read this section *before* viewing the vignette on *Enthusiasm, Animation, and Volume.*)

Advance Organizer

Topic: Enthusiasm, animation, and volume in the therapeutic process.

Purpose: To help clinicians understand the importance of enthusiasm, animation, and volume for work in therapy.

SLP Action: Portray vocal styles for pitch and volume, movements, zest, and a general demeanor indicative of enthusiasm in therapy.

Background: Children, particularly those under 10 years of age, answered more questions and attended better to teachers described as using expanded pitch and vocal ranges.

Links to Prior Learning: Which of your prior teachers held your interest, created engagement, and inspired you to want to learn more: teachers with low affect, or those who were enthusiastic about their work? Clients make the same assessments: enthusiasm in the SLP promotes more attending, focus, and engagement for the client.

Objective and Clarification of Skill to be Learned: The objective is for the SLP to learn and display traits characteristic of enthusiasm and animation during therapy.

Rationale: SLP needs to exhibit enthusiasm, animation, effective manipulations of volume, and even nonverbal skills such as proximity and facial expressions, to increase attending, focus, and engagement in client behavior during therapy.

New Vocabulary: Enthusiasm—strong excitement or feeling for something; animation—spirit, movement, zest, and vigor.

Individualized SLP Outcomes/Performance Objectives: As a result of experiences in this workshop on motivation, I will: (Indicate information you would like to learn during this workshop.)

_____

_____

Section C

(Read this section *before* viewing the vignette on *Enthusiasm, Animation, and Volume*.)

Description/Demonstration

Enthusiasm was defined as a strong excitement or feeling for something. Animation is spirit, movement, zest, and vigor. An enthusiastic SLP inspires clients to engage in communication attempts more often. Enthusiasm has a positive impact on interest, attending, and academic engagement. These skills are all important to speech-language learning. Note the following examples:

Example 1: Young Client: "Yeah, Carl, you did it! You said, 'Dogie run fast.' Way to go!" (accompanied by hand claps, high five, or getting up from chair to do a wiggle dance, etc.)

Example 2: Adolescent Client: "Awesome, Roger. When you control your stuttering that well, it sounds like you really have it together! Way to go!" (accompanied by two thumbs-up)

Section D

(Complete this section *before* the viewing vignette on
Enthusiasm, Animation, and Volume.)

Think-Out-Loud Questions

☑   Read questions aloud.

☑   Verbalize answers to help with cognitive processing.

☑   Write short answers in spaces provided.

1.   What is the first thing that I must do in order to show enthusiasm and animation toward my client?

_____

2.   What is/are the next step(s) that I must take in order to show enthusiasm and animation toward my client?

_____

3.   What vocabulary must I use in order to communicate enthusiasm and animation to my client?

_____

4.   What should I say or do in interactions with my client to motivate him/her?
     (To help with authenticity, give your client an imaginary name!)

_____

_____

_____

5.   How will I know that I am appropriately showing enthusiasm and animation to my client?

_____

Section E

(View the vignette on *Enthusiasm, Animation, and Volume before* completing this section.)

Prompts for Practice Opportunity

Practice the skills discussed in Sections A–D above and demonstrated in Vignette #2. Revisit the DVD demonstrations and Sections A–D as needed to increase comfort with this section. *Use SLP peers, friends, parents, other relatives, large dolls positioned in a chair in front of you to pose as the "client(s)," etc., for your practices. If no one is available to serve as your client(s), use yourself as the client(s) by standing or sitting in front of a large mirror as you practice; the effect of "using yourself as client(s)" is the same, and sometimes more powerful, than having another pose as client(s).* Repeat practices until therapeutic features 1–3 *below* are accomplished. (You may require more or less than the practice check boxes provided.) Check one box each time a feature is practiced. Enter date each feature is accomplished to your satisfaction in the date spaces provided. (Dates may/may not be the same for each feature accomplishment.)

1.   ☐ ☐ ☐ ☐   Accuracy in the skill sequence accomplished.   Date: _____

2.   ☐ ☐ ☐ ☐   Personal comfort in the skill sequence accomplished.   Date: _____

3.   ☐ ☐ ☐ ☐   Adequate speed/fluency in the skill sequence accomplished.   Date: _____

Section F

(View the vignette on *Enthusiasm, Animation, and Volume before* completing this section.)

Post Organizer

Review of Related Content: Enthusiasm was defined as a strong excitement, or feeling for something. Animation is spirit, movement, zest, and vigor. These skills are all important to speech-language learning. Enthusiasm has a positive impact on interest, attending, and academic engagement. These skills are all important to speech-language learning.

What I Accomplished in this Workshop: _____

_____

_____

Importance of My Accomplishment(s) to My Therapy: _____

_____

My Assessment of My Performance of the Skill(s) Presented in this Workshop:

The Easiest Parts for Me: _____

The Most Difficult Parts for Me: _____

Thought Processes/Emotions I Experienced Learning the Skill(s) Presented in this Workshop Compared to What I Ultimately Learned from this Effort (Reflection Exercise):

_____

_____

_____

_____

Date Post Organizer Completed (Enter here and in upper right corner of page 1): _____

Form 4

(DVD Vignette 3)

Therapeutic-Specific Workshop Form: Seating Arrangements, Proximity, and Touch in the Therapeutic Process

Name: _____ Date Post Organizer Completed: _____

Section A

(Read this section *and* the section on *Seating Arrangements, Proximity, and Touch in the Therapeutic Process* in Chapter 6 of your textbook *before* viewing the vignette on *Seating Arrangements, Proximity, and Touch in the Therapeutic Process*.)

Definition	Rationale	Relevance to SLP Profession
Proximity is degree of closeness.	SLPs must become comfortable with therapeutic touch, touching the client on the face, neck, shoulder, upper arm, and upper back because of the "teaching" aspects of therapy.	Appropriate "therapeutic space" for SLP-client(s) interaction is the lower limits of personal space, approximately 2 feet between the SLP's face and the client's face during the "teaching" phases of therapy which require placements, visual demonstrations, etc.

Section B

(Read this section *before* viewing the vignette on *Seating Arrangements, Proximity, and Touch in the Therapeutic Process*.)

Advance Organizer

Topic: Seating Arrangements, Proximity, and Touch in the Therapeutic Process.

Purpose: To help clinicians explore seating arrangements, and become aware of appropriate proximity and touch for therapy.

SLP Action: Determine appropriate seating arrangements, proximity, and touch based on client goals and tolerances.

Background: Physical distance between the teacher and student must be considered because learning is predicated on interaction between the two. The physical distance between SLP and client is extremely important for therapeutic success.

Links to Prior Learning: Have you ever attended a gathering (class, banquet, wedding, concert, etc.) and found that either your enjoyment or your ability to benefit from the information or activity was lessened because you were too far away from the focal point of the event? The lack of proximity was a negative impact for your experience. Similarly, the lack of appropriate proximity negatively impacts the client's learning in therapy.

Objective and Clarification of Skill to be Learned: The objective is for the SLP to determine and establish appropriate seating, proximity, and touch for the client's best performances in therapy.

Rationale: The nature of speech-language intervention dictates both proximity and touch for intervention; SLPs need to become comfortable with establishing appropriate seating, proximity, and touch during therapy.

New Vocabulary: Proximity—degree of closeness.

Individual SLP Outcomes/Performance Objectives: As a result of experiences in this workshop on seating arrangements, proximity, and touch, I will: (Indicate information you would like to learn during this workshop.)

_____

_____

Section C

(Read this section *before* viewing the vignette on *Seating Arrangements, Proximity, and Touch in the Therapeutic Process*.)

Description/Demonstration

Proximity is degree of closeness between the SLP and the client. SLPs must become comfortable with therapeutic touch, touching the client on the face, neck, shoulder, upper arm, and upper back because of the "teaching" aspects of therapy. Appropriate "therapeutic space" for SLP-to-client(s) interaction is the lower limits of personal space: approximately 2 feet between the SLP's face and the client's face during the "teaching" phases of therapy which require placements, visual demonstrations, etc. Of course, individual and cultural responses to proximity and touch may require variation in the SLP's customary practices for proximity and touch in the therapeutic process.

Example 1: "Lydia, pull your chair a little closer so that I can easily touch your throat to feel for your voiced sounds."

Example 2: "Juan, put your hand near my mouth to feel the puff of air on your hand when I make the /p/ sound." (SLP takes Juan's hand and positions it within three inches of his/her mouth as the sound is produced.)

Section D

(Complete this section *before* viewing the vignette on *Seating Arrangements, Proximity, and Touch in the Therapeutic Process*.)

Think-Out-Loud Questions

☑   **Read questions aloud.**

☑   Verbalize answers to help with cognitive processing.

☑   Write short answers in spaces provided.

1.   What is the first thing that I must do in order to establish appropriate therapeutic proximity and touch for my client?

_____

2.   What is/are the next step(s) that I must take in order to establish appropriate therapeutic proximity and touch for my client?

_____

3.   What vocabulary must I use in order to establish appropriate therapeutic proximity and touch for my client?

_____

4.   What should I say or do in interactions with my client to establish appropriate proximity and touch for therapy?
(To help with authenticity, give your client an imaginary name!)

_____

_____

_____

5.   How will I know that I am appropriately establishing therapeutic proximity and touch for my client?

_____

Section E

(View the vignette on *Seating Arrangements, Proximity, and Touch in the Therapeutic Process before* completing this section.)

Prompts for Practice Opportunity

Practice the skills discussed in Sections A–D above and demonstrated in Vignette #3. Revisit the DVD demonstrations and Sections A–D as needed to increase comfort with this section. *Use SLP peers, friends, parents, other relatives, large dolls positioned in a chair in front of you to pose as the "client(s)," etc., for your practices. If no one is available to serve as your client(s), use yourself as the client(s) by standing or sitting in front of a large mirror as you practice; the effect of "using yourself as client(s)" is the same, and sometimes more powerful, than having another pose as client(s).* Repeat practices until therapeutic features 1–3 *below* are accomplished. (You may require more or less than the practice check boxes provided.) Check one box each time a feature is practiced. Enter date each feature is accomplished to your satisfaction in the date spaces provided. (Dates may/may not be the same for each feature accomplishment.)

1. ❑ ❑ ❑ ❑ Accuracy in the skill sequence accomplished.   Date: _____

2. ❑ ❑ ❑ ❑ Personal comfort in the skill sequence accomplished.   Date: _____

3. ❑ ❑ ❑ ❑ Adequate speed/fluency in the skill sequence accomplished.   Date: _____

Section F

(View the vignette on *Seating Arrangements, Proximity, and Touch in the Therapeutic Process before* completing this section.)

Post Organizer

Review of Related Content: SLPs must become comfortable with therapeutic touch, touching the client on the face, neck, shoulder, upper arm, and upper back because of the "teaching" aspects of therapy, and must become comfortable with establishing an appropriate working distance (proximity) for therapy.

What I Accomplished in this Workshop: _____

_____

_____

Importance of My Accomplishment(s) to My Therapy: _____

_____

My Assessment of My Performance of the Skill(s) Presented in this Workshop:

The Easiest Parts for Me: _____

The Most Difficult Parts for Me: _____

Thought Processes/Emotions I Experienced Learning the Skill(s) Presented in this Workshop Compared to What I Ultimately Learned from this Effort (Reflection Exercise):

_____

_____

_____

_____

Date Post Organizer Completed (Enter here and in upper right corner of page 1): _____

Form 5

(DVD Vignette 4)

Therapeutic-Specific Workshop Form: Preparation, Pacing, and Fluency for Therapeutic Momentum

Name: _____ Date Post Organizer Completed: _____

Section A

(Read this section *and* the section on *Preparation, Pacing, and Fluency for Therapeutic Momentum* in Chapter 6 of your textbook *before* viewing the vignette on *Preparation, Pacing, and Fluency for Therapeutic Momentum*.)

Definition	Rationale	Relevance to SLP Profession
Therapeutic momentum is the speed, thrust, or force of moving between segments of the session. Momentum is established through use of pace and fluency in therapy.	It is difficult to maintain proper momentum in therapy if proper pace and fluency are not evident in therapy.	Therapy should move fluidly between segments over the duration of the session. This fluid movement is possible when appropriate preparation, planning, and execution of techniques of therapy are present.

Section B

(Read this section *before* the viewing vignette on *Preparation, Pacing, and Fluency for Therapeutic Momentum*.)

Advance Organizer

Topic: Preparation, Pacing, and Fluency for Therapeutic Momentum.

Purpose: To help clinicians understand the importance of *Preparation, Pacing, and Fluency* in therapy.

SLP Action: Plan effectively, and practice for pace and fluency *before* initial contact with the client.

Background: It is possible for the SLP to be knowledgeable of the information related to needs of the client (the theories and specific techniques of therapy) and still experience difficulty executing therapy. Often, false starts and nonsemantic fillers are present, and the general appearance is that the SLP failed to plan well. Planning well and practicing all aspects of therapy for pace and fluency significantly increase the SLPs skills in maintaining appropriate therapeutic momentum.

Links to Prior Learning: What would be your level of comfort with a dentist who picks up a utensil, then nervously replaces it with a second one several times before beginning treatment? What if the dentist also added occasionally, "Um, let me see; I think it's this one. No, no, it's this one. Yes, I'm sure now, it's this one." Likely both your confidence and comfort levels for the dentist's knowledge and skills would diminish. The same is true for SLPs who exhibit uncertainty in moving from one moment to the next during therapy: the client's confidence and comfort levels for the SLP's knowledge and skills diminish.

Objective and Clarification of Skill to be Learned: The objective is for the SLP to learn to prepare well for therapy and to practice the techniques and progressions of therapy.

Rationale: Nonfluent behaviors in the form of false starts, forgetting to bring needed materials to the setting, and generally fumbling through materials and techniques within the session significantly negatively impact therapeutic momentum.

New Vocabulary: Pace—the presentation rate within the therapy session.

Individualized SLP Outcomes/Performance Objectives: As a result of experiences in this workshop on preparation, pacing, and fluency for therapeutic momentum, I will: (Indicate information you would like to learn during this workshop.)

_____

_____

Section C

(Read this section *before* viewing vignette on *Preparation, Pacing, and Fluency for Therapeutic Momentum.*)

Description/Demonstration

Therapeutic momentum is the speed, or thrust, or force of moving between segments of the session. Momentum is established through use of pace and fluency in therapy. Therapy should move fluidly between segments over the duration of the session. This fluid movement is possible when appropriate preparation, planning, and execution of techniques of therapy are present. It is difficult to maintain proper momentum in therapy if proper pace and fluency are not evident in therapy. Note the following examples:

Example 1: "Sue Li, first we will work on vocabulary words and short-term memory; then, we will work on sentence constructions. Listen to these words and try to remember what you hear: *apple, apricot, banana, peach, pear.* Tell me the first two fruits named on my list."

Example 2: "Everyone, watch. I have a stack of cards that shows one-syllable words or two-syllable words. Choose a card and if it shows a one-syllable word, you each construct one sentence. If the card shows a two-syllable word, you each construct two sentences. Remember, one syllable equals one sentence; two syllables equal two sentences. Ready? Let's begin. Maggie, choose a card."

Section D

(Complete this section *before* viewing vignette on *Preparation, Pacing, and Fluency for Therapeutic Momentum.*)

Think-Out-Loud Questions

☑   Read questions aloud.

☑   Verbalize answers to help with cognitive processing and the practice effect.

☑   Write short answers in spaces provided.

1. What is the first thing that I must do for Preparation, Pacing, and Fluency for Therapeutic Momentum with my client?

   _____

2. What is/are the next step(s) that I must take for Preparation, Pacing, and Fluency for Therapeutic Momentum with my client?

   _____

3. What vocabulary must I use for Preparation, Pacing, and Fluency for Therapeutic Momentum with my client?

   _____

4. What should I say or do in interactions with my client to achieve Preparation, Pacing, and Fluency for Therapeutic Momentum with him/her?
   (To help with authenticity, give your client an imaginary name!)

   _____

   _____

   _____

5. How will I know that I am appropriately showing Preparation, Pacing, and Fluency for Therapeutic Momentum with my client?

   _____

Section E

(View the vignette on *Preparation, Pacing, and Fluency for Therapeutic Momentum* before completing this section.)

Prompts for Practice Opportunity

Practice the skills discussed in Sections A–D above and demonstrated in Vignette #4. Revisit the DVD demonstrations and Sections A–D as needed to increase comfort with this section. *Use SLP peers, friends, parents, other relatives, large dolls positioned in a chair in front of you to pose as the "client(s)," etc., for your practices. If no one is available to serve as your client(s), use yourself as the client(s) by standing or sitting in front of a large mirror as you practice; the effect of "using yourself as client(s)" is the same, and sometimes more powerful, than having another pose as client(s).* Repeat practices until therapeutic features 1–3 *below* are accomplished. (You may require more or less than the practice check boxes provided.) Check one box each time a feature is practiced. Enter date each feature is accomplished to your satisfaction in the date spaces provided. (Dates may/may not be the same for each feature accomplishment.)

1. ❏ ❏ ❏ ❏ Accuracy in the skill sequence accomplished.   Date: _____

2. ❏ ❏ ❏ ❏ Personal comfort in the skill sequence accomplished. Date: _____

3. ❏ ❏ ❏ ❏ Adequate speed/fluency in the skill sequence accomplished. Date: _____

Section F

(View the vignette on *Preparation, Pacing, and Fluency for Therapeutic Momentum before* completing this section.)

Post Organizer

Review of Related Content: Therapy should move fluidly between segments over the duration of the session. This fluid movement is possible when appropriate preparation, planning, and execution of techniques of therapy are present. It is difficult to maintain proper momentum in therapy when proper preparation, pace, and fluency are not evident in therapy.

What I Accomplished in this Workshop: _____

_____

_____

Importance of My Accomplishment(s) to My Therapy: _____

_____

My Assessment of My Performance of the Skill(s) Presented in this Workshop:

The Easiest Parts for Me: _____

The Most Difficult Parts for Me: _____

Thought Processes/Emotions I Experienced Learning the Skill(s) Presented in this Workshop Compared to What I Ultimately Learned from this Effort (Reflection Exercise):

_____

_____

_____

_____

Date Post Organizer Completed (Enter here and in upper right corner of page 1): _____

Form 6

(DVD Vignette 5)

Therapeutic-Specific Workshop Form: Antecedents: Alerting Stimuli, Cueing, Modeling, and Prompting

Name: _____ Date Post Organizer Completed: _____

Definition	Rationale	Relevance to SLP Profession
Antecedents are events that occur before client responses. Any number of actions may serve as antecedents including various alerting behaviors, cueing, modeling, and prompting.	Clients with communication disorders often need help in knowing when to focus on important information that helps them correctly produce targeted objectives. Antecedents offer clients the "heads-up" needed for proper focus on the stimulus.	SLPs should ensure that clients focus on important aspects of therapy, particularly models, by bringing the client's attention to those important aspects. Often, a simple "Watch me" promotes client focus.

Section B

(Read this section *before* viewing the vignette on *Antecedents: Alerting Stimuli, Cueing, Modeling, and Prompting*.)

Advance Organizer

Topic: Antecedents: Alerting Stimuli, Cueing, Modeling, and Prompting.

Purpose: To help clinicians understand the importance of Antecedents: Alerting Stimuli, Cueing, Modeling, and Prompting in therapy.

SLP Action: Learn to effectively use Antecedents: Alerting Stimuli, Cueing, Modeling, and Prompting during therapy.

Background: Antecedents are relatively simple techniques that add significantly to clinical effectiveness. It helps little for the SLP to use good techniques in absence of client focus. Alerting stimuli, cueing , modeling, and prompting all serve to increase client accuracy in therapy.

Links to Prior Learning: Remember when elementary teachers used cues such as turning off lights or raising a hand to signify that students needed to be silent? Those simple alerting behaviors served to give students a "heads-up," which meant they should attend because something important was about to happen. Alerting stimuli in therapy serve the same purpose; these behaviors signify to the client that something important is about to happen.

Objective and Clarification of Skill to be Learned: The objective is for the SLP to learn to use simple alerting stimuli, cueing, modeling, and prompting skills in therapy.

Rationale: Speakers able to benefit maximally from typical communication interactions without cues, models, and prompts, etc. likely do not need to be served by an SLP. Conversely, those clients who do need the services of the SLP often need exaggerated or modified stimuli to bring to their attention the important aspects of speech to which they are asked to respond.

New Vocabulary: Antecedents—events that occur before client responses.

Individualized SLP Outcomes/Performance Objectives: As a result of experiences in this workshop on Antecedents: Alerting Stimuli, Cueing, Modeling, and Prompting, I will: (Indicate information you would like to learn during this workshop.)

_____

_____

Section C

(Read this section *before* viewing the vignette on *Antecedents: Alerting Stimuli, Cueing, Modeling, and Prompting*.)

Description/Demonstration

Antecedents are events that occur before client responses. Any number of actions may serve as antecedents including various alerting behaviors, cueing, modeling, and prompting. Clients with communication disorders often need help in knowing when to focus on important information that helps them correctly produce speech and language targets. Antecedents offer the "heads-up" needed for proper focus on the appropriate stimulus. Note the following examples:

Example 1: "Watch my mouth, while also pointing to the mouth."

Example 2: "Ben." (SLP calls child's name while touching the back portion of his or her face, near the ear as an alerting stimuli to let Ben know that he should prepare to make the /k/ sound toward the back of the mouth.)

Section D

(Complete this section *before* viewing the vignette on *Antecedents: Alerting Stimuli, Cueing, Modeling, and Prompting*.)

Think-Out-Loud Questions

☑   **Read questions aloud.**

☑   **Verbalize answers to help with cognitive processing and the practice effect.**

☑   **Write short answers in spaces provided.**

1. What is the first thing that I must do to use Antecedents: Alerting Stimuli, Cueing, Modeling, and Prompting with my client?

   _____

2. What is/are the next step(s) that I must take to use Antecedents: Alerting Stimuli, Cueing, Modeling, and Prompting with my client?

   _____

3. What vocabulary must I use for Antecedents: Alerting Stimuli, Cueing, Modeling, and Prompting with my client?

   _____

4. What should I say or do in interactions with my client to use Antecedents: Alerting Stimuli, Cueing, Modeling, and Prompting with him/her?
   (To help with authenticity, give your client an imaginary name!)

   _____

   _____

   _____

5. How will I know that I am appropriately using Antecedents: Alerting Stimuli, Cueing, Modeling, and Prompting with my client?

   _____

Section E

(View the vignette on *Antecedents: Alerting Stimuli, Cueing, Modeling, and Prompting* before completing this section.)

Prompts for Practice Opportunity

Practice the skills discussed in Sections A–D above and demonstrated in Vignette #5. Revisit the DVD demonstrations and Sections A–D as needed to increase comfort with this section. *Use SLP peers, friends, parents, other relatives, large dolls positioned in a chair in front of you to pose as the "client(s)," etc., for your practices. If no one is available to serve as your client(s), use yourself as the client(s) by standing or sitting in front of a large mirror as you practice; the effect of "using yourself as client(s)" is the same, and sometimes more powerful, than having another pose as client(s). Repeat practices until therapeutic features 1–3 below are accomplished.* (You may require more or less than the practice check boxes provided.) Check one box each time a feature is practiced. Enter date each feature is accomplished to your satisfaction in the date spaces provided. (Dates may/may not be the same for each feature accomplishment.)

1. ❑ ❑ ❑ ❑   Accuracy in the skill sequence accomplished.   Date: _____

2. ❑ ❑ ❑ ❑   Personal comfort in the skill sequence accomplished.   Date: _____

3. ❑ ❑ ❑ ❑   Adequate speed/fluency in the skill sequence accomplished.   Date: _____

Section F

(View the vignette on *Antecedents: Alerting Stimuli, Cueing, Modeling, and Prompting* before completing this section.)

Post Organizer

Review of Related Content: Antecedents are events that occur before client responses. Any number of actions may serve as antecedents including various alerting behaviors, cueing, modeling, and prompting. SLPs should ensure that clients focus on important aspects of therapy, particularly models, by bringing the client's attention to those important aspects. Often, a simple "Watch me" or "Watch my mouth" promotes client focus.

What I Accomplished in this Workshop: _____

_____

_____

Importance of My Accomplishment(s) to My Therapy: _____

_____

My Assessment of My Performance of the Skill(s) Presented in this Workshop:

The Easiest Parts for Me: _____

The Most Difficult Parts for Me: _____

Thought Processes/Emotions I Experienced Learning the Skill(s) Presented in this Workshop Compared to What I Ultimately Learned from this Effort (Reflection Exercise):

_____

_____

_____

_____

Date Post Organizer Completed (Enter here and in upper right corner of page 1): _____

Form 7

(DVD Vignette 6)

Therapeutic-Specific Workshop Form: Direct Teaching: Learning Modalities, Describing/Demonstrating, Questioning, and Wait-Time

Name: _____ Date Post Organizer Completed: _____

Section A

(Read this section *and* the section on *Direct Teaching: Learning Modalities, Describing/Demonstrating, Questioning, and Wait-Time* in Chapter 6 *before* viewing the vignette on *Direct Teaching: Learning Modalities, Describing/Demonstrating, Questioning, and Wait-Time.*)

Definition	Rationale	Relevance to SLP Profession
Direct teaching is teaching, instructing, or training a client in new skills.	Regardless of techniques used, there are times with concepts or information must be taught, described or demonstrated. SLPs need skills in using learning modalities for direct teaching, describing/demonstrating, questioning, and a related area, wait-time.	Learning modalities such as auditory, visual, or tactile/kinesthetic modalities for teaching, describing, demonstrating, and questioning are integral to speech-language therapy. Additionally, once information is shared with the client, proper use of wait-time becomes a powerful tool for giving the client processing time.

Section B

(Read this section *before* viewing the vignette on *Direct Teaching: Learning Modalities, Describing/Demonstrating, Questioning, and Wait-Time.*)

Advance Organizer

Topic: Direct Teaching: Learning Modalities, Describing/Demonstrating, Questioning, and Wait-Time

Purpose: To help clinicians understand the importance of Direct Teaching: Learning Modalities, Describing/Demonstrating, Questioning, and Wait-Time in therapy.

SLP Action: Learn to effectively use Direct Teaching: Learning Modalities, Describing/Demonstrating, Questioning, and Wait-Time during therapy.

Background: Teaching is fundamental to helping clients understand and institute new skills into their repertoire of new communication abilities. Describing, demonstrating, questioning, and wait-time are skills which, used well, support client learning. Leaning modalities address the methods by which the SLP chooses to present information to clients: visual, auditory, or tactile-kinesthetic. Most people are able to learn through either modality, but most prefer one modality over the others for learning new information.

Links to Prior Learning: Most people have a preferred way of learning materials: visual, auditory, or tactile-kinesthetic. Often to the degree that new information is presented in our preferred modality of learning, that information may be easier learned. For example, think about how you learned the letters of the alphabet. Did you prefer looking at the letters written in some form, or did you prefer hearing someone say the letter names for you? You may have preferred marching to the *alphabet song*. One modality may be stronger in your memory. Clients typically have preferred learning modalities for receiving new information. It may not be possible to always know a client's preferred learning modality, so SLPs are encouraged to use all learning modalities in presenting new information to clients. This way, the likelihood is high that the preferred modality for each client will be addressed at some point in the teaching and learning cycle.

Objective and Clarification of Skill to be Learned: The objective is for the SLP to learn to use Direct Teaching: Learning Modalities, Describing/Demonstrating, Questioning, and Wait-Time in therapy.

Rationale: Because clients in speech-language therapy have not benefited as much as desired from typical communication interactions, more attention must be given to teaching and learning in therapy. SLPs must, therefore, maximize all direct teaching opportunities by properly using learning modalities, describing/demonstrating, questioning, and wait-time during therapy.

New Vocabulary: Learning modalities—visual, auditory, or tactile-kinesthetic; wait-time—the amount of time between a question and the expectation of a response (should be a minimum of 5 seconds).

Individualized SLP Outcomes/Performance Objectives: As a result of experiences in this workshop on Direct Teaching: Learning Modalities, Describing/Demonstrating, Questioning, and Wait-Time, I will: (Indicate information you would like to learn during this workshop.)

_____

_____

Section C

(Read this section *before* viewing the vignette on *Direct Teaching: Learning Modalities, Describing/Demonstrating, Questioning, and Wait-Time*.)

Description/Demonstration

Direct teaching is teaching, instructing, or training a client in new skills. Learning modalities for teaching, describing/demonstrating, questioning, and wait-time are integral to speech-language therapy. Honor all learning modalities by presenting parts of each concept in each of the preferred modality. For example, plan a visual, an auditory, and a tactile/kinesthetic component of all concepts taught. Note the following examples:

Example 1: "Renee, look at this red ball, and listen to the word *ball*. Hold out your hand and feel the ball."

Example 2: "Al, you're working on /t/ today. Look at how we write /t/. Now, trace the letter *t* with your finger. Repeat the sound after me, /t/."

Section D

(Complete this section *before* viewing the vignette on *Direct Teaching: Learning Modalities, Describing/Demonstrating, Questioning, and Wait-Time*.)

Think-Out-Loud Questions

☑ Read questions aloud.

☑ Verbalize answers to help with cognitive processing and the practice effect.

☑ Write short answers in spaces provided.

1. What is the first thing that I must do to use Direct Teaching: Learning Modalities, Describing/ Demonstrating, Questioning, and Wait-Time with my client?

    _____

2. What is/are the next step(s) that I must take to use Direct Teaching: Learning Modalities, Describing/Demonstrating, Questioning, and Wait-Time my client?

    _____

3. What vocabulary must I use for Direct Teaching: Learning Modalities, Describing/Demonstrating, Questioning, and Wait-Time with my client?

    _____

4. What should I say or do in interactions with my client to use Direct Teaching: Learning Modalities, Describing/Demonstrating, Questioning, and Wait-Time with him/her? **(To help with authenticity, give your client an imaginary name!)**

    _____

    _____

    _____

5. How will I know that I am appropriately using Direct Teaching: Learning Modalities, Describing/ Demonstrating, Questioning, and Wait-Time with my client?

    _____

Section E

(View the vignette on *Direct Teaching: Learning Modalities, Describing/ Demonstrating, Questioning, and Wait-Time before* completing this section.)

Prompts for Practice Opportunity

Practice the skills discussed in Sections A–D above and demonstrated in Vignette #6. Revisit the DVD demonstrations and Sections A–D as needed to increase comfort with this section. *Use SLP peers, friends, parents, other relatives, large dolls positioned in a chair in front of you to pose as the "client(s)," etc., for your* practices. *If no one is available to serve as your client(s), use yourself as the client(s) by standing or sitting in front of a large mirror as you practice; the effect of "using yourself as client(s)" is the same, and sometimes more powerful, than having another pose as client(s).* Repeat practices until therapeutic features 1–3 *below* are accomplished. (You may require more or less than the practice check boxes provided.) Check one box each time a feature is practiced. Enter date each feature is accomplished to your satisfaction in the date spaces provided. (Dates may/may not be the same for each feature accomplishment.)

1. ❑ ❑ ❑ ❑   Accuracy in the skill sequence accomplished.   Date: _____

2. ❑ ❑ ❑ ❑   Personal comfort in the skill sequence accomplished.   Date: _____

3. ❑ ❑ ❑ ❑   Adequate speed/fluency in the skill sequence accomplished.   Date: _____

Section F
(View the vignette on *Direct Teaching: Learning Modalities, Describing/Demonstrating, Questioning, and Wait-Time* before completing this section.)

Post Organizer

Review of Related Content: Regardless of techniques used, there are times when concepts or information must be taught, described or demonstrated. SLPs need skills in using learning modalities for direct teaching, describing/demonstrating, questioning, and a related area, wait-time. Although it seems easy enough to ask a question and wait for an answer, oddly, waiting for a client response, especially language clients, often proves challenging for SLPs. Wait time should be practiced following questions and commands.

What I Accomplished in this Workshop: _____

_____

_____

Importance of My Accomplishment(s) to My Therapy: _____

_____

My Assessment of My Performance of the Skill(s) Presented in this Workshop:

The Easiest Parts for Me: _____

The Most Difficult Parts for Me: _____

Thought Processes/Emotions I Experienced Learning the Skill(s) Presented in this Workshop Compared to What I Ultimately Learned from this Effort (Reflection Exercise):

_____

_____

_____

_____

Date Post Organizer Completed (Enter here and in upper right corner of page 1): _____

Form 8

(DVD Vignette 7)

Therapeutic-Specific Workshop Form: Stimulus Presentation (Successive Approximations)

Name: _____ Date Post Organizer Completed: _____

Section A

(Read this section *and* the section on *Stimulus Presentation: Shaping [Successive Approximations]* in Chapter 6 of your textbook *before* viewing the vignette on *Stimulus Presentation: Shaping [Successive Approximations].*)

Definition	Rationale	Relevance to SLP Profession
Shaping, or successive approximations, is a stimulus presentation method for obtaining responses that are not in the client's repertoire. This method requires segmenting the desired response into component parts in order to help a client "bridge" to the new skill.	The SLP needs primary skills in obtaining responses in situations in which the client is unable to give a response remotely close to the desired target. In these situations, the SLP shapes the target through use of systematic approximations, or tiny steps toward the desired target.	A significant part of the SLP's work will focus on helping clients acquire skills not yet in his/her repertoire. Successive approximations, a technique for breaking difficult skills into smaller components, is an appropriate place for beginning that work.

Section B

(Read this section *before* viewing the vignette on *Stimulus Presentation: Shaping [Successive Approximations].*)

Advance Organizer

Topic: Stimulus Presentation: Shaping (Successive Approximations).

Purpose: To help clinicians understand the importance of Stimulus Presentation: Shaping (Successive Approximations) in therapy.

SLP Action: Learn to effectively use shaping (successive approximations) during therapy.

Background: Logically, SLPs use techniques designed to help clients address skills not yet familiar as part of their repertoire. Successive approximations techniques are designed to help the SLP accomplish this task.

Links to Prior Learning: You may have taken lessons in an area for which you were previously unfamiliar such as piano lessons. The teacher may have introduced you to simple mechanics such as where to place the fingers on the keyboard. Then, you may have been asked to "play" a simple scale, one note at a time, with the teacher understanding that, eventually, these simple maneuvers would develop into musical skills. Shaping, or successive approximations, serve a similar function: skills sequences are broken into discrete segments, executed one at a time, then placed in a sequence very slowly in order to achieve productions "approximating" the eventual desired target sequence. Successive approximations are no longer needed when correct productions are possible for the client.

Objective and Clarification of Skill to be Learned: The objective is for the SLP to learn to use Stimulus Presentation: Shaping (Successive Approximations) in therapy.

Rationale: The SLP must have specific and proven ways to effect client productions, even when the client does not yet have the target under controlled production; successive approximations allow the SLP to elicit such productions.

New Vocabulary: Shaping (successive approximations)—a stimulus presentation method for obtaining responses that are not in the client's repertoire through production of slowed, broken-down components of the target skill.

Individualized SLP Outcomes/Performance Objectives: As a result of experiences in this workshop on Stimulus Presentation: Shaping (Successive Approximations), I will: (Indicate information you would like to learn during this workshop.)

_____

_____

Section C

(Read this section *before* viewing the vignette on *Stimulus Presentation: Shaping [Successive Approximations]*.)

Description/Demonstration

The SLP needs primary skills in obtaining responses in situations in which the client may not yet be functioning close to the desired target. In these situations, the SLP shapes the target through use of systematic approximation of the desired target. Shaping, or successive approximations, is a stimulus presentation method for obtaining responses that are not in the client's repertoire. This method requires segmenting the desired response into component parts. Note the following examples:

Example 1: "Lois let's put your /m/ sound back into the word, *man.* Let me hear m-------an." (Lois' response is good.) "Wonderful, now let's put the sounds a little closer, m—an." (Lois' response is again good.) "Excellent, now, let's blend your sound into a complete word, *man.*" (Lois' response is perfect.)

Example 2: "Joyce, tell me your sentence one word at a time. "Let me hear 'I' (response) 'like' (response) 'cookies' (response). Good, easy for you! Now, let's put the words together. Tell me 'I like' (response), great, 'I like cookies' (response). Very nice work, Joyce. 'I like cookies.'"

Section D

(Complete this section *before* viewing the vignette on *Stimulus Presentation: Shaping [Successive Approximations].*)

Think-Out-Loud Questions

☑ Read questions aloud.

☑ Verbalize answers to help with cognitive processing and the practice effect.

☑ Write short answers in spaces provided.

1. What is the first thing that I must do to use Stimulus Presentation: Shaping (Successive Approximations) with my client?

   _____

2. What is/are the next step(s) that I must take to use Stimulus Presentation: Shaping (Successive Approximations) with my client?

   _____

3. What vocabulary must I use for Stimulus Presentation: Shaping (Successive Approximations) with my client?

   _____

4. What should I say or do in interactions with my client to use Stimulus Presentation: Shaping (Successive Approximations) with him/her?
   (To help with authenticity, give your client an imaginary name!)

   _____

   _____

   _____

5. How will I know that I am appropriately using Stimulus Presentation: Shaping (Successive Approximations) with my client?

   _____

Section E

(View the vignette on *Stimulus Presentation: Shaping [Successive Approximations] before* completing this section.)

Prompts for Practice Opportunity

Practice the skills discussed in Sections A–D above and demonstrated in Vignette #7. Revisit the DVD demonstrations and Sections A–D as needed to increase comfort with this section. *Use SLP peers, friends, parents, other relatives, large dolls positioned in a chair in front of you to pose as the "client(s)," etc., for your* practices. *If no one is available to serve as your client(s), use yourself as the client(s) by standing or sitting in front of a large mirror as you practice; the effect of "using yourself as client(s)" is the same, and sometimes more powerful, than having another pose as client(s).* Repeat practices until therapeutic features 1–3 *below* are accomplished. (You may require more or less than the practice check boxes provided.) Check one box each time a feature is practiced. Enter date each feature is accomplished to your satisfaction in the date spaces provided. (Dates may/may not be the same for each feature accomplishment.)

1. ❑ ❑ ❑ ❑   Accuracy in the skill sequence accomplished.   Date: _____

2. ❑ ❑ ❑ ❑   Personal comfort in the skill sequence accomplished.   Date: _____

3. ❑ ❑ ❑ ❑   Adequate speed/fluency in the skill sequence accomplished.   Date: _____

Section F

(View the vignette on *Stimulus Presentation: Shaping [Successive Approximations] before* completing this section.)

Post Organizer

Review of Related Content: The SLP needs primary skills in obtaining responses in situations in which the client may not be functioning close to the desired target. In these situations, the SLP shapes the target through use of systematic approximation of the desired target, successive approximations.

What I Accomplished in this Workshop: _____

_____

_____

Importance of My Accomplishment(s) to My Therapy: _____

_____

My Assessment of My Performance of the Skill(s) Presented in this Workshop:

The Easiest Parts for Me: _____

The Most Difficult Parts for Me: _____

Thought Processes/Emotions I Experienced Learning the Skill(s) Presented in this Workshop Compared to What I Ultimately Learned from this Effort (Reflection Exercise):

_____

_____

_____

_____

Date Post Organizer Completed (Enter here and in upper right corner of page 1): _____

Form 9

(DVD Vignette 8)

Therapeutic-Specific Workshop Form: Positive Reinforcers: Verbal Praise, Tokens, and Primary Reinforcers

Name: _____ Date Post Organizer Completed: _____

Section A

(Read this section *and* the section on *Positive Reinforcers: Verbal Praise, Tokens, and Primary Reinforcers* in Chapter 6 of your textbook *before* viewing the vignette on *Positive Reinforcers: Verbal Praise, Tokens, and Primary Reinforcers*.)

Definition	Rationale	Relevance to SLP Profession
Positive reinforcers are anything, following a response, which increases the frequency of that response. Reinforcers may be verbal or nonverbal such as tokens or other items desired by the client.	SLPs use operant conditioning techniques (reward or reinforcer following correct productions) to increase client's correct productions. As such, SLPs need to understand the nature of rewards and reinforcers for increasing desired client behavior.	The eventual goal is for clients to produce correct products for intrinsic rewards. However, until that time, positive reinforcers, verbal praise, tokens, and primary reinforcers help support correct client productions.

Section B

(Read this section *before* viewing the vignette on *Positive Reinforcers: Verbal Praise, Tokens, and Primary Reinforcers*.)

Advance Organizer

Topic: Positive Reinforcers: Verbal Praise, Tokens, and Primary Reinforcers.

Purpose: To help clinicians understand the importance of Positive Reinforcers: Verbal Praise, Tokens, and Primary Reinforcers in therapy.

SLP Action: Learn to effectively use Positive Reinforcers: Verbal Praise, Tokens, and Primary Reinforcers during therapy.

Background: Positive Reinforcers: Verbal Praise, Tokens, and Primary Reinforcers are founded in behavioral orientations to learning. Operant procedures, whereby positive rewards (verbal praise, tokens, etc.) are used to increase the likelihood of continued correct responses, are important.

Links to Prior Learning: You are, no doubt, able to remember receiving positive reinforcements for jobs well done. Perhaps, verbal praises from parents for a good report card, or other incentives for helping around the house. Positive reinforcers increased the likelihood that you continued the task. The same is true for clients receiving operant conditioning using positive reinforcers; positive reinforcers (verbal praise, tokens, etc.) help increase the occurrences of desired client productions.

Objective and Clarification of Skill to be Learned: The objective is for the SLP to learn to use Positive Reinforcers: Verbal Praise, Tokens, and Primary Reinforcers in therapy.

Rationale: SLPs use operant conditioning techniques (rewards or reinforcers following correct productions) to increase the client's correct productions.

New Vocabulary: Operant conditioning—reward or positive reinforcer following correct production to increase client's correct productions. SLPs, therefore, need to learn as much as possible about the use of positive reinforcers in therapy.

Individualized SLP Outcomes/Performance Objectives: As a result of experiences in this workshop on Positive Reinforcers: Verbal Praise, Tokens, and Primary Reinforcers, I will: (Indicate information you would like to learn during this workshop.)

_____

_____

Section C

(Read this section *before* viewing the vignette on *Positive Reinforcers: Verbal Praise, Tokens, and Primary Reinforcers*.)

Description/Demonstration

Positive reinforcers are anything, following a response, which increases the frequency of that response. The eventual goal is for clients to produce correct products for intrinsic rewards. However, until that time, positive reinforcers such as verbal praise, tokens, and primary reinforcers help support correct client productions. Note the following examples:

Example 1: "Julius, that was a perfect /r/ sound! Your tongue was in exactly the right place. Ten gold stars for you!"

Example 2: "Joe, what a great sentence. You put all the words together to make a sentence. Wow! Wonderful work, Joe!"

Section D

(Complete this section *before* viewing the vignette on *Positive Reinforcers: Verbal Praise, Tokens, and Primary Reinforcers*.)

Think-Out-Loud Questions

☑ Read questions aloud.

☑ Verbalize answers to help with cognitive processing and the practice effect.

☑ Write short answers in spaces provided.

1. What is the first thing that I must do to use Positive Reinforcers: Verbal Praise, Tokens, and Primary Reinforcers with my client?

    _____

2. What is/are the next step(s) that I must take to use Positive Reinforcers: Verbal Praise, Tokens, and Primary Reinforcers with my client?

    _____

3. What vocabulary must I use to implement Positive Reinforcers: Verbal Praise, Tokens, and Primary Reinforcers with my client?

    _____

4. What should I say or do in interactions with my client to use Positive Reinforcers: Verbal Praise, Tokens, and Primary Reinforcers with him/her?
    (To help with authenticity, give your client an imaginary name!)

    _____

    _____

    _____

5. How will I know that I am appropriately using Positive Reinforcers: Verbal Praise, Tokens, and Primary Reinforcers with my client?

    _____

Section E

(View the vignette on *Positive Reinforcers: Verbal Praise, Tokens, and Primary Reinforcers before* completing this section.)

Prompts for Practice Opportunity

Practice the skills discussed in Sections A–D above and demonstrated in Vignette #8. Revisit the DVD demonstrations and Sections A–D as needed to increase comfort with this section. *Use SLP peers, friends, parents, other relatives, large dolls positioned in a chair in front of you to pose as the "client(s)," etc., for your practices. If no one is available to serve as your client(s), use yourself as the client(s) by standing or sitting in front of a large mirror as you practice; the effect of "using yourself as client(s)" is the same, and sometimes more powerful, than having another pose as client(s). Repeat practices until therapeutic features 1–3 below* are accomplished. (You may require more or less than the practice check boxes provided.) Check one box each time a feature is practiced. Enter date each feature is accomplished to your satisfaction in the date spaces provided. (Dates may/may not be the same for each feature accomplishment.)

1. ❑ ❑ ❑ ❑   Accuracy in the skill sequence accomplished.   Date: _____

2. ❑ ❑ ❑ ❑   Personal comfort in the skill sequence accomplished. Date: _____

3. ❑ ❑ ❑ ❑   Adequate speed/fluency in the skill sequence accomplished. Date: _____

Section F

(View the vignette on Positive Reinforcers: Verbal Praise, Tokens, and Primary Reinforcers before completing this section.)

Post Organizer

Review of Related Content: Positive reinforcers are anything, following a response, which increases the frequency of that response. SLPs use operant conditioning techniques (rewards or reinforcers following correct productions) to increase client's correct productions. SLPs use both verbal and nonverbal (tangible) reinforcers to help increase the likelihood of continued correct responses from clients.

What I Accomplished in this Workshop: _____

_____

_____

Importance of My Accomplishment(s) to My Therapy: _____

_____

My Assessment of My Performance of the Skill(s) Presented in this Workshop:

   The Easiest Parts for Me: _____

   The Most Difficult Parts for Me: _____

Thought Processes/Emotions I Experienced Learning the Skill(s) Presented in this Workshop Compared to What I Ultimately Learned from this Effort (Reflection Exercise):

_____

_____

_____

_____

Date Post Organizer Completed (Enter here and in upper right corner of page 1): _____

Form 10

(DVD Vignette 9)

Therapeutic-Specific Workshop Form:
Corrective Feedback in the Therapeutic Process

Name: _____ Date Post Organizer Completed: _____

Section A
(Read this section *and* the section on *Corrective Feedback in the Therapeutic Process* in Chapter 6 of your textbook *before* viewing the vignette on *Corrective Feedback in the Therapeutic Process*.)

Definition	Rationale	Relevance to SLP Profession
Corrective feedback is the information the clinician gives the client regarding the quality, feature, or correctness of a preceding response.	Clients learn to produce targets in speech-language therapy based, in part, on the quality of feedback received from the SLP.	Because of the use of operant conditioning in therapy (use of rewards following a desired response), it is extremely important for the SLP to give clients specific feedback regarding responses in therapy.

Section B
(Read this section *before* viewing the vignette on *Corrective Feedback in the Therapeutic Process*.)

Advance Organizer

Topic: Corrective Feedback in the Therapeutic Process.

Purpose: To help clinicians understand the importance of Corrective Feedback in the Therapeutic Process.

SLP Action: Learn to effectively use Corrective Feedback in the Therapeutic Process.

Background: According to behaviorists, feedback is a major contributor to learning. Clients who are given corrective feedback that is specific, and accurate, tend to learn quicker than clients who simply are given verbal rewards, such as "good job!" "Good job" tells the client that something was done to the SLP's satisfaction, but it doesn't tell *what* was done well. Corrective feedback is specific feedback, for both correct and incorrect responses.

Links to Prior Learning: You are already familiar with verbal reinforcers such as "Great work!" and tangible rewards such as stickers. These reinforcers are important and they serve to promote sustained effort and interest in therapy. However, reinforcers do not *teach* the way that corrective feedback does. SLPs should seek to maintain client interest in therapy through use of reinforcers and rewards.

Additionally, SLPs should develop skills in corrective feedback designed to teach specifics for both correct and incorrect aspects of client responses.

Objective and Clarification of Skill to be Learned: The objective is for the SLP to learn to appropriately use Corrective Feedback in the Therapeutic Process.

Rationale: SLPs use operant conditioning techniques (rewards or reinforcers following correct productions) to increase the client's correct productions; corrective feedback is used to teach specific aspects of client responses that are correct and incorrect. For example, "Your top teeth touched your bottom lip exactly right for that /f/" or "You needed to make a /t/ with your tongue tip up behind the front top teeth, but instead, your tongue humped up in the back and you made a /k/."

New Vocabulary: Corrective feedback—the information the clinician gives the client regarding the quality, feature, or correctness of a preceding response.

Individualized SLP Outcomes/Performance Objectives: As a result of experiences in this workshop on Corrective Feedback in the Therapeutic Process, I will: (Indicate information you would like to learn during this workshop.)

_____

_____

Section C

(Read this section *before* viewing the vignette on *Corrective Feedback in the Therapeutic Process*.)

Description/Demonstration

Because of the use of operant conditioning in therapy (use of rewards following desired responses), it is extremely important for the SLP to give clients specific feedback regarding responses in therapy. Clients learn to produce targets in speech-language therapy based, in part, on the quality of feedback received from the SLP.

Example 1: "Anthony, that was a perfect /k/ sound! Your tongue tip was down in the front and your tongue was humped in the back. I heard the air flow right over the hump for a perfect /k/ sound. Easy for you."

Example 2: "Samuel, you're working hard to say all those words, and I heard two good words: *I* and *want*. But, you left off the last word, *juice*. We need all three words, 'I want juice' to make a complete sentence. If you leave off 'juice,' I don't know what you want. Tell me all three words, 'I want juice.' (Response). Excellent, Samuel. You said all three words, 'I want juice.' Wonderful!"

Section D

(Complete this section *before* viewing the vignette on *Corrective Feedback in the Therapeutic Process*.)

Think-Out-Loud Questions

☑   **Read questions aloud.**

☑   **Verbalize answers to help with cognitive processing and the practice effect.**

☑   **Write short answers in spaces provided.**

1. What is the first thing that I must do to use Corrective Feedback in the Therapeutic Process with my client?

    _____

2. What is/are the next step(s) that I must take to use Corrective Feedback in the Therapeutic Process with my client?

    _____

3. What vocabulary must I use for Corrective Feedback in the Therapeutic Process with my client?

    _____

4. What should I say or do in interactions with my client to use Corrective Feedback in the Therapeutic Process with him/her?
    (To help with authenticity, give your client an imaginary name!)

    _____

    _____

    _____

5. How will I know that I am appropriately using Corrective Feedback in the Therapeutic Process with my client?

    _____

Section E

(View the vignette on Corrective Feedback in the Therapeutic Process before completing this section.)

Prompts for Practice Opportunity

Practice the skills discussed in Sections A–D above and demonstrated in Vignette #9. Revisit the DVD demonstrations and Sections A–D as needed to increase comfort with this section. *Use SLP peers, friends, parents, other relatives, large dolls positioned in a chair in front of you to pose as the "client(s)," etc., for your practices. If no one is available to serve as your client(s), use yourself as the client(s) by standing or sitting in front of a large mirror as you practice; the effect of "using yourself as client(s)" is the same, and sometimes more powerful, than having another pose as client(s).* Repeat practices until therapeutic features 1–3 *below* are accomplished. (You may require more or less than the practice check boxes provided.) Check one box each time a feature is practiced. Enter date each feature is accomplished to your satisfaction in the date spaces provided. (Dates may/may not be the same for each feature accomplishment.)

1. ❑ ❑ ❑ ❑ Accuracy in the skill sequence accomplished.   Date: _____

2. ❑ ❑ ❑ ❑ Personal comfort in the skill sequence accomplished.   Date: _____

3. ❑ ❑ ❑ ❑ Adequate speed/fluency in the skill sequence accomplished.   Date: _____

Section F

(View the vignette on *Corrective Feedback in the Therapeutic Process before* completing this section.)

Post Organizer

Review of Related Conent: Corrective feedback is the information the clinician gives the client regarding the quality, feature, or correctness of a preceding response. Because of the use of operant conditioning in therapy (use of rewards following desired responses), it is extremely important for the SLP to give clients specific feedback regarding responses in therapy. Regardless of whether responses are correct or incorrect, clients learn best when the feedback they receive is specific.

What I Accomplished in this Workshop: _____

_____

_____

Importance of My Accomplishment(s) to My Therapy: _____

_____

My Assessment of My Performance of the Skill(s) Presented in this Workshop:

    The Easiest Parts for Me: _____

    The Most Difficult Parts for Me: _____

Thought Processes/Emotions I Experienced Learning the Skill(s) Presented in this Workshop Compared to What I Ultimately Learned from this Effort (Reflection Exercise):

_____

_____

_____

_____

Date Post Organizer Completed (Enter here and in upper right corner of page 1): _____

Form 11

(DVD Vignette 10)

Therapeutic-Specific Workshop Form:
Data Collection in the Therapeutic Process

Name: _____ Date Post Organizer Completed: _____

Section A

(Read this section *and* the section on *Data Collection in the Therapeutic Process* in Chapter 6 of your textbook *before* viewing the vignette on *Data Collection in the Therapeutic Process*.)

Definition	Rationale	Relevance to SLP Profession
Data collection is recording (making notations of) client responses during the therapeutic session.	Data is needed to make decisions in therapy for basic feedback to clients as to how well they are doing on a regular basis and for making management decisions such as when to consider moving the client to more difficult (or less difficult) levels of therapy. Eventually, data is needed to determine whether to dismiss a client or to refer the client for additional services from other professions.	Many decisions regarding the therapy program instituted for a client will be made based on available data.

Section B

(Read this section *before* viewing the vignette on *Data Collection in the Therapeutic Process*.)

Advance Organizer

Topic: Data Collection in the Therapeutic Process.

Purpose: To help clinicians understand the importance of Data Collection in the Therapeutic Process.

SLP Action: Learn to effectively use Data Collection in the Therapeutic Process.

Background: We are essentially in a data-driven society; the numbers make a difference for countless daily decisions across all professions. Speech-language pathology is no exception. SLPs must become comfortable collecting data on a systematic and routine basis for each client served.

Links to Prior Learning: You are already familiar with skills in corrective feedback designed to teach specifics for both correct and incorrect aspects of client responses. As specific feedback is given to the client, accounts of client productions are also made in the form of data collection. It's good to hear that the SLP thinks a client is doing well in therapy; it's better to know that the client is achieving 86% correct production of the targeted goal!

Objective and Clarification of Skill to be Learned: The objective is for the SLP to learn to use Data Collection in the Therapeutic Process.

Rationale: SLPs use corrective feedback to teach specific aspects of client responses that are correct and incorrect. Data collection accompanies that feedback as written evidence of client performances.

New Vocabulary: Data collection—recording (notating or writing down) client responses during the therapeutic session.

Individualized SLP Outcomes/Performance Objectives: As a result of experiences in this workshop on Data Collection in the Therapeutic Process, I will: (Indicate information you would like to learn during this workshop.)

_____

_____

Section C

(Read this section *before* viewing the vignette on *Data Collection in the Therapeutic Process*.)

Description/Demonstration

Data consists of the numerical accounts of the correct and incorrect responses the client makes during therapy. The numerical accounts are often interpreted in terms of percentages of correct productions for client performances in therapy. Data is collected and compared to the goals and objectives established for the client as a way to determine progress toward goals. SLPs should always know exactly how clients are performing in therapy based on the data taken during therapy sessions. Terms such as "the client performed at an 80% correct production level by correctly producing 8 of 10 sounds" are common.

Example 1: "Valeria, you got 91% correction production of /l/ at the ends of words today. That's wonderful. If your percentages are that high the next time you come to therapy, we'll be able to move you to medial positions of /l/ in words in just a few more sessions. Great work!"

Example 2: "Jerry, you got 84% correction production for subject-verb agreement and 79% correct production for topic maintenance skills. That's great for both of your goals because your percentages are a lot higher now than they were a month ago. Way to go, Jerry!"

Section D

(Complete this section *before* viewing the vignette on *Data Collection in the Therapeutic Process*.)

Think-Out-Loud Questions

☑   **Read questions aloud.**

☑   Verbalize answers to help with cognitive processing and the practice effect.

☑   Write short answers in spaces provided.

1.   What is the first thing that I must do to use Data Collection in the Therapeutic Process with my client?

_____

2.   What is/are the next step(s) that I must take to use Data Collection in the Therapeutic Process with my client?

_____

3.   What vocabulary must I use for discussing Data Collection in the Therapeutic Process with my client?

_____

4.   What should I say or do in interactions with my client to use Data Collection in the Therapeutic Process with him/her?
     (To help with authenticity, give your client an imaginary name!)

_____

_____

_____

5.   How will I know that I am appropriately using Data Collection in the Therapeutic Process with my client?

_____

Section E

(View the vignette on *Data Collection in the Therapeutic Process before* completing this section.)

Prompts for Practice Opportunity

Practice the skills discussed in Sections A–D above and demonstrated in Vignette 10. Revisit the DVD demonstrations and Sections A–D as needed to increase comfort with this section. *Use SLP peers, friends, parents, other relatives, large dolls positioned in a chair in front of you to pose as the "client(s)," etc., for your practices. If no one is available to serve as your client(s), use yourself as the client(s) by standing or sitting in front of a large mirror as you practice; the effect of "using yourself as client(s)" is the same, and sometimes more powerful, than having another pose as client(s). Repeat practices until therapeutic features 1–3 below* are accomplished. (You may require more or less than the practice check boxes provided.) Check one box each time a feature is practiced. Enter date each feature is accomplished to your satisfaction in the date spaces provided. (Dates may/may not be the same for each feature accomplishment.)

1. ❑ ❑ ❑ ❑   Accuracy in the skill sequence accomplished.   Date: _____

2. ❑ ❑ ❑ ❑   Personal comfort in the skill sequence accomplished.   Date: _____

3. ❑ ❑ ❑ ❑   Adequate speed/fluency in the skill sequence accomplished.   Date: _____

Section F

(View the vignette on *Data Collection in the Therapeutic Process* before completing this section.)

Post Organizer

Review of Related Content: Data is needed to make decisions in therapy for basic feedback to clients as to how well they are doing on a regular basis and for making management decisions such as when to consider moving the client to more difficult (or less difficult) levels of therapy. Eventually, data is needed to determine whether to dismiss a client or to refer the client for additional services from other professions.

What I Accomplished in this Workshop: _____

_____

_____

Importance of My Accomplishment(s) to My Therapy: _____

_____

My Assessment of My Performance of the Skill(s) Presented in this Workshop:

The Easiest Parts for Me: _____

The Most Difficult Parts for Me: _____

Thought Processes/Emotions I Experienced Learning the Skill(s) Presented in this Workshop Compared to What I Ultimately Learned from this Effort (Reflection Exercise):

_____

_____

_____

_____

Date Post Organizer Completed (Enter here and in upper right corner of page 1): _____

Form 12

(No DVD Accompaniment for this Workshop)

Therapeutic-Specific Workshop Form:
Probing in the Therapeutic Process

Name: _____ Date Post Organizer Completed: _____

Section A

(Read this section and the section on Probing in the Therapeutic Process in Chapter 6 of your textbook before proceeding to Section B.)

Definition	Rationale	Relevance to SLP Profession
Probing is investigating a client's skills in producing nontargeted responses on the basis of generalization. It is the act of investigating the client's skills in productions not targeted for intervention prior to the probe.	Probes are valuable because of the concept of generalized learning, learning that occurs in a nontargeted area as a result of similarities between the targeted and nontargeted units.	It is important for the SLP to be aware of the client's functioning for targeted as well as nontargeted areas to the degree possible. Probing provides evidence of productions based on generalizations.

Section B

(Read this section before proceeding to Section C.)

Advance Organizer

Topic: Probing in the Therapeutic Process.

Purpose: To help the SLP learn to use Probing in the Therapeutic Process.

SLP Action: Study and use Probing in the Therapeutic Process.

Background: Probing may occur across broad areas of speech-language functioning: voice, fluency, language, phonology, semantics, syntax, morphology, resonance, etc. In most cases probing is used to help determine a client's skills in the accomplishment of therapy goals based on generalization. Probes are used to determine a client's current level of performances and to determine the client's readiness to move on to higher levels of work.

Links to Prior Learning: Sometimes when engaging in an exercise program to address upper body strength, you may find that, perhaps the legs become stronger as well, not because of emphasis on leg strength, but as a function of lower body muscular use in association with upper body training. The strengthened leg muscles in this example equate to generalized functioning of large muscles of the body. The same generalized functioning may occur in speech and language as well. In this regard, the SLP may check for generalized production of speech through use of probes. Remember, however, probes may occur in all areas of speech-language functioning.

Objective and Clarification of Skill to be Learned: The objective is for the SLP to learn to use Probing in the Therapeutic Process

Rationale: Probing helps the SLP determine a more accurate status of client progress and functioning for both targeted and nontargeted skills.

New Vocabulary: Probing—investigating a client's skills in producing nontargeted responses on the basis of generalization.

Individual SLP Outcomes/Performance Objectives: As a result of experiences in this workshop on Probing in the Therapeutic Process, I will: (Indicate information you would like to learn during this workshop.)

_____

_____

Section C

(Read this section *before* proceeding to Section D.)

Description/Demonstration

Probes are valuable because of the concept of generalized learning, learning that occurs in a nontarget area as a result of similarities in muscle movements, generalized comprehension and use, and so forth, for the nontargeted area. It is important for the SLP to be aware of the client's functioning for targeted as well as nontargeted areas. Note the following examples:

Example 1: "Jared, you've been working on /t/ in initial positions of words. Let's do a quick probe to determine if any progress was made on a few words made with /t/ that we haven't worked on yet." (SLP stimulates the client using pre-selected words, with no correction, and no teaching needed for this effort. The SLP may choose all new /t/ words for a pure probe or may intersperse new /t/ words with a few previously addressed /t/ words for an intermixed probe.)

Example 2: "Mr. Nardo, we've been working on categorizing for clothing, but let me check to see quickly how you are doing with categorizing foods. Name at least five vegetables for me."

Section D

(Complete this section *before* proceeding to Section E.)

Think-Out-Loud Questions

☑   **Read questions aloud.**

☑   **Verbalize answers to help with cognitive processing and the practice effect.**

☑   **Write short answers in spaces provided.**

1. What is the first thing that I must do in order to use Probing in the Therapeutic Process with my client?

    _____

2. What is/are the next step(s) that I must take to use Probing in the Therapeutic Process with my client?

    _____

3. What vocabulary must I use for Probing in the Therapeutic Process with my client?

    _____

4. What should I say or do in interactions with my client to use Probing in the Therapeutic Process? **(To help with authenticity, give your client an imaginary name!)**

    _____

    _____

    _____

5. How will I know that I am appropriately using Probes in the Therapeutic Process with my client?

    _____

Section E

(Complete this section *before* proceeding to Section F.)

Prompts for Practice Opportunity

Practice the skills discussed in Sections A–D above. Revisit Sections A–D as needed to increase comfort with this section. *Use SLP peers, friends, parents, other relatives, large dolls positioned in a chair in front of you to pose as the "client(s)," etc., for your practices. If no one is available to serve as your client(s), use yourself as the client(s) by standing or sitting in front of a large mirror as you practice; the effect of "using yourself as client(s)" is the same, and sometimes more powerful, than having another pose as client(s).* Repeat practices until therapeutic features 1–3 *below* are accomplished. (You may require more or less than the practice check boxes provided.) Check one box each time a feature is practiced. Enter date each feature is accomplished to your satisfaction in the date spaces provided. (Dates may/may not be the same for each feature accomplishment.)

1. ❑ ❑ ❑ ❑   Accuracy in the skill sequence accomplished.   Date: _____

2. ❑ ❑ ❑ ❑   Personal comfort in the skill sequence accomplished.   Date: _____

3. ❑ ❑ ❑ ❑   Adequate speed/fluency in the skill sequence accomplished.   Date: _____

Section F

(Complete this section *before* entering the date for *Date Post Organizer Completed*, upper right, page 1.)

Post Organizer

Review of Related Content: Probing is investigating a client's skills in producing nontargeted responses on the basis of generalization. It is the act of investigating client's skills in productions not targeted for intervention prior to the probe. Probes are valuable because of the concept of generalized learning, learning that occurs in a target area as a result of similarities, generalized comprehension and use, and so forth, of the nontargeted area.

What I Accomplished in this Workshop: _____

_____

_____

Importance of My Accomplishment(s) to My Therapy: _____

_____

My Assessment of My Performance of the Skill(s) Presented in this Workshop:

The Easiest Parts for Me: _____

The Most Difficult Parts for Me: _____

Thought Processes/Emotions I Experienced Learning the Skill(s) Presented in this Workshop Compared to What I Ultimately Learned from this Effort (Reflection Exercise):

_____

_____

_____

_____

Date Post Organizer Completed (Enter here and in upper right corner of page 1): _____

Form 13

(No DVD Accompaniment for this Workshop)

Therapeutic-Specific Workshop Form: Behavioral Management in the Therapeutic Process

Name: _____ Date Post Organizer Completed: _____

Section A

(Read this section *and* the section on *Behavioral Management in the Therapeutic Process* in Chapter 6 of your textbook *before* proceeding to Section B.)

Definition	Rationale	Relevance to SLP Profession
Behavioral management is a system used to establish and maintain appropriate client behavior for therapeutic intervention.	Behavior management should be viewed as an integral part of the SLP's program of services.	If the SLP is not able to establish appropriate behavioral parameters for clients, progress in therapy is negatively impacted.

Section B

(Read this section *before* proceeding to Section C.)

Advance Organizer

Topic: Behavioral Management in the Therapeutic Process.

Purpose: To help the SLP learn to use Behavioral Management in the Therapeutic Process.

SLP Action: Study and use Behavioral Management appropriate for the Therapeutic Process.

Background: Whether in the classroom, summer camp, or speech-language therapy sessions, behavioral management is important. Without appropriate behavioral management, chaos threatens to destroy the client's progress in achieving desired goals and objectives.

Links to Prior Learning: Think of the child or adult who constantly disrupts academic or social events. Often entire programs are rendered ineffective because of defiance, noncompliance, or overactivity. The same happens in speech-language therapy; when a client presents with difficult-to-manage behavior, the speech-language session is rendered ineffective unless the SLP is able to appropriately manage undesirable behaviors.

Objective and Clarification of Skill to be Learned: The objective is for the SLP to learn to use Behavioral Management in the Therapeutic Process.

Rationale: Behavioral management should be viewed as an integral part of the SLP's program of services because without appropriate behaviors, the goals and objectives of the session can not be accomplished.

New Vocabulary: Behavioral management—a system used to establish and maintain appropriate client behavior for therapeutic intervention.

Individual SLP Outcomes/Performance Objectives: As a result of experiences in this workshop on Behavioral Management in the Therapeutic Process, I will: (Indicate information you would like to learn during this workshop.)

_____

_____

Section C

(Read this section *before* proceeding to Section D.)

Description/Demonstration

Behavior management should be viewed as an integral part of the SLP's program of services. If the SLP is not able to establish appropriate behavioral parameters for clients, progress in therapy is negatively impacted.

Example 1: "Karen, you seem to be having difficulty controlling your behavior today. I'll let you sit close to me until you are able to sit independently." (SLP pulls child's chair near to monitor and control behavior more closely.)

Example 2: "Willie, you may not run about the room while we're in therapy. You may sit at the table or you may sit on the floor for therapy. Running about the room is not a choice."

Section D

(Complete this section *before* proceeding to Section E.)

Think-Out-Loud Questions

☑   **Read questions aloud.**

☑   **Verbalize answers to help with cognitive processing and the practice effect.**

☑   **Write short answers in spaces provided.**

1.   What is the first thing that I must do in order to use Behavioral Management in the Therapeutic Process with my client?

_____

2. What is/are the next step(s) that I must take in order to use Behavioral Management in the Therapeutic Process with my client?

_____

3. What vocabulary must I use for Behavioral Management in the Therapeutic Process with my client?

_____

4. What should I say or do in interactions with my client to use Behavioral Management in the Therapeutic Process?
   (To help with authenticity, give your client an imaginary name!)

_____

_____

_____

5. How will I know that I am appropriately using Behavioral Management in the Therapeutic Process with my client?

_____

Section E

(Complete this section *before* proceeding to Section F.)

Prompts for Practice Opportunity

Practice the skills discussed in Sections A–D above. Revisit Sections A–D as needed to increase comfort with this section. *Use SLP peers, friends, parents, other relatives, large dolls positioned in a chair in front of you to pose as the "client(s)," etc., for your practices. If no one is available to serve as your client(s), use yourself as the client(s) by standing or sitting in front of a large mirror as you practice; the effect of "using yourself as client(s)" is the same, and sometimes more powerful, than having another pose as client(s).* Repeat practices until therapeutic features 1–3 *below* are accomplished. (You may require more or less than the practice check boxes provided.) Check one box each time a feature is practiced. Enter date each feature is accomplished to your satisfaction in the date spaces provided. (Dates may/may not be the same for each feature accomplishment.)

1. ❏ ❏ ❏ ❏   Accuracy in the skill sequence accomplished.   Date: _____

2. ❏ ❏ ❏ ❏   Personal comfort in the skill sequence accomplished.   Date: _____

3. ❏ ❏ ❏ ❏   Adequate speed/fluency in the skill sequence accomplished.   Date: _____

Section F

(Complete this section *before* entering the date for *Date Post Organizer Completed*, upper right, page 1.)

Post Organizer

Review of Related Content: Behavioral management is a system used to establish and maintain appropriate client behaviors during therapy and should be viewed as an integral part of therapeutic intervention. Inappropriate client behaviors range from overactivity to noncompliance and defiance. SLPs must appropriately manage client behaviors to promote adequate client progress in therapy.

What I Accomplished in this Workshop: _____

_____

_____

Importance of My Accomplishment(s) to My Therapy: _____

_____

My Assessment of My Performance of the Skill(s) Presented in this Workshop:

    The Easiest Parts for Me: _____

    The Most Difficult Parts for Me: _____

Thought Processes/Emotions I Experienced Learning the Skill(s) Presented in this Workshop Compared to What I Ultimately Learned from this Effort (Reflection Exercise):

_____

_____

_____

_____

Date Post Organizer Completed (Enter here and in upper right corner of page 1): _____

Form 14

(No DVD Accompaniment for this Workshop)

Therapeutic-Specific Workshop Form: Troubleshooting in the Therapeutic Process

Name: _____ Date Post Organizer Completed: _____

Section A

(Read this section *and* the section on *Troubleshooting in the Therapeutic Process* in Chapter 6 of your textbook *before* proceeding to Section B.)

Definition	Rationale	Relevance to SLP Profession
Troubleshooting refers to the concept of *constant mental scanning*, whereby the SLP constantly looks for indicators of difficulty when therapy is not proceeding well.	The SLP needs to be aware of all parameters that impact a client's progress in therapy at all times.	Often, clients are unable to make adequate progress in therapy due to extraneous reason (inappropriately applied techniques, errors in scheduling for frequency of service, etc.). SLPs must constantly scan for possibilities to explain lack of progress in therapy and make the necessary corrections.

Section B

(Read this section *before* proceeding to Section C.)

Advance Organizer

Topic: Troubleshooting in the Therapeutic Process.

Purpose: To help the SLP learn Troubleshooting in the Therapeutic Process.

SLP Action: Learn and apply Troubleshooting in the Therapeutic Process

Background: Occasionally SLPs recognize that therapy is not progressing as well as expected. However, often it is difficult to determine what is causing the lags in progress. As SLPs gain more professional experience, skills in Troubleshooting are expected to increase.

Links to Prior Learning: Planning for therapy, implementing it, and evaluating client progress are familiar. Troubleshooting simply means that the SLP systematically seeks to determine cause(s) of less-than-expected results in therapy, particularly when planning and implementation skills appear to be appropriate.

Objective and Clarification of Skill to be Learned: The objective is for the SLP to learn Troubleshooting in the Therapeutic Process.

Rationale: Troubleshooting should be viewed as an integral to the SLP's program of services because when sessions or clients' progressions do not meet expectations, significantly more lack of progress may follow if the SLP fails to correct the cause of the difficulty.

New Vocabulary: Troubleshooting—the concept of constant mental scanning, whereby the SLP constantly looks for indicators of difficulty when therapy is not proceeding well.

Individual SLP Outcomes/Performance Objectives: As a result of experiences in this workshop on Troubleshooting in the Therapeutic Process, I will: (Indicate information you would like to learn during this workshop.)

_____

_____

Section C

(Read this section *before* proceeding to Section D.)

Description/Demonstration

Troubleshooting refers to the concept of *constant mental scanning*, whereby the SLP is constantly attuned to and looking for indicators of whether therapy is perceived as proceeding well. Often, clients are unable to make adequate progress in therapy due to extraneous reasons (inappropriately applied techniques, errors in scheduling for frequency of service, etc.). SLPs must constantly scan for possibilities to explain lack of progress in therapy and make the necessary corrections.

Example 1: "Etta, you seem to be having more difficulty with two of your sounds than expected. Let's take a look at those sounds a little closer." (SLP begins asking questions related to stimulus presentation, techniques used to teach the sound, etc. in an effort to determine causes of difficulty with the sounds.)

Example 2: "Jake, I think we need to change the order of activities for you on this objective. I think doing so will make it easier for you to complete your tasks each day during therapy."

Section D

(Complete this section *before* proceeding to Section E.)

Think-Out-Loud Questions

☑   Read questions aloud.

☑   Verbalize answers to help with cognitive processing and the practice effect.

☑   Write short answers in spaces provided.

1. What is the first thing that I must do in order to use Troubleshooting in the Therapeutic Process with my client?

   _____

2. What is/are the next step(s) that I must take in order to use Troubleshooting in the Therapeutic Process with my client?

   _____

3. What vocabulary must I use during Troubleshooting in the Therapeutic Process with my client?

   _____

4. What should I say or do in interactions with my client to use Troubleshooting in the Therapeutic Process?
   (To help with authenticity, give your client an imaginary name!)

   _____

   _____

   _____

5. How will I know that I am appropriately using Troubleshooting in the Therapeutic Process my client?

Section E

(Complete this section *before* proceeding to Section F.)

Prompts for Practice Opportunity

Practice the skills discussed in Sections A–D above. Revisit Sections A–D as needed to increase comfort with this section. *Use SLP peers, friends, parents, other relatives, large dolls positioned in a chair in front of you to pose as the "client(s)," etc., for your practices. If no one is available to serve as your client(s), use yourself as the client(s) by standing or sitting in front of a large mirror as you practice; the effect of "using yourself as client(s)" is the same, and sometimes more powerful, than having another pose as client(s).* Repeat practices until therapeutic features 1–3 *below* are accomplished. (You may require more or less than the practice check boxes provided.) Check one box each time a feature is practiced. Enter date each feature is accomplished to your satisfaction in the date spaces provided. (Dates may/may not be the same for each feature accomplishment.)

1. ❏ ❏ ❏ ❏   Accuracy in the skill sequence accomplished.   Date: _____

2. ❏ ❏ ❏ ❏   Personal comfort in the skill sequence accomplished.   Date: _____

3. ❏ ❏ ❏ ❏   Adequate speed/fluency in the skill sequence accomplished.   Date: _____

Section F

(Complete this section *before* entering the date for *Date Post Organizer Completed*, upper right, page 1.)

Post Organizer

Review of Related Content: Troubleshooting refers to the concept of *constant mental scanning*, whereby the SLP is constantly attuned to and looking for indicators of whether therapy is perceived as proceeding well. The SLP needs to be aware of all parameters that impact client's progress in therapy at all times. Often, clients are unable to make adequate progress in therapy due to extraneous reasons (inappropriately applied techniques, errors in scheduling for frequency of service, etc.). SLPs must constantly scan for possibilities to explain lack of progress in therapy and make the necessary corrections.

What I Accomplished in this Workshop: _____

_____

_____

Importance of My Accomplishment(s) to My Therapy: _____

_____

My Assessment of My Performance of the Skill(s) Presented in this Workshop:

The Easiest Parts for Me: _____

The Most Difficult Parts for Me: _____

Thought Processes/Emotions I Experienced Learning the Skill(s) Presented in this Workshop Compared to What I Ultimately Learned from this Effort (Reflection Exercise):

_____

_____

_____

_____

Date Post Organizer Completed (Enter here and in upper right corner of page 1): _____

Glossary

Accommodation. The way in which a person adapts his or her way of thinking regarding new experiences.

Advance organizer. Information introduced in advance of the new skill to be learned; designed to bridge the gap between current knowledge and knowledge to be acquired.

Affect. The feeling, emotion, mood, and temperament associated with a thought.

Alerting stimuli. The various means of drawing the client's attention to the coming treatment stimuli.

Analytical learners. People who prefer to learn in a step-by-step fashion, sequentially.

Animation. Relating to spirit, movement, zest, and vigor.

Antecedents. Events that occur before responses; stimuli or events the clinician presents in treatment before a required response.

Articulation. A series of overlapping ballistic movements, articulation is often likened to a fine motor skill in that very small and specific muscle movements are required to produce phonemes.

Artistry. The artistic quality, or effect, on workmanship.

Assimilation (cognitive). A person's ability to transform incoming information so that it fits with his or her existing way of thinking.

Assimilative nasality. Excessive nasality on sounds adjacent to the three normally nasalized consonants due to extended time that the velopharyngeal port is opened when making the three nasalized sounds; any sound following the production of the nasal phonemes is perceived as being nasal also because the port remains open long enough for the sounds to be emitted nasally rather than orally.

Attributes. The primary characteristics or features of the item being described.

Autism. A developmental disability significantly affecting verbal and nonverbal communication and social interaction, generally evident before age three years, which adversely affects a child's educational performance.

Backup reinforcer. Tangible or nontangible items, activities, events for which a client is willing to collect tokens, stars, and so forth for a later exchange, (i.e., markers, book or video checkouts, etc.).

Base-10 forms. Recording forms for notating client responses in multiples of 10.

Behavior management. A system that the SLP uses to establish and maintain appropriate client behavior for therapeutic intervention.

Body of the session. The component of therapy in which the client is introduced to, practices, and masters the relevant aspects and skills for improving communication abilities.

Client-focused difficulties. Difficulties that arise in therapy as a result of the client behaviors that negatively impact progress in therapy.

Clinical trial.   Structured opportunities for the client to produce a response in therapy.

Clinician-focused difficulties.   Difficulties the SLP experiences in therapy that result in ineffective therapy and lack of client progress.

Closing of the session.   The activities at the end of the session designed to review and reiterate objectives and end the session.

Cluster seating.   Semicircle seating for groups in which the SLP's knees are close to the clients' knees, either sitting in chairs, or sitting on the floor without a table between clinician and clients.

Cognitive or **graphic organizers.**   Pictorial or physical presentations of a concept designed to give the learner a visual organizer of information to be addressed.

Cognitive skills.   Abilities in broad areas of perception, memory, imagination, conceptualization, and reasoning.

Collaborative model.   A model of services whereby the SLP serves clients in their respective classrooms as a collaborative effort with the classroom teacher.

Collection of or mentioning of homework.   A brief reminder of tasks related to therapy that clients are asked to complete outside of therapy.

Communication.   A response-seeking, two-way symbolic, yet real-life process; a receiver phenomenon, complex, transitory, continuous, and contextually based event.

Concepts.   The constructs being taught in therapy, including any specific required underlying mental or physical actions or processes needed to change communication behavior.

Concrete Operations Period.   Piagetian stage that ranges from 7 years to 12 years of age, during which time the child learns mental transformations for quantity and time.

Consultative model.   A model of services in which the SLP works with the client's teachers, parents, or other professionals to address the communication needs of the client.

Contingency contracting.   An agreement (verbal or written) between the client and the SLP regarding expected client behavior within the therapeutic setting; part of behavior management strategies.

Continuous schedule of reinforcement.   The client receives a reinforcer following each response.

Cooperative learning.   The instructional use of small groups so that students work together to maximize their own and each other's learning.

Corrective feedback.   The information the clinician gives the client regarding the quality, feature, or correctness of a preceding response.

Critical incidents.   Positive or negative experiences recognized by students as significant because of the influence on the student's development in learning how to do therapy.

Cueing.   An aid to promote correct responses.

Cul-de-sac resonance.   A hollow, muffled sounding voice often caused by posterior tongue retraction, or an anterior nasal airway obstruction.

Data collection.   All actions of the SLP for gathering information that indicates the client's levels of performances for various tasks in therapy.

Data collection forms.   Forms used to (a) notate the individual and specific responses of clients during therapy, or (b) report the overall totals for correct performances on objectives at the end of the session.

Data mixing.   Collecting data on more than one task, task level, or task objective within the same data batch.

Data reporting.   An indication of the total percentages of productions for the session.

Deaf-blindness.   Refers to concomitant hearing and visual impairments, the combination of which causes such severe communication and other developmental and educational needs that they cannot be accommodated in special education programs solely for children with deafness or children with blindness.

Deafness.   A hearing impairment that is so severe that the child is impaired in pro-cessing linguistic information through hearing, with or without amplification, which adversely affects a child's educational performance.

Demonstrating.   Using well organized, step-by-step explanations in language that is easily understood.

Demonstrations.   Written or visual presentations of skills implemented by the SLP; also serve to help students acquire the skills presented.

Dependent contingencies.   All group members share in the reinforcement if one individual achieves a goal.

Describing.   Refers to telling or detailing the major features, functions, characteristics, or aspects of an item or concept deemed important.

Descriptions.   Well-organized explanations of the skills to be learned and the steps taken in learning the new skill; in early child language, elementary communicative interactions in which the adult labels or describes what he or she believes the child is *seeing*.

Development.   The process of natural progression from a previous, lower stage of functioning to a more complex or adult-like stage.

Developmental milestones.   Those "markers" or skills that serve to indicate the client's functioning level compared to age expected levels across various areas of functioning. Developmental milestones are typical for motor, communication, adaptive/self-help, social-emotional, and cognitive skills.

Developmental stages.   Periods of time during the growth process in which thoughts, behaviors, and feelings of an individual remain relatively the same.

Direct language therapy.   Therapy for clients who routinely use verbal expression as the primary mode of communication, but with significant delays or disorders in language skills.

Direct teaching.   Refers to instances when the SLP's task is to *teach, instruct, or train* the client in a new skill.

Dismissal criteria.   The standard used to determine if a client should be dismissed from therapy.

Documentation.   Notations regarding activities associated with daily intervention and management of the client that often serve as an official record of professional-client interactions.

Due process.   Documentation that the child's parents, or guardians, were informed, and gave their informed consent for the child to be assessed, labeled, and placed in speech-language therapy (or other special education services) as prescribed by law.

Duration of therapy.   How much time, typically, in minutes, the client should be seen in therapy during each session.

Edible reinforcers.   Food given as a *positive reinforcer* to increase the frequency of a desired response. *SLPs are encouraged to avoid edible reinforcers.*

Eliciting.   A bringing forth or drawing out.

Emotional disturbance.   A condition exhibiting one or more of the following characteristics over a long period and to a marked degree that adversely affects a child's educational performance: (a) an inability to learn that cannot be explained by intellectual, sensory, or health factors; (b) an inability to build or maintain satisfactory interpersonal relationships with peers and teachers; (c) inappropriate types of behavior or feelings under normal circumstances; (d) a general pervasive mood of unhappiness or depression; and (e) a tendency to develop physical symptoms or fears associated with personal or school problems.

Enthusiasm.   A strong excitement or feeling for something; a zest or zeal for a subject.

Equilibration.   Encompasses both assimilation and accommodation (from Piaget's work), and refers to the overall interaction between existing ways of thinking and new experiences.

Establishment phase.   The first phase within the body of the session used to determine whether planned or intended levels of work for the current session may be addressed.

Excellence.   As applied to speech-language therapy, it is the achievement of therapy to a level of exceptional quality.

Exemplars.   Examples of the phonemes, concepts, and so forth under discussion.

Expansions.   Additions to the child's one to two word utterances to approach more *grammatical correctness*.

Explicit Instruction Model.   An instruction model that is both highly organized and task-oriented.

Expressive language.   The use of conventional symbols (words, signs, etc.) to communicate one's ideas, thoughts, or intentions toward others.

Extensions.   Expansions of the child's simple utterance, plus the expression of an additional unit of information (sometimes referred to as *expansions-plus*).

Extrinsic motivation.   Motivation derived from an external force or stimulus.

Facilitation skills.   Skills that promote or accentuate client learning.

Fine motor skills.   The smaller muscles of the body; often impact hands, fingers, feet, toes, and so forth, with some classifying speech as a fine motor skill.

Fluency.   In terms of the therapy session, it is the smooth movement or transition between various parts of therapy.

Formal Operations Period.   The Piagetian stage that begins at around 12 years and continues throughout life. The characterizing achievement in this stage is the child's ability to reason on the basis of theoretical possibilities as well as concrete realities.

Frequency of therapy.   How often the client is seen in therapy weekly.

Global or synergetic learners.   People who prefer learning from a whole-part-whole format, seeing the whole unit, breaking the unit into parts as needed, then reconstructing back to the whole.

Greeting and rapport.   The initial portion of the therapy session, designed to set an amicable, amenable learning atmosphere for therapy.

Gross motor skills.   Refers to the large muscles and torso skills associated with kicking, rolling, sitting, crawling, standing, walking, running, climbing, throwing, diving, and so forth.

Hand-to-chin rule.   A proximity span whereby, when the clinician's upturned palm is extended to touch under the client's chin, there is a comfortable reach without overextension of the elbow to achieve the touch.

Health Insurance Portability and Accountability Act of 1996 (HIPAA).   National standards designed to protect individuals' medical records and other personal health information and to give patients more control over their health information.

Hearing impairment.   An impairment in hearing, whether permanent or fluctuating, that adversely affects a child's educational performance but that is not included under the definition of deafness.

Heterogeneous groups.   Therapy groups in which clients are working on different objectives, often from different disability categories (e.g., /s/, semantics for body parts, fluency).

High-intensity behavioral management techniques.   Highly structured behavioral programs and classrooms that may require the involvement of multiple individuals.

Homogeneous groups.   Therapy groups in which all clients are working on the same or similar objectives (e.g., /s/, or /k/).

Homorganic phonemes.   Phonemes made in the same anatomical area, but different by one feature; often are different in the manner of production, e.g., /s/ and /t/ are homorganic phonemes; they are made in the same anatomical place, but in a different manner.

Horizontal notations.   A left-to-right progression in taking data across the page (e.g., ⫫ ⎮⎮⎮⎮Ⅹ ⎮ⅩⅢ).

Hypernasality.   Excessive and undesirable amount of perceived nasal cavity resonance during phonation of normally nonnasal vowels and nonnasal voiced consonants.

Hyponasality.   Reduced nasal resonance for the production of the nasal sounds /m/, /n/, and /ŋ/.

Ignoring undesirable behaviors.   A behavior management skill that is *planned* and used to negate a disruptive behavior each time it occurs.

Imitative verbal task.   Verbal response following a modeled verbal stimulus that takes the same form as the stimulus.

Independent contingencies.   Individuals within the group are reinforced for individual achievements toward a goal.

Indirect language therapy.   Therapy designed for very young children and other clients who operate essentially as nonverbal, even if the client uses a few one-word utterances occasionally.

Individual therapy in a group.   A phenomenon often seen when SLPs fail to facilitate the interaction needed within the structure of group therapy, whereby, the SLP works with one child for a few minutes while the other children color, cut, paste, and so forth awaiting their turn.

Individual therapy session.   The SLP works with only one client at a time.

Interactive group therapy.   A therapy structure in which each member of the group serves as a peer model or evaluator for the productions of others in the group in a fashion similar to conversational exchanges such that it is often difficult to determine whose turn it is at the moment.

Interactive nature of learning.   A concept whereby learning occurs through the give and take transfer of information from one person to another.

Interdependent contingencies. All group members are reinforced if all collectively (or all individually) achieve the stated goal.

Intermittent schedule of reinforcement. The client receives a reinforcer after a certain predetermined number of responses, for example, after 3, 5, or even 10 responses.

Interpersonal communication skills. The personal behaviors or interactions used for engaging others.

Intimate space. The zone reserved for close relationships, sharing, protecting, and comforting, typically, up to 1½ feet.

Intrinsic motivation. Motivation derived from an internal force or stimulus.

Introduction of the session. The opening or beginning of the speech-language therapy session.

Kinesthetic. Relating to a sense of movement originating from sensory end organs in muscles, tendons, joints, and sometimes the ear canals.

Language and speech classroom. A speech classroom established as one of the instructional periods of the day.

Learning. The processes and mental structures by which people accumulate experiences and make them into new meanings.

Learning style. The way in which an individual receives, processes, and internalizes new and challenging information.

Loquaciousness. The tendency for the SLP to talk too much.

Low-intensity behavioral management techniques. Typical management parameters; include establishing class rules, using specific praise, and ignoring behaviors.

Medium-intensity behavioral management techniques. Require somewhat more management parameters; include contingency contracting, token economy systems, and self-management strategies.

Mental retardation. Significantly subaverage general intellectual functioning, existing concurrently with deficits in adaptive behavior, and manifested during the developmental period, that adversely affects the child's educational performance.

Minutes matter attitude. A way of thinking about time-on-task during speech-language therapeutic intervention.

Modality/Modalities. Any sensory avenue(s) through which information may be received (e.g., visual, auditory, tactile/kinesthetic).

Modeling. The clinician's production of a target behavior for the client to imitate.

Model of services. The management strategies used in scheduling clients for therapy.

Morphology. The smallest meaning units in language.

Motivation. A stimulus or force that causes a person to act; may be intrinsic or extrinsic.

Mounted mirror seating. Seating arrangement in which the SLP places clients in front of a large mirror that is mounted on the wall, and the SLP sits behind the clients.

Multiple disabilities. Concomitant impairments (such as mental retardation-blindness, mental retardation-orthopedic impairments, etc.), the combination of which causes such severe educational needs that they cannot be accommodated in special education programs solely for one of the impairments. The term does not include deaf-blind.

Nonproductive time. Time that is wasted during therapy.

Nonsemantic fillers. The "ahs," "ums," and "let me sees" often characteristic of those unsure of what should happen next in therapy.

Nontangible reinforcers. Reinforcers that constitute actions or activities as a reward.

Nonthreatening therapeutic touch. Touching the client's shoulder, upper arm, upper back, neck and facial areas in order to support clinical instruction.

OK syndrome. The overuse by the SLP of the word *"OK."*

Operant conditioning. A method of changing behavior in which a reinforcer/reward is offered the subject immediately following the production of a desired response (e.g., verbal praise following the correct production of a phoneme).

Oral defensiveness. Difficulties with different textures, tastes, touch, or temperatures in the mouth.

Orthopedic impairment. A severe difficulty with the skeletal systems (bones, joints, limbs, and associated muscles) to a degree that adversely affects a child's educational performance.

Other health impairment. Limited strength, vitality or alertness, including a heightened alertness to environmental stimuli, that results in limited alertness to the educational environment and adversely affects a child's educational performance.

Parallel-talk. Describing or commenting on what the *child* is doing during indirect therapy.

Pedagogy. The underlying philosophical beliefs and concepts that serve as foundations or guiding principles for the education of students.

Peer evaluators. Clients within a heterogeneous therapy group who are called upon by the SLP to give the target client feedback regarding the accuracy of his or her productions.

Peer models. Clients within a heterogeneous therapy group who are called upon by the SLP to give the target client models, or examples, of how sounds or other structures are produced.

Personal space. Space required for informal conversations between friends, typically 1½ to 4 feet.

Phonology. Study of the sound system associated with language.

Positive reinforcers. Anything, following a response, which increases the frequency of that response; may be extrinsic, such as a token, money, or social, in the form of praise.

Post organizer. A concluding activity that helps students further conceptualize new material.

Pragmatics. The appropriate use of language in context.

Preferred learning modality. The sensory modality through which information appears to be easiest learned.

Preoperational Period. Piagetian stage from 2 years to 7 years and characterized by acquisition of representational skills in areas of language, mental imagery, and drawing.

Primary reinforcers. Reinforcers that do not depend on prior learning and typically satisfy a biological need (e.g., hunger or thirst).

Probing. Investigating a client's skills in producing nontargeted responses on the basis of generalization.

Professionalism. A characteristic style, practice, or habit for personal and professional presentation, representation, and general demeanor.

Prompting. Using special stimuli, verbal or nonverbal, to increase the probability that the client will respond in a desired manner.

Prompts for practice opportunities. Designated points in learning to practice new skills with help from prompts.

Proximity. Degree of closeness in physical distance between persons.

Pseudo-interaction. Interaction in which the clinician talks to another person who poses as a "client" for the SLP's learning purposes.

Public space. One-way communication as exhibited by lecturers, typically 12 to 25 feet.

Pull-in model. A model of services in which the SLP goes into the client's classroom and works with the student individually or in a small group, thereby "pulling-in" the student.

Pull-out model. A model of services in which clients are taken from their typical setting (pulled-out) and served in a designated "speech room."

Questioning. A technique of direct teaching designed to assess learning and facilitate further learning.

Quick-paced lessons. The *presentation rate* used in teaching, not the number of minutes or total amount of time spent in teaching a skill.

Recast. The SLP changes the child's utterance into a different *type* of utterance.

Receptive language. The spoken or visual (signed or written) words one understands.

Recording. Writing down a tally of correct and incorrect client responses, or collecting data.

Regression-recoupment. A phenomena, whereby the level of success obtained in therapy in a previous session no longer exists due to the time between therapy sessions, and the amount of time it takes to again reach the prior level of performance.

Remote associations. Distal times, locations, or activities when the client may have encountered the item being described.

Review of the previous session. A brief questioning by the clinician of what the client worked on in the previous session.

Scanning. Asking the right questions about clinical skills and performances (related to efforts to determine the nature of difficulty experienced in obtaining desired results in therapy).

Schedule of reinforcement. How often the clinician reinforces following client responses.

Schema. A cognitive structure, whereby new information is compared to existing cognitive structures.

Scope. The range or depth of activities of the session (e.g., how many times the client will be asked to repeat a phrase, or how many examples need to be given to help the client understand a concept).

Scripted therapy guides. Written samples or examples of what the student SLP says in a therapeutic situation.

Self-evaluation. Students compare their behavior to a preset standard to determine whether the criterion is being accomplished.

Self-help/adaptive skills. Skills that demonstrate requirements of personal independence, social responsibilities, and environmental demands.

Self-management strategies. Behavioral techniques that are student-directed and typically instituted once teacher-directed behavior management strategies are demonstrated consistently; include *self-monitoring*, *self-evaluation*, and *self-reinforcement* techniques.

Self-monitoring. Students record the frequency of a particular behavior, usually on a card or other form.

Self-reinforcement. Students reward or reinforce themselves following appropriate behavior.

Self-talk. An indirect language technique in which the SLP describes what *he* or *she* is doing as the child looks on.

Semantics. The concepts, vocabulary, relationships, events, and so forth related to an object, idea, person, or place.

Sensorimotor Period. Piagetian stage that ranges from birth to age 2 years.

Sequence. The order in which activities occur within the session.

Shaping (successive approximations). A technique used for obtaining responses that are not in the client's repertoire.

Showtime. An underlying guiding concept whereby clinicians come to understand the significance of the therapy provided to clients.

Social-emotional skills. Skills related to levels of maturation for expressions of affect (feelings), control of emotions, basic self-concept, and social roles.

Social space. A communicating distance of 4 to 12 feet, generally accepted for interactions among strangers, business acquaintances, and teachers and students.

Specific learning disability. A disorder in one or more of the basic psychological processes involved in understanding or in using language, spoken or written, that may manifest itself in an imperfect ability to listen, think, speak, read, write, spell, or to do mathematical calculations, including conditions such as perceptual disabilities, brain injury, minimal brain dysfunction, dyslexia, and developmental aphasia. The term does not include learning problems that are primarily the result of visual, hearing, or motor disabilities, of mental retardation, of emotional disturbance, or of environmental, cultural, or economic disadvantage.

Specific praise. Verbalizing the specific aspect of behavior the client is performing well.

Speech or language impairment. A communication disorder, such as stuttering, impaired articulation, a language impairment, or a voice impairment, that adversely affects a child's educational performance.

Stimulus presentations. The methods used for presenting stimuli during therapy.

Syntax. Rules governing the order of words in a sentence.

Tactile. Relating to a sense of touch.

Tangible reinforcers. Nonedible items that are reinforcing, are used as rewards on occasion to provide variety in reward routines so that the effectiveness of a verbal (social) reinforcer is not diminished (for example, using stickers occasionally in addition to verbal praise).

Task-analysis. A behavioral concept, whereby tasks, or skills, are broken down into component parts in order to learn the parts separately; then the parts are put back together to demonstrate the entire target/required sequence.

Teaching phase of the body. The segment of therapy in which the concepts associated with the target are taught.

Thematic unit. A topic selected as the foundation for broad-based discussion and presentation in language therapy.

Therapeutic environment. The physical and psychological climate designed for the client's maximal benefit from the intervention process.

Therapeutic interaction. A highly responsive and fluid exchange between clinician and clients during therapy.

Therapeutic mindset. The mental disposition or attitude that predetermines the SLP's responses to and interpretations of situations that occur within therapy sessions.

Therapeutic momentum. The speed, thrust, or force of moving between segments of the session.

Therapeutic process. Broad-based professional procedures, activities, and interactions with clients designed for the intervention of communication disorders.

Therapeutic-specific skills. Fundamental, core professional skills necessary for effective speech-language therapy.

Therapeutic-Specific Workshop Form (TSW **Form**). A form that serves as a *learning tool* to guide students through the activities associated with learning new therapy skills; accompanies each skill to be learned.

Think-Out-Loud questions. Questions that the learner verbalizes to him- or herself to help process new skills or information.

Time-on-Task. The time when students are attending to a learning task and are attempting to learn.

Token economy. A system of behavioral management involving nonsocial conditioned reinforcers earned for exhibiting desired academic or social behaviors that may be exchanged for backup reinforcers of predetermined token value.

Tokens. Items that have little inherent value (chips, tickets, stars, marks on a tally sheet, etc.), but which may be given as a temporary reinforcer to be later exchanged for something that the client does value.

Tolerance level. The level of work at which the client experiences success.

Traumatic brain injury. An acquired injury to the brain caused by an external physical force, resulting in total or partial functional disability or psychosocial impairment, or both, that adversely affects a child's educational performance.

Troubleshooting. Constant *mental scanning*, whereby the SLP constantly looks for indicators of difficulty when therapy is not proceeding well.

Ungrammatical utterances. The use of grammatically incorrect language during therapy.

Unnatural productions. Pronunciations presented to the client in which unnatural stress, syllabification, or other abnormalities in modeled presentations occur.

Verbal praise. A type of reinforcement in which the client is praised for giving correct responses or for imitating modeled responses.

Vertical notations. A top-to-bottom orientation and method of data collection.

Vision impairment including blindness. Impairment in vision that, even with correction, adversely affects a child's educational performance. The term includes both partial sight and blindness.

Vocal resonance. The perceptual increases in loudness of the laryngeal tone due to the concentration and reflection of soundwaves by the oral, pharyngeal, and nasal cavities during voice production.

Wait-time. The amount of time the SLP waits for a response from a client after asking a question or giving a command.

Index

Note: Page numbers in **bold** reference non-text material.